Statistical Tools for
Epidemiologic Research

Statistical Tools for Epidemiologic Research

STEVE SELVIN

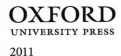

UNIVERSITY PRESS

2011

OXFORD
UNIVERSITY PRESS

Oxford University Press, Inc., publishes works that further
Oxford University's objective of excellence
in research, scholarship, and education.

Oxford   New York
Auckland   Cape Town   Dar es Salaam   Hong Kong   Karachi
Kuala Lumpur   Madrid   Melbourne   Mexico City   Nairobi
New Delhi   Shanghai   Taipei   Toronto

With offices in
Argentina   Austria   Brazil   Chile   Czech Republic   France   Greece
Guatemala   Hungary   Italy   Japan   Poland   Portugal   Singapore
South Korea   Switzerland   Thailand   Turkey   Ukraine   Vietnam

Published by Oxford University Press, Inc.
198 Madison Avenue, New York, New York 10016
www.oup.com

Oxford is a registered trademark of Oxford University Press

Library of Congress Cataloging-in-Publication Data

Selvin, S.
Statistical tools for epidemiologic research / Steve Selvin.
p. ; cm.
ISBN 978-0-19-975596-7
1. Epidemiology—Statistical methods.   I. Title.
[DNLM: 1. Epidemiologic Methods. WA 950 S469sd 2010]
RA652.2.M3S453 2010
614.402′1—dc22
2010013555

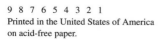

9 8 7 6 5 4 3 2 1
Printed in the United States of America
on acid-free paper.

for David, Liz, Ben, and, especially, Nancy

PREFACE

This text answers the question: After a typical first-year course in statistical methods, what next? One answer is a description of "second-year" methods that provide an introduction to intermediate biostatistical techniques without advanced mathematics or extensive statistical theory (for example, no Bayesian statistics, no causal inference, no linear algebra, and only a slight hint of calculus). Intuitive explanations richly supported with numerous examples produce an accessible presentation for readers interested in the analysis of data relevant to epidemiologic or medical research.

STATISTICAL TOOLS

A common and important statistical technique, called *smoothing*, removes the unimportant details and minimizes the influences of extraneous variation to expose the true underlying and frequently simple relationships within sampled data. This text is a kind of "smoothing." Apparently complicated statistical methods are frequently rather simple conceptually but are obscured by a forest of technical details and are often described with a specialized and sometimes confusing statistical language. The following material, however, is a blend of nonmathematical explanations, symbols, data, examples, and graphics applied to case study data. The goal is simply to explain how statistical methods work.

In most statistical texts, statistical methods are illustrated with examples. In reality, the situation is reversed. The data and questions under investigation dictate the statistical methods. A case study approach describes and illustrates statistical tools that are useful in the quest for answers to specific questions generated from sampled data. The case studies come from published research papers, doctoral dissertations, routinely reported government disease/mortality data, and clinical experimentation. The analysis of actual data leads to descriptions of statistical logic in a realistic context. For example, data collected to identify the role of lifestyle behavior in the likelihood of coronary heart disease are used to illustrate how statistical tools provide answers to important biologic/medical questions about risk and risk factors. Frequently, small subsets of the original data are analyzed for convenience of space and to allow the reader to easily repeat the calculations or explore different approaches. As part of communicating an understanding of the statistical process, minor sacrifices in rigor and notation yield important gains in accessibility to the material. For example, to avoid general notation, all confidence intervals have a level of significance of 95% because other levels are almost never used.

The text is divided into a sequence of 15 chapters starting with analysis of the fundamental 2×2 table. From this foundation, the topics gradually increase in sophistication, with particular emphasis on regression techniques (logistic, Poisson, conditional logistic, and log-linear) and then beyond to useful techniques that are not typically discussed in an applied context. Topics are chosen for two reasons. They describe widely used statistical methods particularly suitable for the analysis of epidemiologic/medical data and contribute to what might be call a "statistical tool box." These topics also illustrate basic concepts that are necessary for an understanding of data analysis in general. For example, *bootstrap estimation* is a topic that introduces an extremely useful statistical tool and, at the same time, clearly illustrates the fundamental concept of sampling variation. In addition, a concerted effort is made to trace the threads of statistical logic throughout the entire book. The same statistical issues are explored in different contexts, links among similar approaches are identified (a road map), extensions of previous methods are always noted, and the same data are occasionally analyzed from different perspectives. Thus, every attempt is made to avoid a "cookbook" kind of presentation of a series of statistical tools.

The presented material evolved from a second-year masters' degree course in epidemiologic data analysis taught over the last decade at the University of California, Berkeley, and also taught as part of the Summer Institute for Biostatistics and Epidemiology at The Johns Hopkins Bloomberg School of Public Health. Parts of the text have also been included in courses presented at the Graduate Summer Session in Epidemiology at the University of Michigan, School of Public Health. In other words, the material has been throughly "classroom tested."

The 15 chapters of this text are a confluence of two sources. Ten chapters consist of new material. The other five chapters are a substantial revision and streamlining of the key elements from my text *Statistical Analysis of Epidemiologic Data*, third edition. They constitute a kind of a "fourth edition." The combination produces an uninterrupted description of statistical logic and methods, so that the reader does not have to refer to other sources for background. That is, the text is largely a self-contained discussion of statistical tools beyond the first-year introductory level.

COMPUTER TOOLS

In keeping with the practical rather than the theoretical nature of the text, the next question becomes: What are the computer software tools that produced the statistical analyses used to describe the case studies? In this computer-laptop-age, a text about use of statistical tools requires a parallel discussion of the computer software tools. The idea of doing statistical computations "by hand" long ago disappeared.

Although statistical software systems give the same answers, the system called *Stata* (version 10.0) is used. It is a relatively simple and widely available computer system that is certainly adequate for the statistical techniques encountered in the text and takes little investment to use effectively. Stata code (identified by dots) and the resulting output (no dots) are given for the analyses of the case studies presented and are located at www.oup.com/us/statisticaltools. The text, as might be expected, describes and explains statistical methods using only the relevant summaries and selected statistical results. The computer output contains the details. The rigors of executing computer code enhances the understanding of the analytic process and provides additional insight into the properties of statistical methods. For example, it is a simple matter to assemble the Stata commands to calculate approximate confidence interval bounds based on the normal distribution. It is also a simple matter to use a Stata command to calculate exact confidence interval bounds, easily producing an immediate idea of the accuracy of the classic approximation.

A small amount of knowledge of the Stata system is assumed. The introductory tutorial that comes with the purchase of the software (*Getting Started with Stata*) is more than sufficient. The Stata code and output are applications of the statistical tools discussed, not artificial problems. Each component of a statistical analysis system, such as the Stata system, is designed to produce a specific result. The analysis of actual data, however, is rarely an orderly process. Therefore, a Stata command frequently provides exactly the desired result. In other situations, it is necessary to construct a series of commands to get the desired result. Both situations are extensively illustrated, with the Stata statistical system applied to the case studies.

Modern computer systems are extremely user-friendly, and extensive resources exist to deal with the sometimes tedious in-and-outs of using the Stata system. For example, three important commands for the application of the Stata system are:

1. *findit* <searches for character strings>
2. *help* <Stata command>
3. http://statcomp.ats.ucla.edu/stata/

The *findit* command searches the Stata online manual for commands associated with specific words or strings of characters. Often, the user is then able to directly access the appropriate *help* command. The *help* command then produces a detailed and complete online description of any valid Stata command, including several example applications. The third command identifies a link to a website (UCLA) that contains a large number of useful examples of the application of the Stata computer code. This code or pieces of this code frequently serve as a template for the problem at hand. The presented Stata output is slightly edited to focus directly on the analytic results. Bookkeeping messages, such as `frequency weights assumed` or `Iteration 2: log likelihood = -876.52235`, are not included.

Applications of other statistical computer systems follow similar patterns. For example, readers familiar with the major statistical systems SAS, SPSS, Splus, or R should be able to translate the Stata computer code into the system of their choice. The computer implementation is purposely made totally separate from the text material, so that no important statistical issues or methods will be missed by completely ignoring the computer input/output. The chapter topics are about understanding how the statistical tools work, and the Stata results are about how the computer tools accomplish the task.

It is important to acknowledge the debt to those who originated the statistical methods and those who taught them to me, particularly the Department of Statistics at the University of California, Berkeley. A listing of the names of these people is far to extensive to produce here. However, four mentors/colleagues stand-out from the rest, namely Elizabeth Scott, Warren Winkelstein, Nicholas Jewell, and Richard Brand.

Steve Selvin

CONTENTS

3. Two Especially Useful Estimation Tools, 54

4. Linear Logistic Regression: Discrete Data, 67

5. Logistic Regression: Continuous Data, 107

6. Analysis of Count Data: Poisson Regression Model, 131

Statistical Tools for
Epidemiologic Research

1

TWO MEASURES OF RISK: ODDS RATIOS AND AVERAGE RATES

Two fundamental statistical measures of association basic to exploring epidemiologic and medical data are the *odds ratio* and the *average rate*. Both statistics are easily used, but their interpretation is enhanced by an understanding of their sometimes subtle properties. This chapter describes these two measures in detail, outlines some of their important properties, and contrasts them to several other commonly used statistical measures of association.

ODDS RATIO

An odds ratio, as the name indicates, is the ratio of two values called *the odds*. The statistical origin of the odds is *a probability*. Specifically, when the probability of an event is denoted p, the odds associated with the event are $p/(1 - p)$. Odds are best understood in terms of gambling, particularly horse racing. When the probability a chosen horse will win a race is 1/3, the odds are 1 to 2 (1/3 divided by 2/3). The odds indicate the pay-off for a bet and at the same time slightly obscure the underlying probability of winning. A fair pay-off for a bet at these odds is $2 for every $1 bet. However, horse racing is not a fair game. The amount paid for a winning bet is considerably less than would be expected from a fair game. Table 1–1 is a typical racing form description of a five-horse race.

Table 1–1. Bay Meadows Handicap—One mile, four-year-olds and up, purse $9,500 (post time 12:45)

Horse	Jockey	Weight	Odds	Probability
In Love With Loot	R. Baze	119	7–2	0.22
Skip A Wink	J. Lumpkins	121	8–5	0.38
Playing'r Song	R. Gonzalez	121	9–5	0.36
Ms. Dahill	J. Ochoa	121	4–1	0.20
Rare Insight	J. Rosario	119	6–1	0.14

The last column translating the odds into probabilities is not a typical part of a racing form. The sum of these "probabilities" is 1.30. When the odds are based on a fair pay-off, these probabilities add to 1.0. However, the track has to pay the winner's purse, support the cost of the track, and make a profit. For this race and all others, the "probabilities" add to a value greater than one and identify the share of the money bet that goes directly to the track.

In statistical applications, the odds ratio (*or*) is a comparison of odds. The odds calculated under one set of conditions, $p_1/(1 - p_1)$, are compared to the odds calculated under another set of conditions, $p_2/(1 - p_2)$ by the ratio

$$odds\ ratio = or = \frac{odds\ under\ conditions\ 1}{odds\ under\ conditions\ 2} = \frac{p_1/(1 - p_1)}{p_2/(1 - p_2)}.$$

The central property of an odds ratio is that when no difference exists between the conditions ($p_1 = p_2$), the odds ratio is $or = 1.0$. When $p_1 \neq p_2$, the odds ratio measures the extent of the difference between the two conditions relative to 1.0.

Although the odds ratio applies to a number of situations, a good place to start is a description of the odds ratio used to evaluate an association observed between two binary variables summarized in a 2×2 *table* (such as Tables 1–2 and 1–3).

The symbols a, b, c, and d represent the counts of the four possible outcomes from a sample made up of $a + b + c + d = m_1 + m_2 = n_1 + n_2 = n$ individuals. For example, in the study of a binary risk factor (denoted F) and the presence/absence of a disease (denoted D), the symbol a represents the number of individuals who have both the risk factor and the disease (Table 1–2).

Table 1–2. Notation for a 2×2 table containing the counts from two binary variables (disease: D = present and $\overline{D}$ = absent and risk factor: F = present and $\overline{F}$ = absent)

	D	$\overline{D}$	Total
F	a	b	n_1
$\overline{F}$	c	d	n_2
Total	m_1	m_2	n

Table 1–3. Breast cancer (D) among military women who served in Vietnam (F) and who did not served in Vietnam ($\overline{F}$) during the war years 1965–1973 [1]

	D	$\overline{D}$	**Total**
F	170	3222	3392
$\overline{F}$	126	2912	3038
Total	296	6134	6430

Data from a study of female military veterans published in 1990 [2] produce a 2×2 table (Table 1–3) and an odds ratio contrasting the breast cancer risk between women who served in Vietnam ($n_1 = 3392$) and women who did not served in Vietnam ($n_2 = 3038$) [1]. The odds ratio measure of the association between a disease ($D =$ breast cancer and $\overline{D} =$ no breast cancer) and a risk factor ($F =$ served in Vietnam and $\overline{F} =$ did not served in Vietnam) is

$$odds\ ratio = or = \frac{odds(Vietnam)}{odds(not\ Vietnam)}$$
$$= \frac{P(D|F)/\left[1 - P(D|F)\right]}{P(D|\overline{F})/\left[1 - P(D|\overline{F})\right]} = \frac{P(D|F)/P(\overline{D}|F)}{P(D|\overline{F})/P(\overline{D}|\overline{F})}$$

and contrasts two conditions, namely those women with the risk factor (F) and those without the risk factor ($\overline{F}$).

The odds of breast cancer among women who served in Vietnam (first row, Table 1–3) are

$$odds(F) = \frac{P(D|F)}{P(\overline{D}|F)} \text{ and are estimated by } \frac{a/n_1}{b/n_1} = \frac{a}{b} = \frac{170}{3222}.$$

The odds of breast cancer among women who did not serve in Vietnam (second row, Table 1–3) are

$$odds(\overline{F}) = \frac{P(D|\overline{F})}{P(\overline{D}|\overline{F})} \text{ and are estimated by } \frac{c/n_2}{d/n_2} = \frac{c}{d} = \frac{126}{2912}.$$

The odds ratio is, therefore, estimated by

$$\hat{or} = \frac{a/b}{c/d} = \frac{170/3222}{126/2912} = \frac{ad}{bc} = \frac{170(2912)}{126(3222)} = 1.219.$$

For all estimated values, the assessment of the influence of random variation is basic to their interpretation. For the breast cancer data, an important question becomes: Is the odds ratio estimate of $\hat{or} = 1.219$ substantially different from 1.0 (no association $= or = 1.0$) in light of its associated sampling variation? In other

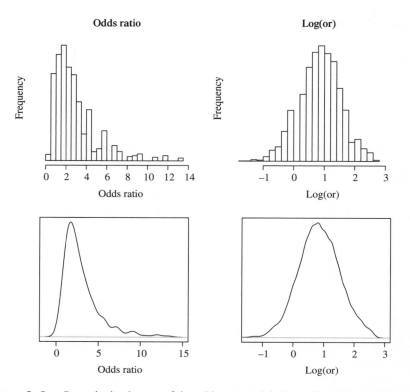

Figure 1–1. Example distributions of the odds ratio and the logarithm of the odds ratio.

words: Does the estimated odds ratio provide clear evidence that the underlying risk of breast cancer differs between military women who served and did not serve in Vietnam?

The vast majority of statistical assessments require either the knowledge or the assumption that the estimated value has at least an approximate normal distribution (more details in Chapter 3). This requirement is frequently not the case for an estimated odds ratio (Figure 1–1, left side).

A typical statistical strategy to assess an estimate with a non-normal distribution begins with a transformation designed so that it has an approximate normal distribution. Then, the usual statistical tools based on the normal distribution apply accurately (for example, statistical tests and confidence intervals). The logarithm of the odds ratio is such an empirically successful transformation (Figure 1–1, right side). *Note*: all logarithms are natural logarithms (base $e = 2.718281828 \ldots$), sometimes called *Napier logarithms* in honor of John Napier (*b.* 1550), who pioneered the use of logarithms. For the example (Figure 1–1) based on 5000 samples of size $n = 30$, the underlying probabilities $p_1 = 0.6$ and $p_2 = 0.4$

($or = 2.250$) produce a mean value of the distribution of the odds ratio of 2.709. This bias (2.250 vs. 2.709) substantially decreases when the logarithm of the odds ratio is used. The mean value of the more normal-like distribution of the $log(or)$ values is 0.841, and the odds ratio becomes $or = e^{0.841} = 2.320$. Furthermore, this bias diminishes as the sample size n increases.

The estimated variance of the distribution of the log-transformed odds ratio is

$$estimated\ variance = variance[log(\hat{or})] = \frac{1}{a} + \frac{1}{b} + \frac{1}{c} + \frac{1}{d}.$$

The origins and some of the theory underlying the determination of this expression are presented in Chapter 3.

A notable property of the estimate of the odds ratio is evident from a close look at the expression for the variance of the logarithm of the odds ratio. The precision of the estimate is determined by the sum of the reciprocal values of each of the four cell frequencies (a, b, c, and d). These frequencies are often not even close to evenly distributed among the four cells of a 2×2 table. Consequently, the precision of the estimated odds ratio is then largely determined by the smallest cell frequencies, and not the entire sample. For the Vietnam example data, because $a = 170$ and $c = 126$ are relatively small cell frequencies, the other two frequencies are not particularly important in determining the variance. The other cell frequencies only slightly increase the variance. That is, the effective "sample size" is close to $a + c = 170 + 126 = 296$ and not $n = 6430$ women.

From the Vietnam breast cancer data (Table 1–3), the estimated variance of the log-transformed odds ratio is

$$variance[log(\hat{or})] = \frac{1}{170} + \frac{1}{3222} + \frac{1}{126} + \frac{1}{2912} = 0.0145,$$

making the standard error equal to 0.120 ($\sqrt{variance[log(\hat{or})]} = \sqrt{0.0145} = 0.120$). The dominate contributions to the variance are from the two smallest frequencies, where $1/170 + 1/120 = 0.0142$. Using this estimated variance and the normal distribution produces an approximate 95% confidence interval calculated from a 2×2 table based on the estimated value, $log(\hat{or})$.

Approximate 95% confidences interval bounds derived from the normal-like distribution of the estimate $log(\hat{or})$ are

$$lower\ bound = \hat{A} = log(\hat{or}) - 1.960\sqrt{variance[log(\hat{or})]}$$

and

$$upper\ bound = \hat{B} = log(\hat{or}) + 1.960\sqrt{variance[log(\hat{or})]}.$$

The approximate 95% confidence interval bounds based on the estimate, $log(\hat{o}r) = log(1.219) = 0.198$, from the breast cancer data are then

$$lower\ bound = \hat{A} = 0.198 - 1.960(0.120) = -0.037$$

and

$$upper\ bound = \hat{B} = 0.198 + 1.960(0.120) = 0.434.$$

These bounds are primarily an intermediate step in constructing a confidence interval for an odds ratio. They directly translate into approximate but generally accurate 95% confidence bounds for the odds ratio estimated by $\hat{o}r = e^{0.198} = 1.219$. The lower bound becomes $e^{\hat{A}} = e^{-0.037} = 0.963$, and the upper bound becomes $e^{\hat{B}} = e^{0.434} = 1.544$, creating the 95% confidence interval (0.963, 1.544).

The process that produces a confidence interval for an odds ratio is a specific application of a general technique. A confidence interval for a function of a summary statistic is typically created by applying the same function to the bounds of the original confidence interval. Specifically, for the odds ratio, when the confidence interval bounds for the summary statistic $log(\hat{o}r)$ are $(\hat{A}, \hat{B})$, then the bounds for the odds ratio based on the function $\hat{o}r = e^{log(\hat{o}r)}$ are $(e^{\hat{A}}, e^{\hat{B}})$.

The confidence interval for the odds creates another example. When the confidence interval bounds for the probability p are $\hat{A}$ and $\hat{B}$, based on the estimated probability $\hat{p}$, then the confidence interval bounds for the odds based on the function $\hat{o} = \hat{p}/(1 - \hat{p})$ are $\hat{A}/(1 - \hat{A})$ and $\hat{B}/(1 - \hat{B})$. In general, when two confidence interval bounds are $\hat{A}$ and $\hat{B}$, based on an estimated value $\hat{g}$, in many cases, the confidence interval bounds for the function $f(\hat{g})$ are the same function of the original bounds, namely $f(\hat{A})$ and $f(\hat{B})$.

Using the same logarithmic transformation, a test statistic to compare the estimated odds ratio to the value $or = 1.0$ (no association between serving in Vietnam and breast cancer) is

$$z = \frac{log(\hat{o}r) - log(1.0)}{\sqrt{variance[log(\hat{o}r)]}} = \frac{0.198 - 0}{0.120} = 1.649.$$

The test statistic z has an approximate standard normal distribution when $log(or) = log(1) = 0$. The probability of a more extreme value occurring by chance alone is the *significance probability* = p-value = $P(|Z| \geq 1.649 | or = 1) = 0.099$. Such a p-value indicates that the elevated value of the observed odds ratio comparing the odds of breast cancer between women who served and did not serve in Vietnam is plausibly due to random variation. From another point of view, the approximate 95% confidence interval (0.963, 1.544) supports the same inference. A 95% confidence interval contains the likely values of the underlying odds ratio estimated by $\hat{or} = 1.219$, and the value 1.0 (exactly no association) is one of these values.

An optimal and general approach to assessing evidence of an association from data classified into a 2×2 table employs the *chi-square distribution*. The Pearson chi-square test statistic is applied to compare the four observed values (denoted o_{ij}) to four values generated as if no association exists (expected values, denoted e_{ij}). For data from a 2×2 table, some algebra produces the short-cut expression

$$X^2 = \sum\sum \frac{(o_{ij} - e_{ij})^2}{e_{ij}} = \frac{n(ad - bc)^2}{n_1 n_2 m_1 m_2}$$

where the expected values are $e_{ij} = n_i m_j / n$ for $i = 1, 2$ and $j = 1, 2$ (Table 1–2). The four expected values represented by e_{ij} are theoretical cell frequencies calculated as if risk factor and disease are exactly independent (details follow in Chapter 2). For the breast cancer data, the four expected values are given in Table 1–4. At this point, note that the ratios of $D/\overline{D}$ counts (expected odds) are identical regardless of Vietnam status ($156.1/3235.9 = 139.9/2898.1 = 296/6134 = 0.048$) indicating exactly no association. Thus, the odds ratio is exactly 1.0 for these theoretical values. In a statistical context, the term *expected value* has a technical meaning. An expected value is a theoretical value calculated to conform exactly to specified conditions and is treated as a fixed (nonrandom) quantity. The test statistic X^2 has a chi-square distribution with one degree of freedom when no association exists ($or = 1$). For the Vietnam/cancer data, the value of the chi-square test statistic is

$$X^2 = \frac{n(ad - bc)^2}{n_1 n_2 m_1 m_2} = \frac{6430[170(2912) - 126(3222)]^2}{3392(3038)(296)6134} = 2.726$$

yielding a p-value $= P(X^2 \geq 2.726 | no\ association) = 0.099$. The parallel statistical test based on the logarithm of the odds ratio is not the same as the

Table 1–4. Expected numbers of breast cancer cases (D) among military women who served in Vietnam (F) and those who did not serve in Vietnam (F) when the odds ratio $or = 1$ (no association*)

	D	$\overline{D}$	Total
F	$e_{11} = 156.1$	$e_{12} = 3235.9$	$n_1 = 3392$
$\overline{F}$	$e_{21} = 139.9$	$e_{22} = 2898.1$	$n_1 = 3038$
Total	$m_1 = 296$	$m_1 = 6134$	$n = 6430$

$$* = or = \frac{156.1/3235.9}{139.9/2898.1} = 1.0.$$

chi-square test but rarely differs by an important amount (previously, $X^2 = (1.649)^2 = 2.719$).

An odds ratio of 1.0 generates a variety of equivalent expressions for the relationships between the probability of a disease D and a risk factor F. Some examples are:

$$P(F|D) = P(F|\overline{D}),\ P(D|F) = P(D|\overline{F}),$$
$$P(D \text{ and } F) = P(D)P(F) \text{ and } P(D|F) = P(D).$$

The last expression shows in concrete terms that an odds ratio of $or = 1$ means that the risk factor (F) is unrelated to the likelihood of disease (D).

An advertisement and a brochure produced by the March of Dimes (1998) states:

> Debbie and Rich Hedding of Pittsford Vt. were devastated when they lost two babies to neural tube defects (NTDs). When Debbie read about folic acid in a March of Dimes brochure, she was astonished when she learned about the role of folic acid in preventing NTDs. "I was in tears by the time I finished reading the material. I haven't been taking folic acid nor had I been told about it. I couldn't believe that I could have reduced the risk of recurrence by 70 percent. I immediately began taking folic acid and telling every women I could about it."

The published odds ratio was $\hat{o}r = 0.28$ (the 95% confidence interval is (0.12, 0.71), *Lancet*, 1996). The 70% reduction in risk refers to $(1 - 0.280) \times 100 = 72\%$. However, the odds ratio, as the name indicates, is a ratio measure of association. It measures association in terms of a multiplicative scale and behaves in an asymmetric way on an additive scale. Odds ratios between zero and 1 indicate a decrease in risk, and odds ratios greater than 1 (1.0 to infinity) indicate an increase in risk. From a more useful point of view, an odds ratio of $1/or$ measures the same degree of association as the odds ratio or, but in the opposite direction, which is a property of a ratio scale. Thus, an odds ratio of 0.28 reduces risk of an NTD by a factor of $1/0.28 = 3.57$, a reduction considerably greater than 70%. Comparisons on a ratio scale are necessarily made in terms of ratios.

From the perspective of a 2×2 table, interchanging the rows (or columns) changes the odds ratio from or to $1/or$ but does not influence the degree of association between variables because the order of the rows (or columns) is purely arbitrary. The result of a statistical test of association, for example, is unchanged (same p-value). It should be noted that the logarithms of values measured on a ratio scale produce values that are directly comparable on an additive scale. An odds ratio of 0.28 is equivalent to an odds ratio of 3.57, relative to 1.0 on a ratio scale. Thus, the value $\log(0.28) = -1.273$ is equivalent to the value $\log(3.57) = 1.273$ relative to $\log(1) = 0$ on an additive scale. The transformation of an odds

Table 1–5. Four measures of association from a 2×2 table and expressions for their estimation

	Measures	Symbols	Estimates*
Difference in probabilities (rows)	$P(D\|F) - P(D\|\overline{F})$	$\hat{p}_1 - \hat{p}_2$	$\dfrac{a}{a+b} - \dfrac{c}{c+d}$
Difference in probabilities (columns)	$P(F\|D) - P(F\|\overline{D})$	$\hat{P}_1 - \hat{P}_2$	$\dfrac{a}{a+c} - \dfrac{c}{b+d}$
Relative risk	$\dfrac{P(D\|F)}{P(D\|\overline{F})}$	$\hat{r}r$	$\dfrac{a/(a+b)}{c/(c+d)}$
Odds ratio	$\dfrac{P(D\|F)/P(\overline{D}\|F)}{P(D\|\overline{F})/P(\overline{D}\|\overline{F})}$	$\hat{o}r$	$\dfrac{a/b}{c/d}$

Note: * = notation from Table 1–2.

ratio to the logarithm of an odds ratio can be viewed as a change from a ratio scale to the more familiar and intuitive additive scale.

The odds ratio is one of a number of possible measures of association between two binary variables described by a 2×2 table. Table 1–5 lists three other common measures of an association where, again, $D/\overline{D}$ could represent the presence/absence of disease and $F/\overline{F}$ could represent the presence/absence of a binary risk factor. Although these summary values reflect the magnitude of an association in different ways, their statistical evaluation follows much the same pattern.

Normal distribution–based statistical tests and 95% confidence intervals associated with the evaluation of measures of association require estimates of their *variances*. Expressions for estimates of the variances of the distributions of these measures of association and their values from the Vietnam/cancer data are given in Table 1–6.

Each measure of association can be assessed with a normal distribution–based test statistic of the form

$$z = \frac{\hat{g} - g_0}{\sqrt{variance(\hat{g})}}$$

where $\hat{g}$ represents any one of the estimated measures of association and g_0 represents a theoretical value. The previous chi-square statistic, however, is easily applied and typically used to evaluate the influence of random variation in a 2×2 table.

Approximate confidence intervals for these measures of association (Tables 1–5 and 1–6) based on the normal distribution are created from a single expression. An approximate but again generally accurate 95% confidence interval is

$$\hat{g} \pm 1.960\sqrt{variance(\hat{g})}.$$

Table 1-6. Expressions for estimates of the variances of the distributions of six measures of association* applied to the comparison of the risk of breast cancer between female veterans who served and did not serve in Vietnam (Table 1-3)

	Symbols	Variances	Std. errors
Difference in proportions (rows)	$\hat{p}_1 - \hat{p}_2$	$\dfrac{\hat{p}_1(1 - \hat{p}_1)}{n_1} + \dfrac{\hat{p}_2(1 - \hat{p}_2)}{n_2}$	0.0052
Difference in proportions (columns)	$\hat{P}_1 - \hat{P}_2$	$\dfrac{\hat{P}_1(1 - \hat{P}_1)}{m_1} + \dfrac{\hat{P}_2(1 - \hat{P}_2)}{m_2}$	0.0294
Relative risk	$\hat{rr}$	$\hat{rr}^2\left[\dfrac{1}{a} - \dfrac{1}{n_1} + \dfrac{1}{c} + \dfrac{1}{n_2}\right]$	0.1388**
Logarithm of the relative risk	$log(\hat{rr})$	$\dfrac{1}{a} - \dfrac{1}{n_1} + \dfrac{1}{c} - \dfrac{1}{n_2}$	0.1149**
Odds ratio	$\hat{or}$	$\hat{or}^2\left[\dfrac{1}{a} + \dfrac{1}{b} + \dfrac{1}{c} + \dfrac{1}{d}\right]$	0.1467
Logarithm of the odds ratio	$log(\hat{or})$	$\dfrac{1}{a} + \dfrac{1}{b} + \dfrac{1}{c} + \dfrac{1}{d}$	0.1203

Note: * = Chapter 3 contains a discussion of the statistical origins of these expressions.

    ** = another version of the estimated variance excludes the terms $1/n_1$ and $1/n_2$ (Chapter 6).

Table 1-7. Six measures of association applied to evaluate the risk of breast cancer among female veterans who served in Vietnam (statistical tests and 95% confidence intervals)

	Symbols	Estimates	p-Values	Lower	Upper
Difference in proportions (rows)*	$\hat{p}_1 - \hat{p}_2$	0.009	0.099	−0.002	0.019
Difference in proportions (columns)*	$\hat{P}_1 - \hat{P}_2$	0.049	0.099	−0.009	0.107
Relative risk	$\hat{rr}$	1.208	0.099	0.964	1.513
Logarithm of the relative risk	$log(\hat{rr})$	0.189	0.099	−0.036	0.414
Odds ratio	$\hat{or}$	1.219	0.099	0.963	1.544
Logarithm of the odds ratio	$log(\hat{or})$	0.198	0.099	−0.037	0.434

Note: * Identical to the previous chi-square test, $X^2 = 2.726$.

As with the odds ratio, approximate tests and 95% confidence intervals for the relative risk measure of association (a ratio measure of association) are more accurate when the logarithm of the relative risk is used (an additive measure of association). Examples from the Vietnam/cancer data are displayed in Table 1–7.

PROPERTIES OF THE ODDS RATIO

The term *relative risk* (denoted rr, Table 1–5) refers to a ratio of two probabilities and is a natural multiplicative measure to compare the probability of disease between a group with the risk factor to a group without the risk factor (Chapter 6). When the disease is rare [$P(D|F)$ and $P(D|\overline{F})$ are both less than 0.1], the odds ratio is approximately equal to the relative risk ($or \approx rr$). For the Vietnam example data, the estimated odds ratio is $\hat{or} = 1.219$ and the estimated relative risk is $\hat{rr} = 1.208$, because breast cancer is rare in both groups (probability ≈ 0.05).

The results from a survey of 720 primary care physicians conducted by Schulman and colleagues were published in *The New England Journal of Medicine* (1999). These authors pointed out that their data indicate that "women (odds ratio, 0.60; 95% confidence interval 0.4 to 0.9, ...) and blacks (odds ratio, 0.60; 95% confidence interval 0.4 to 0.9, ...) were less likely to be referred to cardiac catheterization than men and whites, respectively." This apparent inequality in care immediately became a topic of the national news coverage and the subject of the television show *Nightline*. Generally, the media reported that a recent study showed that 40% of black patients were less likely than white patients to be referred for appropriate coronary care.

The collected data showed a 84.7% correct response for black and a 90.6% correct response for white patients from physicians managing chest pain. Thus, an odds ratio of

$$odds\ ratio = \hat{or} = \frac{0.847/0.153}{0.906/0.094} = 0.574.$$

For these same data, the estimated relative risk is

$$relative\ risk = \hat{rr} = \frac{P(correct|black)}{P(correct|white)} = \frac{0.847}{0.906} = 0.935.$$

As noted, an odds ratio accurately measures risk (approximates relative risk) only when the "disease" is rare in both compared groups. Although an odds ratio measures the association between race and care, it does not reflect risk because the probability of correct care is not rare in both compared groups.

Following the publication of this article, the editors of *The New England Journal of Medicine* stated that, "we take responsibility for the media over-interpretation of the article by Schulman and colleagues. We should not have allowed the odds ratio in the abstract." Perhaps the most intuitive and easily interpreted contrast between white and black patients is the directly measured difference in proportions, where

$$difference = P(correct|white) - P(correct|black) = 0.906 - 0.847 = 0.059.$$

A small numeric example illustrates the reason for the similarity of the odds ratio to the relative risk as a measure of risk only when the disease is rare. Fictional data simply indicate the role of the "rare disease requirement."

Consider the case in which the probability of disease is $P(disease) = 8/28 = 0.29$ (not rare) and

	Disease	No disease	Total
Risk factor present	3	10	13
Risk factor absent	5	10	15

$$odds\ ratio = \frac{3/10}{5/10} = 0.60 \qquad relative\ risk = \frac{3/13}{5/15} = 0.69$$

Now, consider the case where the probability of disease is $P(disease) = 8/208 = 0.04$ (rare in both groups) and

	Disease	No disease	Total
Risk factor present	3	100	103
Risk factor absent	5	100	105

$$odds\ ratio = \frac{3/100}{5/100} = 0.60 \qquad relative\ risk = \frac{3/103}{5/105} = 0.61$$

In symbols, for the second case, both measures of association are similar because $b \approx a+b$ and $d \approx c+d$ making

$$\hat{r} = \frac{a/(a+b)}{c/(c+d)} \approx \frac{a/b}{c/d} = \hat{o}r \qquad \text{(Table 1–5)}$$

That is, the number of cases of disease 3 and 5 are not particularly small relative to 13 and 15 (approximately 40%) but are substantially smaller than 103 and 105 (approximately 5%).

At the beginning of the 18th century, Sir Thomas Bayes (*b.* 1702) noted that, for two events, denoted A and B,

$$P(A \text{ and } B) = P(A|B)P(B) \qquad \text{and} \qquad P(A \text{ and } B) = P(B|A)P(A),$$

leading to the historic expression called *Bayes' theorem* where

$$P(A|B) = \frac{P(B|A)P(A)}{P(B)}.$$

Less historic, but important to the study of disease and other binary variables, the odds ratio has the same value whether the association under study is measured by comparing the likelihoods of the risk factor between individuals with and without the disease or is measured by comparing the likelihoods of the disease between individuals with and without the risk factor. Retrospectively and case/control collected data require the comparison of the likelihood of the risk factor between individuals with and without the disease. Prospectively and cross-sectionally collected data require the comparison of the likelihood of the disease among individuals with and without the risk factor. The key to assessing an association using these two kinds of data is the comparison of the probability of the risk factor among those with the disease $P(F|D)$ to those without disease $P(F|\overline{D})$, or the comparison of the probability of the disease among those with the risk factor $P(D|F)$ to those without the risk factor $P(D|\overline{F})$.

An application of Bayes' theorem shows that, regardless of the kind of data collected, the odds ratio measure of association is the same. Specifically, four applications of Bayes' theorem give

$$or = \frac{P(D|F)/P(\overline{D}|F)}{P(D|\overline{F})/P(\overline{D}|\overline{F})} = \frac{\left[\dfrac{P(F|D)P(D)}{P(F)} \Big/ \dfrac{P(F|\overline{D})P(\overline{D})}{P(F)}\right]}{\left[\dfrac{P(\overline{F}|D)P(D)}{P(\overline{F})} \Big/ \dfrac{P(\overline{F}|\overline{D})P(\overline{D})}{P(\overline{F})}\right]}$$

$$= \frac{P(F|D)/P(F|\overline{D})}{P(\overline{F}|D)/P(\overline{F}|\overline{D})} = or.$$

The estimated odds ratio follows the same pattern, where

$$\hat{or} = \frac{a/b}{c/d} = \frac{ad}{bc} = \frac{a/c}{b/d} = \hat{or}.$$

The property that the odds ratio and its estimate are the same for both kinds of data is also a property of comparing two proportions from a 2×2 table. That is, the test statistics produce exactly the same result. Specifically, the evaluation of the difference $P(D|F) - P(D|\overline{F})$ or $P(F|D) - P(F|\overline{D})$ produces

$$\text{difference in proportions (rows)} = \frac{\hat{p}_1 - \hat{p}_2}{\sqrt{\dfrac{\hat{p}_1(1-\hat{p}_1)}{n_1} + \dfrac{\hat{p}_2(1-\hat{p}_2)}{n_2}}}$$

$$= \frac{\hat{P}_1 - \hat{P}_2}{\sqrt{\dfrac{\hat{P}_1(1-\hat{P}_1)}{m_1} + \dfrac{\hat{P}_2(1-\hat{P}_2)}{m_2}}} = \text{difference in proportions (columns)}.$$

Another notable property of the odds ratio is that it is always further from 1.0 (no association) than the relative risk calculated from the same 2×2 table. In symbols,

$$\text{when } rr \geq 1.0, \text{ then } or \geq rr \geq 1.0$$

and

$$\text{when } rr \leq 1.0, \text{then } or \leq rr \leq 1.0.$$

In this sense, the relative risk is conservative, because any association measured by relative risk is more extreme when measured by an odds ratio.

THREE STATISTICAL TERMS

A discussion of the odds ratio calculated from a 2×2 table presents an opportunity to introduce three fundamental concepts relevant to many statistical analyses. These concepts are properties of summary values calculated from data and are not properties of the sampled population. This extremely important distinction is frequently not made clear. The concepts are: *interaction, confounding*, and *independence*. These three general properties of summary values are defined and discussed for the simplest possible case, three binary variables classified into two 2×2 tables, where associations are measured by odds ratios. The example binary variables are discussed in terms of a disease D, a risk factor F, and a third variable labeled C. This introductory description is expanded in subsequent chapters.

When the odds ratios calculated from each of two tables differ, the question arises: Do the estimated values differ by chance alone or does a systematic difference exist? The failure of a measure of association to be the same within each subtable is an example of an *interaction* (Table 1–8A). An interaction, in simple terms, is the failure of the values measured by a summary statistic to be the same under different conditions.

The existence of an interaction is a central element in addressing the issues involved in combining estimates. In the case of two 2×2 tables, the first issue is the choice between describing an association with two separate odds ratios (denoted $or_{DF|C}$ and $or_{DF|\overline{C}}$) or a single summary odds ratio (denoted or_{DF}). When odds ratios systematically differ, a single summary odds ratio is usually not meaningful and, in fact, such a single value can be misleading (an example follows). However, when the odds ratios measuring association differ only by chance alone,

Table 1–8A. An odds ratio measure of association between the risk factor F and disease D that differs at the two levels of the variable C (an interaction)

C	D	$\overline{D}$	Total		$\overline{C}$	D	$\overline{D}$	Total
F	20	20	40		F	60	20	80
$\overline{F}$	10	40	50		$\overline{F}$	10	20	30
Total	30	60	90		**Total**	70	40	110

$$or_{DF|C} = 4 \qquad\qquad or_{DF|\overline{C}} = 6$$

Table 1–8B. The odds ratios between the risk factor F and disease D at the two levels of the variable C (no interaction) and a single odds ratio from the combined table.

C	D	$\overline{D}$	Total
F	40	20	60
$\overline{F}$	10	40	50
Total	50	60	110

$$or_{DF|C} = 8$$

$\overline{C}$	D	$\overline{D}$	Total
F	80	20	160
$\overline{F}$	10	20	30
Total	90	40	130

$$or_{DF|\overline{C}} = 8$$

$C + \overline{C}$	D	$\overline{D}$	Total
F	120	40	160
$\overline{F}$	20	60	80
Total	140	100	240

$$or_{DF|(C+\overline{C})} = or_{DF} = 9$$

the opposite is true. A single odds ratio is not only a meaningful summary but provides a useful, simpler, and more precise measure of the association between the risk factor and disease.

When a single odds ratio is a useful summary (no interaction), the second issue becomes the choice of how the summary value is calculated. The choice is between a summary value calculated by combining the two odds ratios or by combining the data into a single table and then calculating a summary odds ratio. When the table created by adding two subtables does not reflect the relationship within each subtable, it is said that the variable used to create the subtables has a *confounding influence*. Specifically (Table 1–8B), the odds ratio in the combined table $or_{DF|(C+\overline{C})} = or_{DF} = 9.0$ is not equal to odds ratios in each subtable where $or_{DF|C} = or_{DF|\overline{C}} = 8.0$, identifying the fact that the variable C has a confounding influence. Consequently, to accurately estimate the risk/disease association it is necessary to account for the variable C by combining the odds ratios from each subtable. Otherwise, combining the data into a single table fails to account for the influence of the variable C, producing a biased estimate.

When the variable C is unrelated to the disease or the risk factor. The odds ratio calculated from the 2×2 table formed by combining the data then accurately reflects the risk factor/disease relationship. Table 1–8C illustrates the case where all three odds ratios equal 4.0 ($or_{DF|C} = or_{DF|\overline{C}} = or_{DF|C+\overline{C}} = or_{DF} = 4.0$). The variable C is then said to be an *independent* summary of the risk/disease association. The collapsed table (C-table + $\overline{C}$-table) eliminates the variable C and accurately produces a simpler and more precise measure of the association.

This description of the terms interaction, confounding, and independence does not account for random variation of observed values, but consists of simple and fictional data that perfectly reflect the three concepts. However, important properties are illustrated. Namely, the presence or absence of an interaction determines

Table 1–8C. The odds ratios between the risk factor *F* and disease *D* at the two levels of the variable *C*, and a single odds ratio from the combined table (independence)

C	*D*	$\overline{D}$	**Total**
F	20	20	40
$\overline{F}$	10	40	50
Total	30	60	90

$$or_{DF|C} = 4$$

$\overline{C}$	*D*	$\overline{D}$	**Total**
F	40	40	80
$\overline{F}$	20	80	100
Total	60	120	180

$$or_{DF|\overline{C}} = 4$$

$C+\overline{C}$	*D*	$\overline{D}$	**Total**
F	60	60	120
$\overline{F}$	30	120	150
Total	90	180	270

$$or_{DF|(C+\overline{C})} = or_{DF} = 4$$

whether or not a single summary value is useful. When a single summary is useful, the presence or absence of a confounding influence from a third variable determines the way in which a summary value is calculated. When a confounding influence exists, the values calculated from each subtable are combined to form a summary value. When a confounding influence does not exist, the summary value is more effectively and simply calculated from a single table created by adding the subtables. That is, the third variable is ignored. The topic of creating accurate summary values in applied situations is continued in detail in Chapter 2 and beyond.

A classic statistical example [3], called *Simpson's paradox*, is not really a paradox but an illustration of the consequences of ignoring an interaction. Simpson's original "cancer treatment data" are presented in Table 1–9.

Simpson created "data" in which the summary values from each subtable have the opposite relationship from the summary value calculated from the combined data. A new treatment (denoted *F*) appears more successful than the usual treatment (denoted $\overline{F}$) for two kinds of cancer patients, but when the data are combined into a single table, the new treatment appears less effective.

The three relevant odds ratios are:

$$or_{SF|C} = 2.38, \quad or_{SF|\overline{C}} = 39.0 \quad \text{and} \quad or_{SF|C+\overline{C}} = or_{SF} = 0.45.$$

The stage I cancer patients (*C*) and stage II cancer patients ($\overline{C}$) clearly differ with respect to the new treatment, reflected by their extremely different odds ratios (2.38 and 39.0). Technically, it is said that the treatment and stage measures of survival (odds ratios) have a strong (a very strong) interaction with the treatment classification. Therefore, combining the data and calculating a single summary value produces a result that has no useful interpretation. The point is, when

Table 1–9. The "data" used to demonstrate Simpson's paradox

S = Survived and $\overline{S}$ = died
F = New treatment and $\overline{F}$ = usual treatment
C = Stage I cancer (not severe) and $\overline{C}$ = stage IV cancer (severe)

C	F	$\overline{F}$	Total
S	95	800	895
$\overline{S}$	5	100	105
Total	100	900	1000

$P(survived|new) = P(S|F) = 0.95$
$P(survived|usual) = P(S|\overline{F}) = 0.88$

$\overline{C}$	F	$\overline{F}$	Total
F	400	5	405
$\overline{F}$	400	195	595
Total	800	200	1000

$P(survived|new) = P(S|F) = 0.50$
$P(survived|usual) = P(S|\overline{F}) = 0.025$

$C + \overline{C}$	F	$\overline{F}$	Total
S	495	805	1300
$\overline{S}$	405	295	700
Total	900	1100	2000

$P(survived|new) = P(S|F) = 0.55$
$P(survived|usual) = P(S|\overline{F}) = 0.73$

measures of association that reflect two different relationships are combined, any value of a summary statistic is possible and is rarely meaningful.

AVERAGE RATES

Disease and mortality rates are familiar and extensively used summaries of risk, particularly in public health, medicine, and epidemiology. The United States 1940 cancer mortality rate among individuals 60–64 years old was 88.7 deaths per 100,000 person-years, and 60 years later the cancer mortality rate for the same age group has decreased to 75.9 deaths per 100,000 person-years. One gets a sense of the change in risk by comparing two such rates, but the answers to a number of questions are not apparent. Some examples are: Why report the number of deaths per person-years? How do these rates differ from probabilities? What is their relationship to the mean survival time? Or, more fundamentally: Why does such a rate reflect risk? The following is a less than casual but short of rigorous description of the statistical origins and properties of an average rate. To simplify the terminology, rates from this point on are referred to as *mortality rates*, but the description applies to disease incidence rates, as well as to many other kinds of average rates.

An average rate is a ratio of two mean values. For a mortality rate, the mean number of deaths divided by the mean survival time experienced by those individuals at risk forms the average rate.

The mean number of deaths is also the *proportion* of deaths. A proportion is another name for a mean value calculated from zeros and ones. In symbols and denoted q,

$$mean\ value = proportion = \frac{0+1+0+0+\cdots+1}{n} = \frac{\sum x_i}{n} = \frac{d}{n} = q$$

where x_i represents a binary variable that takes on only the values zero or one among n individuals and d represents the sum of these n values of zeros and ones. In the language of baseball, this mean value is called a *batting average* but elsewhere it is usually referred to as a proportion or an estimated probability (Chapter 3).

The mean survival time, similar to any mean value, is the total time at risk experienced by the n individuals who accumulated the relevant survival time divided by n. In symbols, the estimated mean survival time is

$$\bar{t} = \frac{total\ time\ at\text{-}risk}{total\ number\ individuals\ at\text{-}risk} = \frac{\sum t_i}{n}$$

where t_i represents the time at risk for each of n at-risk individuals ($i = 1, 2, \cdots, n$). Then, the expression for an average rate (denoted R) becomes

$$R = average\ rate = \frac{mean\ number\ of\ deaths}{mean\ survival\ time} = \frac{q}{\bar{t}} = \frac{d/n}{\sum t_i/n} = \frac{d}{\sum t_i}.$$

Equivalently, but less intuitively, an average rate is usually defined as the total number of deaths (d) divided by the total time-at-risk ($\sum t_i$).

An average rate can be viewed as the reciprocal of a mean value. When a trip takes 4 hours to go 120 miles, the mean travel time is 2 minutes per mile ($\bar{t} = 240/120 = 2$ minutes per mile, or $\bar{t} = 4/120 = 1/30$ of an hour per mile). Also, a trip of 120 miles traveled in 4 hours yields an average rate of speed of $120/4 = 30$ miles per hour. The reciprocal of the mean time of 1/30 of an hour per mile is an average rate of 30 miles per hour.

For an average mortality rate, first consider the not very frequently occurring case in which a group of individuals is observed until all at-risk persons have died. The mean survival time is then $\bar{t} = \sum t_i/n$, and the number of deaths is $d = n$ (all died) making

$$average\ rate = R = \frac{d}{\sum t_i} = \frac{n}{\sum t_i} = \frac{1}{\bar{t}} \quad or \quad \bar{t} = \frac{1}{R}.$$

A more realistic case occurs when a group of individuals is observed for a period of time and, at the end of that time, not all at-risk persons have died. A single estimate requires that the value estimated be a single value. Thus, when a single rate is estimated from data collected over a period of time, it is implicitly assumed that the risk described by this single value is constant over the same time period or at least approximately constant. When a mortality rate is constant, then the mean survival time is also constant. Under this condition, the constant mortality rate associated with d deaths among n at-risk individuals is, as before, estimated by the average rate given by $R = d/\sum t_i$, where t_i represents the observed time alive for both individuals who died and survived. The mean time lived (denote $\hat{\mu}$) by all n individuals is again estimated by the reciprocal of this rate or

$$\hat{\mu} = \frac{1}{R} = \frac{\sum t_i}{d}.$$

Naturally, as the rate of death increases, the mean survival time decreases and vice versa.

The estimated mean survival time is the total survival time observed for all n at-risk individuals divided by d (number of deaths) and not n (number of observed individuals) for the following reason. The sum of the survival times ($\sum t_i$) is too small because not all n observed individuals died. The $n - d$ individuals who did not die would contribute additional survival time if the period of observation was extended. Specifically, the amount of "missing time," on average, is $\mu(n - d)$ because each individual who did not die would have contributed, on average, an additional time of μ to the total survival time if he were observed until his death. Including this "missing time," the expression for the mean survival time becomes

$$\hat{\mu} = \frac{total\ time}{total\ number\ individuals\ at\text{-}risk} = \frac{\sum t_i + \hat{\mu}(n - d)}{n},$$

and solving for $\hat{\mu}$ gives $\hat{\mu} = \sum t_i/d$ as the estimated mean survival time. This estimate $\hat{\mu}$ is unbiased in the sense that it compensates for the $n - d$ incomplete survival times (unobserved times to death). As long as the mean survival time μ is the same for those individuals who died during the time period under consideration and those who did not, the mortality rate and the mean survival time are again inversely related or $\hat{\mu} = \sum t_i/d = 1/R$.

Many sources of disease incidence and mortality data consist of individuals classified into categories based on their age at death or time of death. For these kinds of survival data, the exact time of death is not usually available. This is particularly true of publicly available disease and mortality data (see the National Center for Health Statistics or the National Cancer Institute or Center for Disease Control websites http://www.cdc.gov/nchs/ or http://www.nci.nih.gov

or http://www.cdc.gov). However, a generally accurate but approximate average mortality rate can be calculated when the length of the age or time interval considered is not large.

Consider a time interval with limits denoted a_i to a_{i+1} years (length of the interval $= \delta_i = a_{i+1} - a_i$ years), where l_i individuals are alive at the beginning of the interval and d_i of these individuals died during the interval. The total time alive (at-risk) is made up of two distinct contributions. First, the $l_i - d_i$ individuals who survived the entire interval (δ_i years) contribute $\delta_i(l_i - d_i)$ person-years to the total years lived. Second, over a short interval such as 5 or even 10 years, deaths usually occur approximately at random throughout the interval so that, on average, each individual who died contributes $\frac{1}{2}\delta_i$ years to the total years lived. Thus, the d_i individuals who died during the interval contribute $\frac{1}{2}\delta_i d_i$ person-years to the total years lived. Therefore, the approximate total years lived during the ith interval is

$$total\ person\text{-}years\text{-}at\text{-}risk = \delta_i(l_i - d_i) + \frac{1}{2}\delta_i d_i = \delta_i\left(l_i - \frac{1}{2}d_i\right).$$

An approximate average mortality rate for the ith interval (denoted R_i), based on this approximate years-at-risk, is then

$$average\ mortality\ rate = R_i = \frac{number\ of\ deaths\ in\ the\ i^{th}\ interval}{total\ years\text{-}at\text{-}risk\ in\ the\ i^{th}\ interval}$$

$$= \frac{d_i}{\delta_i(l_i - \frac{1}{2}d_i)}\ deaths\ per\ person\text{-}years.$$

This approximate rate is again the mean number of deaths ($q_i = d_i/l_i$) divided by the mean survival time ($\bar{t}_i = \delta_i[l_i - \frac{1}{2}d_i]/l_i$) or, as before, $R_i = q_i/\bar{t}_i$.

The probability of death in a specific interval of time is

$$probability\ of\ death\ in\ the\ i^{th}\ interval = q_i = \frac{d_i}{l_i}.$$

That is, the probability q_i is the number events that have a specific property (for example, deaths $= d_i$) divided by the total number of events that could have occurred (for example, all persons who could have died, at-risk $= l_i$). In human data, disease or death are frequently rare events causing d_i to be much smaller than l_i ($d_i \ll l_i$). In this case, an average rate for a specific age or time interval essentially equals the probability of death divided by the length of the interval.

Or, in symbols,

$$R_i = \frac{mean\ number\ of\ deaths}{mean\ survival\ time} = \frac{d_i/l_i}{\delta_i(l_i - \frac{1}{2}d_i)/l_i}$$

$$= \frac{q_i}{\delta_i(1 - \frac{1}{2}q_i)} \approx \frac{q_i}{\delta_i} \quad \left(1 - \frac{1}{2}q_i \approx 1\right).$$

Therefore, when the interval length considered is 1 year ($\delta_i = 1$), the value of a mortality rate and a probability of death are usually interchangeable ($R_i \approx q_i$). Furthermore, a rate ratio and a ratio of probabilities are also essentially equal when applied to the same time interval. In symbols, the ratios are

$$rate\ ratio = \frac{R_1}{R_2} \approx \frac{q_1/\delta}{q_2/\delta} = \frac{q_1}{q_2} = relative\ risk\ ratio.$$

Geometry of an Average Rate

The exact geometry of an average rate is complicated and requires specialized mathematical tools [4]. However, the approximate geometry is simple and is displayed in Figure 1–2. The key to a geometric description of a rate is the proportion of surviving individuals measured at two points in time. These proportions are called *survival probabilities* and for the time interval a_i to a_{i+1} (length again δ_i) they are

$$P_i = \frac{l_i}{l_0} \quad and \quad P_{i+1} = \frac{l_{i+1}}{l_0}$$

where P_i and P_{i+1} then represent the proportion of individuals alive at times a_i and a_{i+1} among the original population of individuals at-risk (size denoted l_0).

The approximate mean person-years again consists of two parts, namely the mean years lived by those who survived the entire interval (a rectangle) and the mean years lived by those who died during the interval (a triangle). In more detail, for those individuals who lived the entire interval

$$rectangle = width \times height = \delta_i P_{i+1}\ person\text{-}years,$$

and for those individuals who died during the interval

$$triangle = \frac{1}{2}base \times altitude = \frac{1}{2}\delta_i(P_i - P_{i+1}) = \frac{1}{2}\delta_i D_i\ person\text{-}years,$$

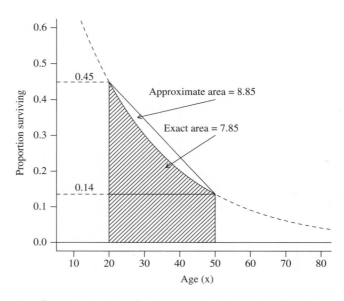

Figure 1–2.   The approximate and exact areas (approximate and exact mean survival times) describing the mortality pattern of a hypothetical population.

where $P_i - P_{i+1} = D_i$ represents the proportion of deaths that occurred in the ith interval. Then,

$$area = approximate\ mean\ survival\ time = rectangle + triangle$$

$$= \delta_i P_{i+1} + \frac{1}{2}\delta_i D_i = \delta_i\left(P_i - \frac{1}{2}D_i\right)\ person\text{-}years.$$

Again, it is necessary to assume that the underlying mortality rate is at least close to constant, so that a single rate R accurately reflects the risk for the entire interval.

From the plot (Figure 1–2), two example survival probabilities are $P_{20} = 0.45$ and $P_{50} = 0.14$ at ages 20 and 50 years and, therefore, the area of the *rectangle* = $30(0.14) = 4.20$ person-years. The mean number of deaths (proportion) is $D_{20} = P_{20} - P_{50} = 0.45 - 0.14 = 0.31$. Therefore, the area of the *triangle* = $\frac{1}{2}30(0.45 - 0.14) = \frac{1}{2}30(0.31) = 4.65$ person-years. The approximate mean survival time then becomes *total area* = $4.20 + 4.65 = 8.85$ person-years for the interval 20 to 50 years ($\delta = 30$). More succinctly, the mean time survived is $30(0.45 - \frac{1}{2}0.31) = 8.85$ years. The average approximate rate is again the ratio of these two mean values or

$$R = \frac{0.31}{8.85} \times 10,000\ person\text{-}years = 350.3\ deaths\ per\ 10,000\ person\text{-}years.$$

From another but equivalent prospective, when $l_0 = 1000$ individuals are at risk, then for the interval age 20 to 50 years

$$total\ years\text{-}at\text{-}risk = l_0(\delta_i P_{i+1}) + l_0 \left(\frac{1}{2}\delta_i D_i \right)$$

$$= 1000(30)(0.14) + 1000 \left(\frac{1}{2} \right)(30)(0.31)$$

$$= 4200 + 4650 = 8850\ person\text{-}years \quad and$$

$$total\ deaths = l_0 D_i = 1000(0.31) = 310\ deaths$$

producing the identical approximate average rate

$$rate = R = \frac{total\ deaths}{total\ person\text{-}years\text{-}at\text{-}risk} \times 10,000$$

$$= \frac{310}{8850} \times 10,000$$

$$= 350.3\ deaths\ per\ 10,000\ person\text{-}years.$$

To calculate the exact area (mean survival time), the survival probability curve (Figure 1–2, dashed line) must be mathematically defined (left to more advanced presentations). However, for the example, the exact rate generated from the survival probabilities (Figure 1–2) is 400 death per 10,000 person-years at risk for any interval (constant mortality rate). As the interval length δ decreases, the approximate rate becomes a more accurate estimate of this constant rate because a straight line (approximate) and a curve (exact) become increasingly similar. That is, a rectangle plus a triangle more accurately estimate the mean person-years at risk (area under the curve). For the example, the approximate average rate is 395 deaths per 10,000 person-years for a 10-year interval, and the rate is 399 deaths per 10,000 person-years for a 5-year interval.

Proportionate Mortality "Rates"

Researchers Coren and Halpren found that the "average age of death for right-handers in the sample was 75 years. For left-handers, it was 66." The authors attributed this difference in age-at-death primarily to a difference in risk from accidents (*New England Journal of Medicine*, 1988).

The study described by the newspaper story is based on a sample of 1,000 death certificates. All individuals sampled are dead. Comparing the frequency of deaths among individuals with different exposures or risk factors is called a *proportionate mortality study*. A fundamental property of proportionate mortality studies in general is that it is not possible to determine from the data whether

San Francisco Chronicle

sfgate.com   415-777-1111

Right-Handers Outlive Lefties By 9-Year Average, Study Says

By Malcolm Gladwell
Washington Post

Boston

In a dramatic and controversial finding, a team of psychologists has reported that left-handed people may live an average of nine years less than right-handers.

The study, based on an analysis of death certificates in the San Bernardino area, is the first to suggest that the well-documented susceptibility of left-handers to a variety of behavioral and physiological disorders can have a substantial effect on life expectancy.

Researchers suspect that left-handers are far more prone to certain kinds of diseases than right-handers and that they are disproportionately represented among those born prematurely and among the mentally retarded. Left-handers are also far more likely to suffer serious accidents.

Speculation

These differences ▸ some researchers ᵗ to speculate ᵗᵗ make uᵖ poᵖᵗ

ence (in left-handers' life expectancy)," said Alan Seariman, a psychologist at St. Lawrence University in New York. "But I certainly can't imagine that there is a nine-year difference. Does it seem reasonable to you that there could have been a difference this large and it would have been unnoticed until 1991?"

Other researchers said Coren and Halpern did not make sure that the difference in death rates

---

'We were astounded. We had no idea that the difference was going to be this huge'

---

very stable data. There is nothing peculiar about this study."

Coren and Halpern offer several explanations for their findings. The first is straightforward: 7.9 percent of left-handers in the sample died in accidents, compared with 1.5 percent of right-handers.

This finding squares with at least one previous study that showed that living in a technological world designed for right-handers has made left-handers five times more likely to get into an accident than their counterparts.

Traffic Peril

As an exam-ᵖ handers hᵉ tage ᵗ

the exposure increased the risk in one group or decreased the risk in another or both. For example, the increased life-time observed in right-handed individuals could be due to a decrease in their risk, or to an increase in the risk of left-handed individuals, or both.

In addition, a frequent problem associated with interpreting proportionate mortality data is that the results are confused with an assessment of the risk of death, as illustrated by the Coren and Halpren report. Rates cannot be calculated from proportionate mortality data. The individuals who did not die are not included in the collected data. From a symbolic point of view, only half of the 2×2 table necessary to estimate a rate is available or

	Exposed	Unexposed	Total
Died	x	$n-x$	n
Alive	?	?	?
Total	?	?	?

In terms of the right- and left-handed mortality data, the frequencies of surviving left- and right-handed individuals are not known. It is likely that the frequency of right-handedness is increased among the older individuals sampled, causing an apparent longer lifetime.   Early in the 20th century, being left-handed was frequently treated as a kind of disability and many naturally left-handed children were trained to be right-handed. As the century progressed, this practice became less frequent. By the end of the 20th century, therefore, the frequency of right-handedness was relative higher among older individuals or conversely, relative lower among younger individuals. The death certificates collected by Coren and Halpren, therefore, likely contain older individuals who are disproportionately right-handed, increasing the observed life-time associated with right-handedness. The absence of the numbers of surviving right- and left-handed individuals makes it impossible to compare the risk of death between these two groups. More simply, to estimate a rate requires an estimate of the person-years at risk accumulated by those who die, as well as by those who survive. Similarly, to estimate the probability of death requires the number of deaths, as well as the number of those who did not die. A study measuring risk based on a sample including individuals who died and who survived allows a comparison between rates that accounts for the influence of the differing distributions of left- and right-handed individuals that is not possible in a proportionate mortality study.

2

TABULAR DATA: THE 2 × *k* TABLE AND SUMMARIZING 2 × 2 TABLES

THE 2 × *k* TABLE

The $2 \times k$ table is a summary description of a binary variable measured at k-levels of another variable. Of more importance, a complete description of the analysis of a $2 \times k$ table provides a valuable foundation for describing a number of general statistical issues that arise in the analysis of data contained in a table (continued in Chapter 13).

As noted (Chapter 1), an epidemiologic analysis frequently begins with classifying data into a 2×2 table. A natural extension is a $2 \times k$ table, in which the frequency of a binary variable, such as the presence/absence of a disease or case/control status, is recorded at k-levels of another variable. The resulting $2 \times k$ table can be viewed from the perspective of the k-level variable (risk factor) or from the perspective of the binary outcome variable (present/absent). In terms of analytic approaches, the two points of view are:

1. *Regression analysis*: What is the relationship between a k-level risk variable and a binary outcome?
2. *Two-sample analysis*: Does the mean value of the k-level risk variable differ between two sampled groups?

Table 2–1. Pancreatic cancer and coffee consumption among male
cases and controls ($n = 523$)

Coffee consumption (cups/days)

	$X = 0$	$X = 1$	$X = 2$	$X \geq 3$	**Total**
$Y = 1$ (cases)	9	94	53	60	216
$Y = 0$ (controls)	32	119	74	82	307
Total	41	213	127	142	523
$\hat{P}_j$	0.220	0.441	0.417	0.423	0.413

These two questions generate different analytic approaches to describing the relationships within a $2 \times k$ table but, as will be seen, result in the same statistical assessment. Both approaches are distribution-free, in the sense that knowledge or assumptions about the distribution that generates the sampled data is not required. A number of texts completely develop the theory, analysis, and interpretation of discrete data classified into multiway tables (for example, [4], [5], and [6]).

Case/control data describing coffee consumption and its relationship to pancreatic cancer [7] provide an example of a $2 \times k$ table and its analysis. Men ($n = 523$) classified as cases (denoted $Y = 1$, row 1) or controls (denoted $Y = 0$, row 2) and by their reported consumption of 0, 1, 2, and 3, or more cups of coffee per day (denoted $X = j$, $j = 0, 1, 2$, or 3, columns) produce a 2×4 table (Table 2–1). For simplicity, more than three cups consumed per day are considered as three, incurring a slight bias.

The analysis of a $2 \times k$ table consists of the answer to three basic questions. A general evaluation of the influence of the risk factor (X) on the binary status (Y) is the first task (Is coffee drinking associated in any way to case/control status?). Second, the kind of relationship between the k-level numeric variable and the binary outcome is explored (How does pancreatic cancer risk change as the amount of coffee consumed increases?). Third, the comparison of the mean value of the variable X among cases ($Y = 1$) to the mean value of the variable X among controls ($Y = 0$) indicates the magnitude of the risk/outcome association (Does the mean amount of coffee consumed differ between cases and controls?).

INDEPENDENCE/HOMOGENEITY

The general notation for a $2 \times k$ table containing n observations classified by two categorical variables (denoted X and Y) is displayed in Table 2–2 (summarized in a variety of forms at the end of this section).

The symbol n_{ij} represents the number of observations falling into both the ith row and the jth column; namely, the count in the $(i, j)^{th}$-cell. For the pancreatic

Table 2–2. Notation for a $2 \times k$ table

	$X = 1$	$X = 2$	$X = 3$	$X = 4$				$X = k$	Total
$Y = 1$	n_{11}	n_{12}	n_{13}	n_{14}	.	.	.	n_{1k}	$n_{1.}$
$Y = 0$	n_{21}	n_{22}	n_{23}	n_{24}	.	.	.	n_{2k}	$n_{2.}$
Total	$n_{.1}$	$n_{.2}$	$n_{.3}$	$n_{.4}$	.	.	.	$n_{.k}$	n

Table 2–3. Notation for the probabilities underlying data classified into a $2 \times k$ table

	$X = 1$	$X = 2$	$X = 3$	$X = 4$				$X = k$	Total
$Y = 1$	p_{11}	p_{12}	p_{13}	p_{14}	.	.	.	p_{1k}	q_1
$Y = 0$	p_{21}	p_{22}	p_{23}	p_{24}	.	.	.	p_{2k}	q_2
Total	p_1	p_2	p_3	p_4	.	.	.	p_k	1.0

cancer data, the cell frequency n_{23} is 74 ($n_{23} = 74$, intersection of the second row and third column of Table 2–1). The *marginal frequencies* are the sums of the columns or the rows and are represented by $n_{.j}$ and $n_{i.}$, respectively. In symbols, the marginal frequencies are

$$n_{.j} = n_{1j} + n_{2j} \quad (k \text{ column sums})$$

and

$$n_{i.} = n_{i1} + n_{i2} + \cdots + n_{ik} = \sum n_{ij} \quad (\text{two row sums})$$

where $i = 1, 2 =$ number of rows and $j = 1, 2, \cdots, k =$ number of columns. For example, the total number of controls among the 523 study subjects (Table 2–1) is the marginal frequency of row 2 or $n_{2.} = 32 + 119 + 74 + 82 = 307$.

The properties of a $2 \times k$ table are determined by the relationships among three kinds of probabilities (Table 2–3). They are: the probability that an observation falls in a specific cell (denoted p_{ij}), the marginal probability that an observation falls in a specific column (denoted p_j, column $= j$), and the marginal probability that an observation falls in a specific row (denoted q_i, row $= i$).

The symbol n_{ij} represents an observed frequency subject to random variation, while the symbols p_{ij}, p_j, and q_i represent unobserved theoretical and fixed population probabilities.

Independence

The first issue to be addressed in the analysis of data classified into a $2 \times k$ table concerns the statistical independence of the row variable (Y) and the column variable (X). When categorical variables X and Y are unrelated, the cell probabilities are completely determined by the marginal probabilities (Table 2–4). Specifically, the probability that $Y = 1$ and $X = j$ simultaneously is then

$$p_{1j} = P(Y = 1 \text{ and } X = j) = P(Y = 1)P(X = j) = q_1 p_j \quad (\text{first row}),$$

Table 2–4. The notation for the expected values when the two categorical variables X and Y are statistically independent

	$X = 1$	$X = 2$	$X = 3$	$X = 4$				$X = k$	Total
$Y = 1$	$nq_1\,p_1$	$nq_1\,p_2$	$nq_1\,p_3$	$nq_1\,p_4$	.	.	.	$nq_1 p_k$	nq_1
$Y = 0$	$nq_2\,p_1$	$nq_2\,p_2$	$nq_2\,p_3$	$nq_2\,p_4$	.	.	.	$nq_2 p_k$	nq_2
Total	np_1	np_2	np_3	np_4	.	.	.	np_k	n

and similarly,

$$p_{2j} = P(Y = 0 \text{ and } X = j) = P(Y = 0)P(X = j) = q_2 p_j \quad \text{(second row)}$$

where $j = 1, 2, \cdots, k$.

The expected number of observations in the $(i, j)^{th}$-cell is $nq_i p_j$ when, to repeat, X and Y are statistically independent. Because the underlying cell probabilities (p_{ij}) are theoretical quantities (population parameters), these values are almost always estimated from the collected data. Under the conditions of independence, the probabilities p_{ij} are estimated from the marginal probabilities (denoted $\hat{p}_{ij}$) where

$$\hat{q}_i = \frac{n_{i.}}{n} \quad \text{and} \quad \hat{p}_j = \frac{n_{.j}}{n}$$

giving the estimate of p_{ij} as $\hat{p}_{ij} = \hat{q}_i \hat{p}_j$. Estimated cell counts follow because $\hat{n}_{ij} = n\hat{p}_{ij} = n\hat{q}_i \hat{p}_j$, which is usually written as $\hat{n}_{ij} = n_{i.} n_{.j}/n$. These expected values are calculated for each cell in the table and are compared to the observed values, typically using a chi-square test statistic to assess the conjecture that the categorical variables X and Y are unrelated.

For the pancreatic cancer case/control data, such expected cell frequencies ($\hat{n}_{ij}$) are given in Table 2–5. The marginal frequencies remain the same as those in the original table (Table 2.1). A consequence of statistical independence is that a table is unnecessary. The marginal probabilities exactly reflect the relationships within the row and column cell frequencies. For the case/control expected values (Table 2–5), the marginal row ratio is $216/307 = 0.706$ and is also the ratio between

Table 2–5. Estimated counts generated under the hypothesis of independence

	Coffee consumption (cups/day)				
	$X = 0$	$X = 1$	$X = 2$	$X \geq 3$	Total
$Y = 1$ (cases)	16.93	87.97	52.45	58.65	216
$Y = 0$ (controls)	24.07	125.03	74.55	83.35	307
Total	41	213	127	142	523
P	0.413	0.413	0.413	0.413	0.413

the row frequencies in every column (Table 2–5). For example, in column 1, the ratio is $16.93/24.07 = 0.706$. Furthermore, the probabilities $P(Y = 1)$ are identical for each value of X ($\hat{P} = 0.413$, Table 2–5).

A Pearson chi-square test statistic effectively summarizes the correspondence between the hypothesis-generated expected values ($\hat{n}_{ij}$) and the observed data values (n_{ij}). The test statistic for the pancreatic cancer 2×4 table becomes

$$X^2 = \sum \sum \frac{(n_{ij} - \hat{n}_{ij})^2}{\hat{n}_{ij}} = \sum \sum \frac{(n_{ij} - n_{i.}n_{.j}/n)^2}{n_{i.}n_{.j}/n}$$
$$= \frac{(9 - 16.93)^2}{16.93} + \cdots + \frac{(82 - 83.35)^2}{83.35} = 7.099$$

where, again, $i = 1$, 2 and $j = 1$, 2, 3, and 4. Thus, the chi-square statistic consists of the sum of eight comparisons, one for each cell in the table. The summary X^2 value has an approximate chi-square distribution with $k - 1$ degrees of freedom when the two categorical variables used to classify the observations into a $2 \times k$ table are unrelated. For the coffee/cancer data, the degrees of freedom are three, and the significance probability (p-value) is $P(X^2 \geq 7.099 | no\ X/Y\text{-}relationship) = 0.069$. A small p-value, say in the neighborhood of 0.05, indicates that the observed cell frequencies estimated as if coffee consumption (X) and case/control status (Y) were statistically independent do not correspond extremely well to the observed values (Table 2–5 compared to Table 2–1), presenting the possibility of an underlying systematic pattern of association.

Homogeneity

Alternatively, data classified into a $2 \times k$ table can be assessed for homogeneity. The primary issue is the consistency of k conditional probabilities (denoted P_j) where P_j represents the probability that $Y = 1$ for a specific level of X or, in symbols, $P_j = P(Y = 1 | X = j) = p_{1j}/p_j$. A natural estimate of the probability P_j is the frequency in the first row of the jth column (n_{1j}) divided by the total in the jth column ($n_{.j}$) or $\hat{P}_j = n_{1j}/n_{.j}$. From the pancreatic cancer data, these estimates are: $\hat{P}_1 = 9/41 = 0.220$, $\hat{P}_2 = 94/213 = 0.441$, $\hat{P}_3 = 53/127 = 0.417$ and $\hat{P}_4 = 60/142 = 0.423$ (Table 2–1).

To begin, a hypothesis is imposed stating that the sampled data are classified into categories (columns) where the underlying probabilities P_j are identical regardless of the level of X. In symbols, homogeneity means

$$homogeneity\ hypothesis: \quad P_1 = P_2 = P_3 = \cdots = P_k = P,$$

or equivalently,

$$homogeneity\ hypothesis: \quad P(Y = 1 | X = j) = P(Y = 1) = P.$$

The k estimated probabilities $\hat{P}_j$ then differ only because of sampling variation. To evaluate this conjecture, a single probability P (ignoring the column variable X) is estimated from the tabled data ($\hat{P} = n_1./n$) and compared to each probability $\hat{P}_j$, estimated from each column of the tabled data ($\hat{P}_j = n_{1j}/n_{.j}$).

For the pancreatic cancer data, the value P is estimated by $\hat{P} = 216/523 = 0.413$. The variability among the estimates $\hat{P}_j$ relative to the estimate $\hat{P}$ reflects the extent of inequality among the column probabilities (homogeneity). A chi-square statistic summarizes this variation. Thus, the test statistic

$$X^2 = \sum \left[\frac{\hat{P}_j - \hat{P}}{\sqrt{variance(\hat{P}_j)}} \right]^2 = \frac{\sum n_{.j}(\hat{P}_j - \hat{P})^2}{\hat{P}(1 - \hat{P})} \qquad j = 1, 2, \cdots, k$$

has an approximate chi-square distribution with $k - 1$ degrees of freedom, when the variation among the estimates $\hat{P}_j$ is due only to chance. For the pancreatic cancer data, the value of the test statistic is again $X^2 = 7.099$.

Notice that the chi-square statistic is a measure of the variability among a series of estimated values. The test statistic X^2, therefore, provides an assessment (p-value) of the likelihood that this variability is due entirely to chance. The purpose of calculating a chi-square statistic is frequently to identify nonrandom variation among a series of estimated values.

It is not a coincidence that the chi-square value to evaluate independence and the chi-square value to evaluate homogeneity are identical. A little algebra shows that these two apparently different assessments produce identical summary values. If P_j is constant for all levels of X, then the variable Y is not influenced by the variable X, which is another way of saying that X and Y are independent ($P = P_j$, Table 2–5). In symbols, the relationship between homogeneity and independence is

$$homogeneity = P(Y = i|X = j) = P(Y = i) \quad \text{implies that}$$
$$P(Y = i|X = j)P(X = j) = P(Y = i)P(X = j) \quad \text{and, therefore,}$$
$$P(Y = i \text{ and } X = j) = P(Y = i)P(X = j) = independence,$$

which is the relationship that generates the expected values for the chi-square test of independence.

REGRESSION

A chi-square test statistic used to assess independence does not require the categorical variables to be numeric or even ordered. Considerable gains (for example, increased statistical power) are achieved by forming and testing specific hypotheses about relationships within a table. One such opportunity arises when the k-level categorical variables are numeric. In this setting, the key to a specific statistical hypothesis becomes k pairs of data values. The k categories of X produce the k pairs of observations $(x_j, \hat{P}_j)$ where, as before, $\hat{P}_j$ represents the estimated conditional probability that $Y = 1$ associated with each numeric value represented by x_j (categories = columns). The pancreatic cancer case/control data yield four pairs of observations. These x/y-pairs are (0, 0.220), (1, 0.441), (2, 0.417) and (3, 0.423) (Table 1–2 and Figure 2–1, circles). The estimates $\hat{P}_j$ are again simply the proportion of cases within each level of coffee consumption (x_j).

One approach to summarizing these k proportions is to estimate a straight line based on the k pairs $(x_j, \hat{P}_j)$ and to use the slope of the estimated line to reflect the strength of the relationship between the row and column categorical variables. Identical to linear regression analysis applied to a continuous variable, three quantities are necessary to estimate this line: the sum of squares of X (S_{XX}), the sum of squares of Y (S_{YY}), and the sum of cross-products of X and Y (S_{XY}).

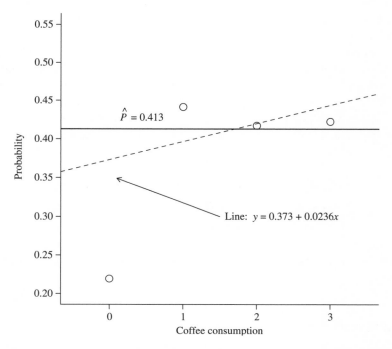

Figure 2–1. Proportion of cases of pancreatic cancer by consumption of 0, 1, 2 and 3 or more cups of coffee per day (circles).

These quantities calculated, from a $2 \times k$ table, are:

$$S_{XX} = \sum n_{.j}(x_j - \bar{x})^2 \quad \text{where} \quad \bar{x} = \sum n_{.j}x_j/n,$$
$$S_{YY} = n_1.n_2./n, \quad \text{and}$$
$$S_{XY} = (\bar{x}_1 - \bar{x}_2) S_{YY} \quad \text{where} \quad \bar{x}_i = \sum n_{ij}x_j/n_i.$$

for $i = 1,\ 2$ and $j = 1,\ 2,\ \cdots,\ k$. The quantity $\bar{x}_1$ represents the mean of the X-values when $Y = 1$ based on $n_1.$ observations (row 1), $\bar{x}_2$ represents the mean of the X-values when $Y = 0$ based on $n_2.$ observations (row 2) and $n = n_1. + n_2.$ represents the total number of observations. It is not necessary to consider the data in terms of a $2 \times k$ table. The mean values and the sums of squares are the same when the data are viewed as n pairs of values $(x_i,\ y_i)$ where the table frequencies are the numbers of identical x/y-pairs (Table 2–1). From either calculation, these values for the pancreatic cancer case/control data are: $\bar{x}_1 = 1.759$, $\bar{x}_2 = 1.671$, $S_{XX} = 474.241$, $S_{YY} = 126.792$, and $S_{XY} = 11.189$.

The ordinary least-squares linear regression estimates of the slope and intercept of a summary line are given by

$$\hat{b} = \frac{S_{XY}}{S_{XX}} \quad \text{and} \quad \hat{a} = \hat{P} - \hat{b}\bar{x},$$

and the estimated line becomes $\tilde{P}_j = \hat{a} + \hat{b}x_j$.

For the pancreatic data, the estimated slope is $\hat{b} = 11.189/474.241 = 0.0236$ and intercept is $\hat{a} = \hat{P} - \hat{b}\bar{x} = 0.413 - 0.0236(1.707) = 0.373$, making the estimated regression line $\tilde{P}_j = 0.373 + 0.0236x_j$. The value $\hat{P} = 216/523 = 0.413$ is again the proportion of cases when the coffee consumption is ignored. Therefore, as before, the estimates $\hat{P}_j$ from the data are

$$\hat{P}_1 = 0.220, \quad \hat{P}_2 = 0.441, \quad \hat{P}_3 = 0.417, \quad \hat{P}_4 = 0.423, \quad \text{and} \quad \hat{P} = 0.413.$$

The corresponding estimates $\tilde{P}_j$ from the summary straight line are

$$\tilde{P}_1 = 0.373, \quad \tilde{P}_2 = 0.396, \quad \tilde{P}_3 = 0.420, \quad \tilde{P}_4 = 0.443, \quad \text{and} \quad \tilde{P} = 0.413.$$

An estimate of the variance of the distribution of the estimated slope $\hat{b}$ is

$$variance(\hat{b}) = \frac{S_{YY}}{nS_{XX}} = \frac{126.792}{523(474.241)} = 0.000512.$$

To evaluate the influence of random variation on the estimated slope, a chi-square test statistic is typically used. The ratio of the squared estimated slope to its estimated variance has an approximate chi-square distribution with one degree of freedom when the column variable X is unrelated to the conditional probabilities P_j. More technically, the hypothesis $b = 0$ generates a test statistic

$$X_L^2 = \frac{(\hat{b} - 0)^2}{variance(\hat{b})} \qquad (L \text{ for } linear)$$

that has an approximate chi-square distribution with one degree of freedom (discussed further in Chapter 3 and beyond).

The estimates necessary to calculate the test statistic from the pancreatic cancer data are: $\hat{b} = 0.0236$ and $variance(\hat{b}) = 0.000512$, giving a chi-square distributed value of

$$X_L^2 = \frac{(0.0236 - 0)^2}{0.000512} = 1.089$$

and a p-value $= P(X_L^2 \geq 1.089 | b = 0) = 0.297$. No strong evidence emerges that the regression coefficient describing a linear response relationship between coffee consumption and the proportion of pancreatic cancer cases is different from zero (Figure 2–1). That is, the estimated line $\tilde{P}_j = 0.373 + 0.0236x_i$ (dashed line) is not remarkably different from the horizontal estimated line $\hat{P} = 0.413$ (solid line) in light of the influence of random variation. Estimating a summary line ($\tilde{P}_i$) and testing the slope $\hat{b}$ as a measure of association is frequently referred to as a *test for linear trend*.

A further refinement of a regression approach is achieved by dividing the total chi-square test statistic, X^2, into two interpretable parts:

- Part 1: Linear $= X_L^2$ (L for linear) has an approximate chi-square distribution with one degree of freedom (Is the straight line describing the relationship between variables X and Y horizontal?), and
- Part 2: Nonlinear $= X_{NL}^2 = X^2 - X_L^2$ (NL for nonlinear) has an approximate chi-square distribution with $k - 2$ degrees of freedom (Is the relationship between variables X and Y accurately described by a straight line?).

The chi-square statistic, X_L^2, measures the extent to which an estimated line deviates from a horizontal line. The chi-square statistic, X_{NL}^2, summarizes the "distance" between the estimated value $\tilde{P}_j$ based on X and the observed values $\hat{P}_j$. That is, the value of X_{NL}^2 measures the degree to which a straight line is a useful summary of the relationship between variables X and $\hat{P}_j$. Calculated directly, the chi-square statistic measuring nonlinearity is

$$X_{NL}^2 = \frac{\sum n_{.j}(\hat{P}_j - \tilde{P}_j)^2}{\hat{P}(1 - \hat{P})}$$

Table 2–6. Summary of partitioned chi-square statistic

	Chi-square	Degrees of freedom	p-Value
Nonlinear $= X^2_{NL} = \dfrac{\Sigma n_{.j}\left(\hat{P}_j - \tilde{P}_j\right)^2}{\hat{P}\left(1 - \hat{P}\right)}$	6.010	2	0.050
Linear $= X^2_L = \dfrac{\Sigma n_{.j}\left(\tilde{P}_j - \hat{P}\right)^2}{\hat{P}\left(1 - \hat{P}\right)}$	1.089	1	0.297*
Overall $= X^2 = \dfrac{\Sigma n_{.j}\left(\hat{P}_j - \hat{P}\right)^2}{\hat{P}\left(1 - \hat{P}\right)}$	7.099	3	0.069

* = Lack of linearity likely makes this p-value meaningless.

where $j = 1, 2, \cdots, k$. The test-statistic X^2_{NL} is again a measure of variability and has a chi-square distribution when the variation is strictly random. The assessment of the variability in this case is measured by the difference between the values estimated from the line ($\tilde{P}_j$) and values estimated from the data ($\hat{P}_j$). These two chi-square test statistics partition the total chi-square value into two interpretable pieces, or $X^2_{NL} + X^2_L = X^2$. A summary of the partitioned chi-square statistic is presented in Table 2–6.

For an assessment of linear trend to be useful, the trend in the probabilities P_j associated with levels of X must be at least approximately linear. Therefore, evaluation of linearity is a critical component of using the slope of a straight line as a summary description of the x/y-relationship. When a straight line does not reflect the data accurately, it makes little sense to compare a nonlinear relationship to a horizontal line. The overall chi-square statistic from the pancreatic cancer data is $X^2 = 7.099$, and the linear component is $X^2_L = 1.089$, leaving the nonlinear component as $X^2_{NL} = 7.099 - 1.089 = 6.010$ with $k - 2 = 4 - 2 = 2$ degrees of freedom (p-value $= 0.050$). This moderately large chi-square value (small p-value) suggests a likely failure of a straight line as an accurate summary of the relationship between pancreatic cancer risk and coffee consumption. The extent to which a summary value fails, an analysis based on that summary equally fails. A potential threshold-like effect of coffee consumption is visible in Figure 2–1. That is, the risk associated with coffee drinkers appears to differ from non–coffee drinkers, but does not appear to increase in a consistent linear pattern.

It is possible that the summary chi-square test statistic (X^2) is not significant (for example, p-value > 0.05), whereas the test for linearity (X^2_L) indicates evidence of a linear relationship. This apparent contradiction occurs because the summary chi-square test is not an extremely powerful test and can fail to detect a specific association between the levels of X and a binary variable Y. Failure to reject the hypothesis of statistical independence does not mean that X and Y are unrelated. It means that the overall chi-square test produces insufficient evidence to declare variables X and Y unrelated. An alternative approach, such as the more powerful and specific tests for linear trend or nonlinearity, can identify relationships not identified by the more general but less powerful summary chi-square test of independence.

The correlation between two categorical variables, X and Y, contained in a $2 \times k$ table is calculated in the usual way, where

$$r_{XY} = \frac{S_{XY}}{\sqrt{S_{XX}S_{YY}}}.$$

The correlation coefficient r_{XY} as always is a summary value between -1 and $+1$ and indicates the effectiveness of a straight line based on X to predict the value Y, even when X takes on discrete values and Y are estimated probabilities. The correlation coefficient between case/control status and coffee consumption is $r_{XY} = 11.819/\sqrt{(474.241)(126.792)} = 0.046$. Not surprisingly, the correlation coefficient is related to the test of significance of the estimated slope because both summary statistics measure the extent to which the variable X predicts the variable Y based on an estimated straight line. The specific relationship is $X_L^2 = nr_{XY}^2$. For the pancreatic cancer data, the linear chi-square statistic once again is $X_L^2 = 523(0.046)^2 \doteq 1.089$.

A purpose of analyzing a $2 \times k$ table for linear trend is frequently to explore a possible dose–response relationship. When the estimated probabilities $\hat{P}_j$ more or less smoothly increase or decrease with increasing values of x_j, it is less likely that the identified association results from bias or artifact and more likely that the observed relationship reflects a systematic association ("real"). The analysis of the coffee consumption and pancreatic cancer data shows visual as well as statistical evidence of a nonlinear relationship, possibly a threshold response. Threshold responses, like the one illustrated, are prone to bias, particularly bias caused by other related variables. For example, perhaps coffee drinkers smoke more cigarettes than non–coffee drinkers and, therefore, at least part of the observed case–control response might be due to an unobserved relationship with smoking.

TWO-SAMPLE: COMPARISON OF TWO MEAN VALUES

Another approach to the analysis of a relationship between a binary variable and k-level numeric variable is the comparison of two mean values. A natural measure of association between a binary variable Y and a numeric variable X is the difference between the two mean values $\bar{x}_1$ and $\bar{x}_2$. As before, the mean value $\bar{x}_1$ is calculated for all values where $Y = 1$ (n_1. observations), and $\bar{x}_2$ is calculated for all values where $Y = 0$ (n_2. observations). For the pancreatic cancer data, the mean level of coffee consumption among the n_1. $= 216$ cases is $\bar{x}_1 = 1.759$ cups per day ($Y = 1 =$ case, row 1), and the mean level among the n_2. $= 307$ controls is $\bar{x}_2 = 1.671$ ($Y = 0 =$ control, row 2), producing an increase of $\bar{x}_1 - \bar{x}_2 = 0.088$ cups of coffee consumed per day associated with the pancreatic cancer cases. The primary question becomes: Is the observed mean increase likely due to random variation, or does it provide evidence of an underlying systematic increase in coffee consumption among the cases?

Parallel to the classic two-sample Student's t-test, an estimate of the variance of the distribution of the differences between two mean values from a $2 \times k$ table is based on the conjecture or knowledge that the variances in both groups are the same. This variance is then estimated by

$$variance(\bar{x}_2 - \bar{x}_1) = V_p^2 \left(\frac{1}{n_1.} + \frac{1}{n_2.} \right)$$

where V_p^2 is a pooled estimate of the variability of the variable X (columns) ignoring the values of Y (rows). Specifically, an expression for the estimate of the common variance is

$$V_p^2 = \frac{S_{XX}}{n}.$$

A t-like statistical test of the difference between mean values is then given by the test statistic

$$Z = \frac{\bar{x}_2 - \bar{x}_1 - 0}{\sqrt{variance(\bar{x}_2 - \bar{x}_1)}} = \frac{\bar{x}_2 - \bar{x}_1}{\sqrt{V_p^2 \left(\frac{1}{n_1.} + \frac{1}{n_2.} \right)}},$$

and Z has an approximate standard normal distribution (mean $=0$ and variance $=1$) when the mean values $\bar{x}_1$ and $\bar{x}_2$ differ only because of sampling variation. For the example pancreatic cancer data, the mean values $\bar{x}_1 = 1.759$ and $\bar{x}_2 = 1.671$, as well as the $variance(\bar{x}_2 - \bar{x}_1) = 0.00717$ produce the test statistic $z = -1.042$, yielding a p-value $= P(|Z| \geq 1.042 \mid no\ difference\ in\ response) = 0.297$. The value $z^2 = (-1.042)^2 = 1.089$ and is same as the chi-square statistic X_L^2 calculated previously from the estimated slope $\hat{b}$ and its variance. The regression approach and the comparison of two mean values always lead to identical chi-square test statistics and significance levels ($X_L^2 = Z^2$).

The estimated regression coefficient ($\hat{b}$), the correlation coefficient (r_{XY}), and the observed mean difference ($\bar{x}_2 - \bar{x}_1$) are algebraically related when calculated from a $2 \times k$ table. For example, each estimate is likely close to zero when the variables X and Y are unrelated. Of more importance, the three statistics are different kinds of summary descriptions of the association between the numeric levels of a risk factor and a binary outcome but, in terms of the statistical evaluation of the influence of sampling variability, lead to the same inference (same p-values).

So far, the choice of the numeric values for X has not been an issue. This choice is, nevertheless, important and careful thought should be given to an appropriate scale for the variable X. Some fields of study almost always use the logarithm of X. In yet other situations, natural units arise, such as the number of cups of coffee consumed per day. Rather complicated polynomial expressions are occasionally used to define a "dose variable" [8]. The results of an analysis of a dose/response relationship can differ, sometimes considerably, depending on the scale chosen for the X-variable (Chapter 13). The choice of scale is essentially nonstatistical and is primarily determined by subject-matter considerations. However, when choices for the numeric X-values differ only by their measurement units ($X_{new} = aX_{old} + b$, where a and b are constants), no change occurs in the chi-square statistic or the associated p-value. For example, using the values $X = 0, 8, 16$, and 24 ounces of coffee consumed per day instead of 0, 1, 2, and 3 cups per day does not change the statistical results from the pancreatic cancer analysis ($X_{new} = 8X_{old}$). The p-values, for example, reflecting any of the three measures of risk associated with coffee consumption remain the same (Table 2–6).

AN EXAMPLE: CHILDHOOD CANCER AND PRENATAL X-RAY EXPOSURE

The Oxford Survey of Childhood Cancer [9] collected data on malignancies in children under 10 years of age (cases/controls) and information on the mother's exposure to prenatal x-rays (six levels). The case/control data in Table 2–7 (a small part of a large study of childhood cancer published in 1953) are the number of prenatal x-rays received by the mothers of children with a malignant disease (cases) and mothers of healthy children who are the same age and sex, from similar areas of residence (controls).

The proportion of cases whose mothers received prenatal x-rays 0, 1, 2, 3, 4, or ≥ 5 times (x_j) are 0.489, 0.546, 0.564, 0.596, 0.678, and 0.691 ($\hat{P}_j = n_{1j}/n_{j.}$), respectively (Table 2–7 and Figure 2–2). For simplicity, the few values greater than five were coded as 5 for these calculations.

The chi-square test statistic that measures independence/homogeneity (*hypothesis*: the proportion of cases is the same regardless of maternal x-ray exposure) is $X^2 = 47.286$. A chi-square value of this magnitude definitely indicates the presence of a strong systematic pattern of response (p-value $= P(X^2 \geq 47.286 | no\ association) < 0.001$).

Table 2–7. Cases of childhood cancer and controls classified by the number of prenatal maternal x-rays received, a 2 × 6 table (Oxford Survey of Childhood Cancer, 1953)

Number of prenatal x-rays

	0	1	2	3	4	≥ 5	Unk	Total
Cases(n_{1j})	7332	287	199	96	59	65	475	8513
Control (n_{2j})	7673	239	154	65	28	29	325	8513
Total ($n_{.j}$)	15005	526	353	161	87	94	800	17026
Proportion ($\hat{P}_j$)	0.489	0.546	0.564	0.596	0.678	0.691	–	0.495
Estimated* ($\tilde{P}_j$)	0.489	0.530	0.572	0.613	0.655	0.696	–	0.495

* = Based on the model estimated linear response $\tilde{P}_j = 0.489 + 0.0415\,x_j$

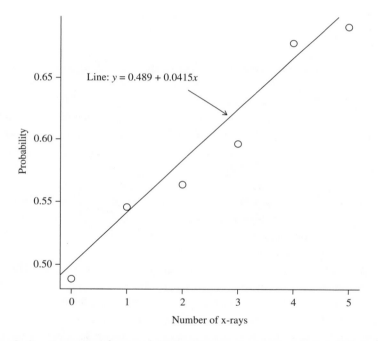

Figure 2–2. Proportion of cases of childhood cancer for exposure to 0, 1, 2, 3, 4, and 5 or more x-rays during pregnancy.

The mean number of x-rays received by the mothers of the cases is $\bar{x}_1 = 0.191$ ($n_{1.} = 8038$) and by the mothers of the controls is $\bar{x}_2 = 0.122$ ($n_{2.} = 8188$). The t-like comparison

$$z = \frac{0.191 - 0.122}{\sqrt{0.415\left(\dfrac{1}{8038} + \dfrac{1}{8188}\right)}} = 6.805$$

indicates that the observed difference in mean number of maternal x-ray exposures between cases and controls is extremely unlikely due to chance variation (p-value $= P(|Z| \geq 6.805|$ *equal mean exposure levels*$) < 0.001$).

Postulating a linear increase in response to x-ray exposure is the simplest possible description of a trend in risk of childhood cancer. A straight line summarizing the proportion of cases (Table 2–7 and Figure 2–2) has an estimated slope of $\hat{b} = 0.0415$. The estimated standard deviation of the distribution of the estimate $\hat{b}$ is $\sqrt{variance(\hat{b})} = 0.00609$. Thus, the chi-square test statistic to evaluate the hypothesis that $b = 0$ (a horizontal line) is

$$X_L^2 = \left[\frac{0.0415}{0.00609} \right]^2 = 46.313$$

producing, as expected, a result identical to the previous comparison of mean values ($z^2 = (-6.805)^2 = 46.313$).

A test of linear trend, as pointed out, has meaning only when the data are effectively summarized by a straight line. A striking feature of these x-ray data is the apparent straight-line dose response. The chi-square test statistic (*NL*) reflecting the nonlinear component of the total chi-square statistic from the childhood cancer data is $X_{NL}^2 = X^2 - X_L^2 = 47.286 - 46.313 = 0.973$ with $6 - 2 = 4$ degrees of freedom, producing the p-value $= 0.914$. The extremely small chi-square value (large p-value) measuring the extent of nonlinearity in the description of x-ray exposure and the risk of childhood cancer is entirely consistent with the linear response clearly seen from the plotted data (Figure 2–2 and Table 2–7, estimates $\hat{P}_j$ versus $\tilde{P}_j$).

The partitioned chi-square values are summarized in Table 2–8. The strong and linear response is convincing evidence of a substantial and consistently increasing risk associated with each additional prenatal x-ray and the subsequent development of cancer in the children of the x-rayed mothers. This observation 60 years ago brought a halt to using x-rays as a routine prenatal diagnostic tool.

Table 2–8. Summary of Partitioned Chi-square Analysis of the Oxford Childhood Cancer X-ray Data

	Chi-square	Degrees of freedom	p-Values
Linear $= X_L^2$	46.313	1	< 0.001
Nonlinear $= X_{NL}^2$	0.973	4	0.914
Overall $= X^2$	47.286	5	< 0.001

SUMMARY OF THE NOTATION FOR A 2 × *k* TABLE

Coffee Consumption Data

	Coffee consumption				
	$X = 0$	$X = 1$	$X = 2$	$X \geq 3$	Total
$Y = 1$ (cases)	9	94	53	60	216
$Y = 0$ (controls)	32	119	74	82	307
Total	41	213	127	142	523
$\hat{P}_j = n_{1j}/n_{.j}$	0.220	0.441	0.417	0.423	0.413

General 2 × *k* Table: Notation n_{ij}

	$X = 1$	$X = 2$	$X = 3$	$X = 4$		$X = k$	Total
$Y = 1$	n_{11}	n_{12}	n_{13}	n_{14}	$\cdots$	n_{1k}	$n_{1.}$
$Y = 0$	n_{21}	n_{22}	n_{23}	n_{24}	$\cdots$	n_{2k}	$n_{2.}$
Total	$n_{.1}$	$n_{.2}$	$n_{.3}$	$n_{.4}$	$\cdots$	$n_{.k}$	n

Underlying Probabilities: Notation p_{ij}

	$X = 1$	$X = 2$	$X = 3$	$X = 4$		$X = k$	Total
$Y = 1$	p_{11}	p_{12}	p_{13}	p_{14}	$\cdots$	p_{1k}	q_1
$Y = 0$	p_{21}	p_{22}	p_{23}	p_{24}	$\cdots$	p_{2k}	q_2
Total	p_1	p_2	p_3	p_4	$\cdots$	p_k	1.0

Null Hypothesis–generated Values: Notation $n_{ij} = q_i \, p_j$

	$X = 1$	$X = 2$	$X = 3$	$X = 4$		$X = k$	Total
$Y = 1$	$nq_1 \, p_1$	$nq_1 \, p_2$	$nq_1 \, p_3$	$nq_1 \, p_4$	$\cdots$	$nq_1 p_k$	nq_1
$Y = 0$	$nq_2 \, p_1$	$nq_2 \, p_2$	$nq_2 \, p_3$	$nq_2 \, p_4$	$\cdots$	$nq_2 p_k$	nq_2
Total	np_1	np_2	np_3	np_4	$\cdots$	np_k	n

Values Generated by the Hypothesis of Independence of Coffee Consumption Data

	Coffee consumption				
	$X = 0$	$X = 1$	$X = 2$	$X \geq 3$	Total
$Y = 1$ (cases)	16.93	87.97	52.45	58.65	216
$Y = 0$ (controls)	24.07	125.03	74.55	83.35	307
Total	41	213	127	142	523
$\hat{P} = \hat{P}_j = \hat{n}_{1j}/n_{.j}$	0.413	0.413	0.413	0.413	0.413

**Values Generated by the Hypothesis of a Linear
Dose–Response from Coffee Consumption**

	Coffee consumption				
	$X = 0$	$X = 1$	$X = 2$	$X \geq 3$	**Total**
$Y = 1$ (cases)	15.28	84.41	53.33	62.98	216
$Y = 0$ (controls)	25.72	128.59	73.67	79.02	307
Total	41	213	127	142	523
$\tilde{P}_j = 0.373 + 0.0236x_j$	0.373	0.396	0.420	0.443	0.413

SUMMARIZING 2 × 2 TABLES: APPLICATION OF
A WEIGHTED AVERAGE

To describe the influence of maternal cigarette smoking during pregnancy and the likelihood of a low-birth-weight infant among four race/ethnicity groups, a series of records of nonobese women were obtained from the University of California, San Francisco Moffitt Hospital perinatal database. The data collected during the period 1980–1990 contain self-reported maternal smoking histories (nonsmoker and smoker), race/ethnicity (white, African-American, Hispanic, and Asian), and the weight of the mother's newborn infant. The birth weight of each infant was classified as low birth weight (<2500 grams) or "normal" birth weight (≥2500 grams). For mothers with more than one delivery during the study period, a delivery was selected at random. After removing newborns with major congenital malformations, multiple births, and missing data, a total of 8,859 mother/infant pairs are available for study (Table 2–9).

Two binary variables produce four counts, denoted a_i, b_i, c_i, and d_i ($n_i = a_i + b_i + c_i + d_i$), for each 2 × 2 table in a series of $i = 1, 2, \cdots, k$ tables (Chapter 1, Table 1–1). The binary variables smoking exposure and risk of a low-birth-weight infant create four ($k = 4$) race-specific 2 × 2 tables (Table 2–9, $i = 1, 2, 3,$ and 4) where

Birth Weight

$Race_i$	$< 2500g$	$\geq 2500g$	**Total**
Smokers	a_i	b_i	$a_i + b_i$
Nonsmokers	c_i	d_i	$c_i + d_i$
Total	$a_i + c_i$	$b_i + d_i$	n_i

Two distinct statistical approaches produce a summary measure of the association between smoking exposure and low birth weight, a model-free (present chapter) and a model-based analysis (Chapter 4).

Table 2–9. Mother/infant pairs classified by smoking exposure, birth weight, and race/ethnicity (four 2 × 2 tables, San Francisco, 1980–1990)

White	< 2500g	≥ 2500g	**Total**
Smokers	98	832	930
Nonsmokers	169	3520	3689
Total	267	4352	4619

African-American	< 2500g	≥ 2500g	**Total**
Smokers	54	227	281
Nonsmokers	55	686	741
Total	109	913	1022

Hispanic	< 2500g	≥ 2500g	**Total**
Smokers	11	85	96
Nonsmokers	61	926	987
Total	72	1011	1083

Asian	< 2500g	≥ 2500g	**Total**
Smokers	7	102	109
Nonsmokers	90	1936	2026
Total	97	2038	2135

To start, a measure of association needs to be chosen. Among several effective measures of association that could be applied to summarize these smoking exposure data, a popular choice is the odds ratio. The odds ratio estimated from a specific 2 × 2 table (the ith table, denoted $\hat{o}r_i$) is

$$\hat{o}r_i = \frac{a_i/b_i}{c_i/d_i} = \frac{a_i/c_i}{b_i/d_i} = \frac{a_i d_i}{b_i c_i}.$$

Four such estimated odds ratios measure the association between smoking exposure and low birth weight for white, African-American, Hispanic, and Asian mothers (Table 2–10). The same statistical tools described in Chapter 1 are applied, once for each race/ethnicity group.

Table 2–10. Odds ratios and their approximate 95% confidence intervals for each race/ethnicity group

Race/ethnicity	n_i	$\hat{o}r_i$	Lower bound	Upper bound
White	4619	2.453	1.892	3.182
African-American	1022	2.967	1.980	4.446
Hispanic	1083	1.965	0.996	3.875
Asian	2135	1.476	0.667	3.267

Table 2–11. Logarithm of the estimated odds ratios and their estimated variances for each race/ethnicity group

Race/ethnicity	n_i	$log(\hat{o}r_i)$	$S^2_{log(\hat{o}r_i)}$	w_i
White	4619	0.897	0.018	56.795
African-American	1022	1.088	0.043	23.494
Hispanic	1083	0.675	0.120	8.323
Asian	2135	0.390	0.164	6.087

As noted (Chapter 1), a direct evaluation of an odds ratio is not very tractable but is easily accomplished using the logarithm of the odds ratio $[log(\hat{o}r)]$ and the normal distribution. For the birth-weight data, the log-transformed estimated odds ratios and their estimated variances for each race/ethnicity group are given in Table 2–11. The estimated variances describing the variability of the logarithm of an estimated odds ratio are calculated from the expression

$$estimated\ variance\ (log\text{-}odds\ ratio) = S^2_{log(\hat{o}r_i)} = \frac{1}{a_i} + \frac{1}{b_i} + \frac{1}{c_i} + \frac{1}{d_i}.$$

A useful estimate of the summary odds ratio depends on the answer to two sequential questions: Do these four measures of association systematically differ among race/ethnicity groups? And, if the measures differ only because of random variation, what is their common value? The first question concerns the presence/absence of an interaction influence of race/ethnicity, and the second question concerns the presence/absence of a confounding influence (Chapter 1).

The question of an interaction is statistically addressed by assessing the amount of variation among the observed log-transformed odds ratios, where this variability is measured relative to the mean log-transformed odds ratio. An effective estimate of this mean value is achieved by a weighted average of the individual estimated values. In symbols, for k observed 2×2 tables,

$$mean\ log\text{-}transformed\ odds\ ratio = \overline{log(or)} = \frac{\sum w_i log(\hat{o}r_i)}{\sum w_i} \qquad i = 1, 2, \cdots, k$$

where the k estimated log-transformed odds ratios are combined using the reciprocal of their estimated variances as weights (denoted w_i, Table 2–11). Reciprocal variances used as weights $w_i = 1/S^2_{log(\hat{o}r_i)}$ emphasize log-transformed odds ratios estimated with high precision (small variances) and deemphasize the less-precise estimates (large variances). Combining a series of estimates weighted by their reciprocal variances produces a single summary mean value. In fact, variance-weighted averages are a fundamental statistical tool producing many kinds of summary values.

From the maternal smoking data, the estimated mean log-transformed odds ratio is

$$\overline{log(or)} = \frac{56.795(0.897) + 23.494(1.088) + 8.323(0.675) + 6.087(0.390)}{94.699}$$

$$= 0.892.$$

This summary value measure of association is easily interpreted only when the averaged quantities each estimate the same underlying value. That is, the log-odds values that make up the estimate only differ because of random variability (homogeneous values).

Comparison of each observed log-odds ratio to the estimated common mean value measures the extent of variation among the k individual log-transformed values. The formal statistical evaluation follows a typical pattern. Quantities with approximate normal distributions are created and squared. Then, the sum of these squared values has an approximate chi-square distribution when the variation among the estimated values is strictly random. For the odds ratio case, the quantity

$$z_i = \frac{log(\hat{or}_i) - \overline{log(or)}}{S_{log(\hat{or}_i)}}$$

has an approximate standard normal distribution when the estimated odds ratios randomly vary from a single value. Therefore, the sum of these values squared

$$X_W^2 = \sum z_i^2 = \sum \left[\frac{log(\hat{or}_i) - \overline{log(or)}}{S_{log(\hat{or}_i)}} \right]^2 = \sum w_i \left[log(\hat{or}_i) - \overline{log(or)} \right]^2$$

has an approximate chi-square distribution with $k - 1$ degrees of freedom when the estimates $log(\hat{or}_i)$ differ only because of random variation ($i = 1, 2, \cdots, k$, and k is again the number of log-transformed odds ratios compared). This version of the Pearson chi-square test statistic is frequently referred to as *Woolf's test for homogeneity* [10]. It is a test for the presence of interaction among k 2×2 tables.

For the birth-weight data, Woolf's test statistic is

$$X_W^2 = 56.795(0.897 - 0.892)^2 + \cdots + 6.087(0.390 - 0.892)^2 = 2.828$$

and has an approximate chi-square distribution with three degrees of freedom when the four underlying race-specific odds ratios are homogeneous. That is, when the underlying odds ratio is the same for the four race/ethnicity groups or, in symbols, $or_1 = or_2 = or_3 = or_4 = or$. Specifically for the low-birth-weight data, the p-value $= P(X_W^2 \geq 2.828 | \text{ random differences only}) = 0.419$. The probability of observing greater variation among the four estimated log-odds ratios by chance alone is likely. Thus, Woolf's chi-square test provides no persuasive evidence that the four odds ratios systematically differ among the four race/ethnicity groups.

When no substantial evidence exists to the contrary, it is usual to proceed as if the underlying odds ratios are homogeneous, producing a potentially useful and a certainly simple description of the risk–disease relationship. It is important to keep in mind that accepting the hypothesis of homogeneity does not mean it is true.

The next step is to estimate the common odds ratio. Behaving as if the four estimated odds ratios differ only because of random variation, three estimates of the common odds ratio are:

1. *Woolf's estimate* [10]: $\hat{o}r_w = e^{\overline{log(or)}} = e^{0.892} = 2.441$ (this chapter),
2. *Maximum likelihood estimate* [8]: $\hat{o}r_{mlk} = 2.423$ (Chapter 4), and
3. *Mantel-Haenszel estimate* [11]: $\hat{o}r_{MH} = 2.448$ (Chapter 7).

No important differences exist among the three kinds of estimates, which is typical for most sets of 2×2 tables, especially when the observed counts are large in all cells of all tables.

The estimated summary odds ratio $\hat{o}r_w = e^{\overline{log(or)}} = e^{0.892} = 2.441$ has the obvious property that it reflects the association between smoking exposure and the risk of a low-birth-weight infant with a single value. In addition, this summary value is "free" of possible influences from race/ethnicity (called *an adjusted estimate*). When an odds ratio is estimated within a race-specific stratum (Tables 2–10 and 2–11), it is not influenced by differences among race/ethnicity groups. The summary odds ratio made up of these strata-specific values is, therefore, equally uninfluenced by race/ethnicity.

The estimated variance associated with the distribution of the weighted average estimate $\overline{log(or)}$ is

$$S^2_{\overline{log(or)}} = \frac{1}{\sum w_i}.$$

The weights w_i are again the reciprocal of the estimated variances of each estimate $log(\hat{o}r_i)$. The smoking/birth-weight data yield a summary estimate of $\overline{log(or)} = 0.892$, with an estimated variance of $S^2_{\overline{log(or)}} = 1/94.699 = 0.011$.

Note: In general, the variance of a weighted average is the reciprocal of the sum of the weights when two conditions hold:

1. The values averaged are independent, and
2. The weights are the reciprocal of the variances of the values averaged.

For a series of k values denoted m_i, a weighted mean value is

$$\overline{m} = \frac{\sum w_i m_i}{\sum w_i} \quad \text{with weights} \quad w_i = \frac{1}{variance(m_i)} \quad i = 1, 2, \cdots, k,$$

then

$$variance(\overline{m}) = variance\left[\frac{\sum w_i m_i}{\sum w_i}\right] = \frac{1}{[\sum w_i]^2}\sum variance(w_i m_i)$$

$$= \frac{1}{[\sum w_i]^2}\sum w_i^2 variance(m_i)$$

$$= \frac{1}{[\sum w_i]^2}\sum w_i = \frac{1}{\sum w_i}$$

since $variance(m_i) = 1/w_i$.

Because estimated summary values tend to have approximate normal distributions, particularly estimates that combine values sampled from approximately symmetric distributions, such as the log-odds ratio, tests of significance and confidence intervals are accurately constructed from weighted average estimates. For example, to compare the estimated summary log-mean value from the birth-weight data to the conjecture that no association exists between smoking exposure and the likelihood of a low-birth-weight infant, then

$$z = \frac{\overline{log(or)} - log(1)}{\sqrt{S_{log(or)}^2}} = \frac{\overline{log(or)} - 0}{\sqrt{1/\sum w_i}} = \frac{0.892 - 0}{\sqrt{0.011}} = 8.685$$

is a random value from a standard normal distribution, when no association exists within all four tables ($log(or) = log(1) = 0$ or $or = 1$). The corresponding p-value of $P(Z \geq 8.683 | no\ association) < 0.001$ leaves little doubt that $\hat{o}r_w = 2.441$ reflects a systematic association.

In addition, an approximate 95% confidence interval based on the estimate $\overline{log(or)} = 0.892$ and the normal distribution is

$$lower\ bound = \hat{A} = log(\hat{o}r) - 1.960S_{\overline{log(\hat{o}r)}} = 0.892 - 1.960\sqrt{0.011} = 0.691$$

and

$$upper\ bound = \hat{B} = log(\hat{o}r) + 1.960S_{\overline{log(\hat{o}r)}} = 0.892 + 1.960\sqrt{0.011} = 1.094,$$

producing the confidence interval of $(0.691, 1.094)$. Because $\hat{o}r_w = e^{\overline{log(or)}} = e^{0.892}$ $= 2.441$, an approximate 95% confidence interval for the underlying summary odds ratio estimated by $\hat{or}_w = 2.441$ is the same function of the confidence interval bounds and

$$(e^{lower\ bound}, e^{upper\ bound}) = (e^{\hat{A}},\ e^{\hat{B}}) = (e^{0.691}, e^{1.094}) = (1.996, 2.986).$$

In other words, the 95% confidence interval indicates that the "true" underlying common odds ratio or, estimated by $\hat{or}_w = 2.441$, is unlikely to be less than 1.996 or greater than 2.986 (probability= 0.05). Plausible candidates for this odds ratio (or), therefore, lie between 1.996 and 2.986. However, like the summary odds ratio itself, statistical tests and confidence intervals based on a single odds ratio are useful assessments of an association only if the strata-specific odds ratios differ because of sampling variation (homogeneous values or no interaction).

ANOTHER SUMMARY MEASURE: DIFFERENCE IN PROPORTIONS

Smoking exposure and its association with the risk of a low-birth-weight infant is naturally assessed by comparing two conditional probabilities, namely

$$p_1 = P(low\ birth\ weight\ infant\ |\ smoking\ mother)\quad \text{and}$$
$$p_2 = P(low\ birth\ weight\ infant\ |\ nonsmoking\ mother).$$

These two probabilities are estimated for each of the four race/ethnicity groups by the observed proportions of low-birth-weight infants delivered by mothers who smoke and mothers who do not smoke (denoted $\hat{p}_{i1}$ and $\hat{p}_{i2}$ for each 2×2 table, $i = 1, 2, 3,$ and 4). Furthermore, each of the four race/ethnicity groups produces a difference between these proportions, $\hat{d}_i = \hat{p}_{i1} - \hat{p}_{i2}$, reflecting the difference in likelihood of a low-birth-weight infant between smoking and nonsmoking mothers (Table 2–12). As with the odds ratio measures, each strata-specific estimate is not influenced by race/ethnicity.

As expected, these proportions show a clear influence of maternal smoking on the likelihood of a low-birth-weight infant. In all four race/ethnicity groups, the race-specific differences in the likelihood of a low-birth-weight infant is higher among mothers who smoke ($\hat{p}_{i1} > \hat{p}_{i2}$).

The process described for combining and assessing the odds ratios from a series of 2×2 tables using a weighted average applies to most measures of association. Similar to the odds ratio summary, the differences in proportions of low-birth-weight infants between smokers and nonsmokers can be combined into a single summary difference and statistically assessed. Using a weighted average,

Table 2–12. Low-birth-weight infants classified by mother's race/ethnicity and smoking exposure (proportions, differences, and variances)

Race/ethnicity	i	Smokers $\hat{p}_{i1}$	Nonsmokers $\hat{p}_{i2}$	Differences $\hat{d}_i$	Variances* $\hat{v}_i^*$	Weights w_i
White	1	0.105	0.046	0.060	0.113	8832.6
African-American	2	0.192	0.074	0.118	0.645	1549.9
Hispanic	3	0.115	0.062	0.053	1.116	896.4
Asian	4	0.064	0.044	0.020	0.572	1747.4

* $= 1000 \times \hat{v}_i = 1000 \times variance(\hat{p}_{i1} - \hat{p}_{i2}) = 1000 \times variance(\hat{d}_i)$ for $i = 1, 2, 3,$ and 4.

the overall summary difference in proportions is

$$\bar{d} = \frac{\sum w_i \hat{d}_i}{\sum w_i} = \frac{8832.6(0.060) + \cdots + 1747.4(0.020)}{8832.6 + \cdots + 1747.4} = 0.061$$

where the weights w_i are again the reciprocal of the variances of the observed differences d_i [$w_i = 1/variance(\hat{d}_i)$]. Specifically, the estimated variance of the distribution of the estimated difference $\hat{d}_i$ is

$$variance(\hat{d}_i) = \frac{\hat{p}_{i1}(1 - \hat{p}_{i1})}{n_{i1}} + \frac{\hat{p}_{i2}(1 - \hat{p}_{i2})}{n_{i2}}$$

where n_{i1} is the number of smoking and n_{i2} is the number of nonsmoking mothers in the ith-race/ethnicity group ($i = 1, 2, 3,$ and 4, Table 2–9).

Because the summary mean value $\bar{d}$ is a single value, the quantity estimated must also be a single value. That is, the underlying difference in the proportions of low-birth-weight infants must be the same for all four race/ethnicity groups or, in other words, the estimated values $\hat{d}_i = \hat{p}_{i1} - \hat{p}_{i2}$ differ by chance alone (homogeneous values or no interaction). The homogeneity of these four differences ($\hat{d}_i$-values) is again a critical issue in creating and interpreting a single summary value. When the d_i-values randomly differ, the estimated summary mean value $\bar{d}$ is both precise and unbiased. When the d_i-values systematically differ, the mean value $\bar{d}$ is a biased and potentially a misleading summary of the influence of smoking exposure on the likelihood of a low-birth-weight infant.

The variability among the estimated differences is again key to the decision to combine or not combine the k differences between proportions of low-birth-weight infants into a single summary estimate (interaction?). This variability is measured by the chi-square test statistic

$$
\begin{aligned}
X^2 &= \sum w_i(\hat{d}_i - \overline{d})^2 \\
&= 8832.6(0.060 - 0.061)^2 + \cdots + 1747.4(0.020 - 0.061)^2 \\
&= 8.070.
\end{aligned}
$$

As before, this summary measure of variability has an approximate chi-square distribution with three degrees of freedom when only random differences exist among the four race-specific strata estimates $\hat{d}_i$ and their mean value $\overline{d}$. The p-value $P(X^2 \geq 8.070 | d_1 = d_2 = d_3 = d_4 = d) = 0.045$, provides a substantial indication of a lack of homogeneity. Therefore, the single summary $\overline{d}$ likely obscures important differences in the assessment of smoking and the likelihood of a low-birth-weight infant among some or all of the four race/ethnicity groups. For example, the underlying difference in the proportion of low-birth-weight infants observed between smokers and nonsmokers in African-Americans ($\hat{d}_2 = 0.118$) is likely to be systematically greater than the difference in Asians ($\hat{d}_4 = 0.020$).

The summary odds ratio produces an apparently useful single summary of low-birth-weight risk associated with smoking. The summary difference in proportions does not. Thus, the presence/absence of an interaction depends on the choice of the measure of association. A question not addressed is: Do the four groups under study systematically differ in their risk–outcome relationships? The question addressed is: Can the four measures of association be combined to create a single unbiased measure of the risk–outcome relationship? This first unanswered question refers to issues concerning the populations sampled. The second answered question refers to the issues concerning the statistical analysis. The answer to the second question, as illustrated, depends on the choice of the measure of association.

Confounding

One measure of the confounding influence of race/ethnicity on the relationship between the risk of a low-birth-weight infant and smoking is the difference between two odds ratios. The odds ratio calculated ignoring the influence of race/ethnicity is compared to the summary odds ratio calculated using a weighted average that accounts for any influences. The first odds ratio is estimated from a table created by combining the data, and the second odds ratio is estimated by combining the table-specific odds ratios. The difference between these two summary odds ratios directly measures the extent of confounding (Chapter 1).

Table 2–13. The smoking/birth weight table ignoring race/ethnicity
(Table 2-9 collapsed into a single table)

Combined	$< 2500g$	$\geq 2500g$	**Total**
Smokers	170	1246	1416
Nonsmokers	375	7068	7443
Total	545	8314	8859

The odds ratio reflecting the influence of smoking on the risk of a low-birth-weight infant, ignoring race/ethnicity is

$$\hat{or} = \frac{\sum a_i / \sum b_i}{\sum c_i / \sum d_i} = \frac{170/1246}{375/7068} = 2.572 \qquad i = 1, 2, 3, \text{ and 4 tables.}$$

The odds ratio estimate $\hat{or} = 2.572$ is calculated from the single 2×2 table created by adding the four race-specific tables (Table 2–13) and, therefore, does not account for possibly differing values of the odds ratio among the race/ethnicity groups.

The second odds ratio, assuming that the underlying association between smoking exposure and low birth weight is the same for all four race/ethnicity groups, is any one of the previously estimated common odds ratios. All three adjusted estimates account for the influence of race/ethnicity. For example, Woolf's weighted average estimate is 2.441 ($\hat{or}_w = 2.441$). The difference between the two summary odds ratios, 2.572 versus 2.441, directly indicates the extent to which the confounding caused by race/ethnicity influences the relationship between smoking exposure and low birth weight, when the association is measured by an odds ratio.

An unequivocal assessment of a confounding influence does not exist. The degree of confounding depends on how it is measured. When the confounding influence of a specific variable is measured by comparing two proportions, or by comparing two odds ratios, or by comparing any two measures of association, the degree of influence will differ. Like a number of situations that arise in statistical analysis, the combining of a series of 2×2 tables demonstrates that both the presence/absence of homogeneity and the extent of a confounding influence depends on the choice of the statistical measure of association. This fact serves as a reminder that interaction and confounding influences are properties of the statistical analysis and not of the population sampled.

3

TWO ESPECIALLY USEFUL ESTIMATION TOOLS

Estimation of the parameters of statistical models and their evaluation are major components of statistical analysis. This chapter outlines two techniques key to statistical estimation in general: namely, maximum likelihood estimation and the derivation of the properties of statistical functions. These somewhat theoretical topics are not critical to understanding the application of statistical methods, but provide valuable insight into the origins of parameter estimates and the variances of their distributions.

MAXIMUM LIKELIHOOD ESTIMATION*

Maximum likelihood estimation is used in the vast majority of statistical analyses to determine values for the parameters of models describing the relationships within sampled data. The complexity of this technique lies in the technical application and not its underlying principle. Maximum likelihood estimation is conceptually simple. A small example introduces the fundamental logic at the heart of this process.

---

* The following four sections have previously appeared in the text *Analysis for Epidemiologic and Medical Data*, Cambridge University Press, 2006.

Suppose a thumb tack tossed in the air has an unknown probability of landing with the point up (denoted p). Furthermore, three tacks are tossed, and one lands point up and the other two land point down. The probability of this result is $3p(1 - p)^2$. When two values are proposed as an estimate of the parameter p, it is not hard to decide the most likely to have produced the observed result (one up and two down) and, therefore, is the better estimate of the unknown probability p. For the example, the likelihood is that one up-tack occurs out of the three tossed when $p = 0.2$ is $3(0.2)(0.8)^2 = 0.384$, and the probability of the same outcome occurs when $p = 0.8$ is $3(0.8)(0.2)^2 = 0.096$. The "maximum-likelihood" question becomes: Which of the two postulated probabilities (0.2 and 0.8) is the best estimate of the unknown underlying value p? Although no unequivocal answer exists, selecting the probability $p = 0.2$ is simply more sensible. The observed data "best" support this answer because $p = 0.2$ makes the observed results four times more likely than $p = 0.8$. Of the two choices, selecting $p = 0.2$ is more consistent with the observed data.

Maximum likelihood estimation is a natural extension of the same logic. The data are considered as fixed, and all possible values of the parameter are examined (not just two values). The parameter that makes the observed data the most likely (maximizes the likelihood of its occurrence) is chosen as the "best" estimate. It is again the value most consistent with the observed data. For the thumb tack example, this value is 0.333. No other choice of p makes the observed data (one up and two down) more likely. For all other possible values of the parameter p, the probability $3p(1 - p)^2$ is less than $3(0.333)(0.667)^2 = 0.444$. The maximum likelihood estimate $\hat{p} = 0.333$ is not the correct value, but is the best choice in light of the observed data.

Expanding this example continues to illustrate the logic of the maximum likelihood estimation process. Say $n = 50$ tacks are tossed in the air and $x = 15$ land point up. That is, the data are

up, up, down, up, down, down, ... , down and up.

The probability that this event occurred is

$$L = p \times p \times (1 - p) \times p \times (1 - p) \times (1 - p) \times \cdots \times (1 - p) \times p,$$

or more succinctly

$$L = p^{15}(1 - p)^{35}.$$

The expression labeled L is called the *likelihood function*. As with the previous examples, the value of the parameter p is unknown. The maximum likelihood question becomes: Among all possible values for p, which value makes the observed result ($x = 15$ up-tacks) most likely to have occurred? The answer is found by calculating the likelihood function L for all possible values of p and identifying the largest value. Because sums are easier to describe conceptually and deal with mathematically, instead of the likelihood L (a product), the logarithm of L (a sum) is typically used [denoted $log(L)$]. For the thumb tack example, the likelihood value L is the product $L = p^{15}(1 - p)^{35}$, and the log-likelihood value is the sum $log(L) = 15\ log(p) + 35\ log(1 - p)$. The value that maximizes the log-likelihood function also maximizes the likelihood function. For the thumb tack data, 12 selected values of the parameter p produce the log-likelihood values in Table 3–1.

In fact, the possible values of p range continuously from 0 to 1. Figure 3–1 displays the log-likelihood values $log(L)$ for a relevant range of p (0.04 to 0.7).

Table 3–1.   Selected values of the parameter p and the corresponding log-likelihood values for x = 15 up-tacks among x = 50 tosses

p	0.05	0.10	0.15	0.20	0.25	0.30	0.35	0.40	0.45	0.50	0.55	0.60
$log(L)$	–46.7	–38.2	–34.1	–32.0	–30.9	–30.5	–30.8	–31.6	–32.9	–34.7	–36.9	–39.7

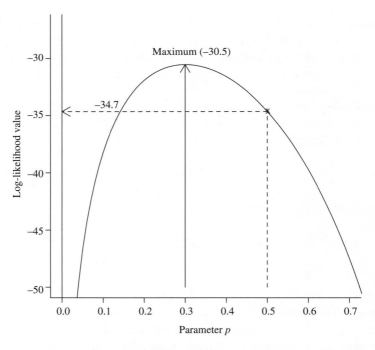

Figure 3–1.   The log-likelihood function for the thumb tack data (n = 50 and x = 15).

The log-likelihood function increases until $p = 0.3$, and then decreases. The value 0.3 is the value of p that maximizes the log-likelihood function $log(L)$ and, therefore, maximizes the likelihood function L. It is denoted $\hat{p}$ and called *the maximum likelihood estimate of the parameter p*. To repeat, no other value is more consistent with the observed data. The occurrence of 15 up-tacks (35 down-tacks) is most likely when p is 0.3, making $\hat{p} = 0.3$ the maximum likelihood estimate. Technically, the log-likelihood value $log(L_{\hat{p}=0.3}) = -30.5$ is greater than $log(L_{\hat{p}\neq0.3})$ for all other possible values of the probability p (Figure 3–1).

A natural and commonly used estimate of the probability that a tack lands up is the proportion of up-tacks observed among the total number tossed or, for the example, $\hat{p} = x/n = 15/50 = 0.3$. An amazing property of maximum likelihood estimation is that it frequently provides a statistically rigorous justification for "everyday" estimates. For example, mean values, proportions, and rates are frequently maximum likelihood estimates.

A maximum likelihood estimate is typically derived with a calculus argument for simple cases and a computer algorithm for more complicated cases. The thumb tack example continues to illustrate. The maximum of a single-valued log-likelihood function is that point at which the derivative is zero. In symbols, the maximum of the function $log(L)$ occurs at the value of p that is the solution to the equation $\frac{d}{dp}log(L) = 0$. For example, when x tacks land up out of n tosses, then

$$\frac{d}{dp}log(L) = \frac{d}{dp}[xlog(p) + (n-x)log(1-p)] = 0.$$

where $log(L) = log[p^x(1-p)^{n-x}] = xlog(p) + (n-x)log(1-p)$ is the value of the log-likelihood function for all possible parameter values p ($0 \leq p \leq 1$). Thus,

$$\frac{d}{dp}log(L) = \frac{x}{\hat{p}} - \frac{n-x}{1-\hat{p}} = 0 \quad \text{and yields the solution} \quad \hat{p} = \frac{x}{n}.$$

Again, the estimated value $\hat{p} = x/n$ maximizes the likelihood function and is also the natural estimate of the parameter p (proportion of up-tacks).

In addition, the variance of a maximum likelihood estimate can be estimated from the log-likelihood function. For the example, the variance of the distribution of the estimate $\hat{p}$ is estimated by $\hat{p}(1 - \hat{p})/n$. In general, maximum likelihood estimates are found with a computer algorithm, so that the details of the numerical estimation process, as well as the derivation of the variance expression, are rarely issues when analyzing data and are left to more theoretical presentations.

When more than one parameter is estimated, the notation and computation become more elaborate but the maximum likelihood logic remains the same. Regardless of the complexity of the likelihood function, the estimates are those values that are most likely to have produced the observed data. Suppose that

l parameters are to be estimated; then the maximum likelihood estimates are the set of l parameter values that make the likelihood function the largest possible. In symbols, the l parameters denoted θ_1, θ_2, θ_3, $\cdots$, θ_l have maximum likelihood estimates $\hat{\theta}_1$, $\hat{\theta}_2$, $\hat{\theta}_3$, $\cdots$, $\hat{\theta}_l$ when the likelihood value L evaluated at these values is larger than the likelihood values calculated from all other possible sets of parameter values θ_1, θ_2, θ_3, $\cdots$, θ_l or, in symbols,

$$L(\hat{\theta}_1, \hat{\theta}_2, \cdots, \hat{\theta}_l | x_1, x_2, \cdots, x_n) > L(\theta_1, \theta_2, \cdots, \theta_l | x_1, x_2, \cdots, x_n).$$

Here x_1, x_2, $\cdots$, x_n represent n observations treated as fixed values. The computer techniques applied to find this set of estimates are sophisticated and complex but the interpretation of the estimated values remains simple. It is the unique set of estimates that are most consistent with the observed data. In other words, among all possible sets of parameters, it is that set that makes the occurrence of the observed data most likely.

For most statistical techniques, the parameter values are thought of as fixed, and the data are subject to sampling variation. Maximum likelihood estimation reverses the situation. The observed data are considered fixed, and the parameters are varied over all possible values to find the specific value or values that maximize the likelihood function.

It is frequently difficult to construct the likelihood function L for a statistical model. Furthermore, the computational process necessary to find estimates and their variances is extremely tedious for more than two parameters. Consequently, a computer algorithm is almost always used to create the likelihood function and to estimate statistical model parameters and their variances.

FOUR PROPERTIES OF MAXIMUM LIKELIHOOD ESTIMATES

1. *Maximum likelihood estimates based on large numbers of observations have approximate normal distributions.*

    Often, as few as 10 or 20 observations are sufficient to produce estimates with approximately normal distributions. Therefore, the evaluation of maximum likelihood estimates in terms of confidence intervals and statistical tests follows typical patterns. For example, when $\hat{\theta}$ represents a maximum likelihood parameter estimate, an approximate 95% confidence interval is $\hat{\theta} \pm 1.960\sqrt{variance(\hat{\theta})}$, based on the normal distribution. Again based on the normal distribution, the test statistic

$$X^2 = z^2 = \frac{(\hat{\theta} - \theta_0)^2}{variance(\hat{\theta})}$$

has an approximate chi-square distribution with one degree of freedom when θ_0 is the "true" underlying parameter estimated by $\hat{\theta}$. The word "true" in this statistical context means that the difference between the estimate $\hat{\theta}$ and the parameter θ_0 is due entirely to random variation. The maximum likelihood estimated variance, denoted by $variance(\hat{\theta})$, serves as an estimate of the variance of the approximate normal distribution that describes the variation of the estimated value $\hat{\theta}$. This chi-square assessment of a maximum likelihood estimated parameter is sometimes called *Wald's test*.

2. *A maximum likelihood estimate is optimal in the sense that it usually has a smaller variance than competing estimates.*

    When the sample size is large, the maximum likelihood estimate is, under general conditions, the most precise estimate available (smallest variance). Thus, for a wide variety of analyses, the estimates that most efficiently utilize the sampled data are those that maximum the likelihood function.

3. *As noted, the estimated variances of a maximum likelihood estimates are necessarily calculated as part of the estimation process.*

    The computer algorithm that produces the estimates produces estimates of their variances.

4. *A function of a maximum likelihood estimate is itself a maximum likelihood estimate and has properties 1, 2, and 3.*

    When the estimate $\hat{\theta}$ represents a maximum likelihood estimate, then, for example, $e^{\hat{\theta}}$ or $\sqrt{\hat{\theta}}$ or $n\hat{\theta}$ or $1/\hat{\theta}$ are also maximum likelihood estimates. These estimates also have minimum variance and approximate normal distributions for large sample sizes. For the thumb tack tossing example, because $\hat{p} = 0.3$ is the maximum likelihood estimate of the probability that a tack lands up, then $n\hat{p} = 100(0.3) = 30$ is the maximum likelihood estimate of the number of up-tacks that would occur among $n = 100$ tosses. Furthermore, the probability $\hat{q} = 1 - \hat{p} = 1 - 0.3 = 0.7$, thus making $\hat{q} = 0.7$ the maximum likelihood estimate of the probability a tack lands point down.

LIKELIHOOD STATISTICS

Producing optimal parameter estimates and their estimated variances from sampled data is only one of the valuable properties of a likelihood function. The likelihood function or the logarithm of the likelihood function (not just the maximum) reflect the probability that the collected data occurred for a specific set of parameters. For example, if $p = 0.8$, then the likelihood of one-up and two-down tacks is $L = 3p(1-p)^2 = 3(0.8)(0.2)^2 = 0.096$ or $log(L) = -2.343$.

    Table 3–1 shows the log-likelihood value $log(L)$ is -34.7 when $p = 0.5$ is postulated as the underlying probability of observing 15 up-tacks among

$n = 50$ tosses. This likelihood value is clearly not the maximum but, nevertheless, reflects the probability that 15 up-tacks occur as if p were equal to 0.5. The maximum value of the log-likelihood occurs at $\hat{p} = 0.3$, where $log(L) = -30.5$. These two log-likelihood values (-34.7 and -30.5) differ for one of two distinct reasons. Because the estimate $\hat{p}$ is subject to sampling variation, the two log-likelihood values possibly differ by chance alone when $p = 0.5$ is the underlying parameter. Alternatively, when the value $p = 0.5$ is not the underlying parameter, the two log-likelihood values then differ systematically. Thus, the question of why $\hat{p} = 0.3$ differs from $p = 0.5$ is addressed by the difference in log-likelihood values. The larger the difference in likelihood values, the smaller the probability that the two values differ by chance alone.

To help choose between these two alternatives (random vs. systematic) based on the observed difference between two log-likelihood values generated from two statistical models, a theorem from theoretical statistics becomes an important analytic tool. The theorem states that the difference between two log-likelihood values multiplied by -2 has an approximate chi-square distribution when three conditions hold. The first condition is that estimates from the two models generating the log-likelihood values must be calculated from exactly the same data. Second, the compared models must be *nested*. Nested means that one model is a special case of the other (examples follow). Third, the two log-likelihood values must differ only because of random variation. When the first two conditions apply, a test statistic with a chi-square distribution (called the *likelihood ratio test statistic*) produces an assessment of the plausibility of the third condition in terms of a significance probability. The question becomes: Is the observed difference between log-likelihood values calculated from the same data likely a systematic difference, or likely due only to the influence of random variation? To help answer this question, the comparison of two log-likelihood values and a chi-square distribution produces a significance probability (p-value). Specifically, the likelihood ratio test statistic is

$$X^2 = -2[log(L_0) - log(L_1)]$$

and has an approximate chi-square distribution with m degrees of freedom when $log(L_0)$ and $log(L_1)$, calculated from two nested models, differ by chance alone. Large values of X^2 (small p-value) indicated that chance is not a plausible explanation of the observed difference. The degrees of freedom, m, are the difference between the number of parameters estimated to calculate each log-likelihood value.

The thumb tack tossing example conforms to all three requirements if the underlying probability that a tack lands up is $p = 0.5$ (hypothesis) and the estimated value $\hat{p} = 0.3$ differs from 0.5 strictly by chance alone. Then, the likelihood ratio test statistic (using the log-likelihood values from Table 3–1 and Figure 3–1)

$$X^2 = -2[log(L_{p=0.5}) - log(L_{p=0.3})]$$
$$= -2[(-34.657) - (-30.543)] = 8.228$$

is a single observation from a chi-square distribution with one degree of freedom. For $log(L_{p=0.3})$, one estimate is made (namely, $\hat{p} = 0.3$) and, for $log(L_{p=0.5})$, no estimate is made ($p = 0.5$ was selected) thus yielding one degree of freedom. The probability that a more extreme difference between the log-likelihood values occurs by chance alone is then p-value $= P(X^2 \geq 8.228 | p = 0.5) = 0.004$ from a chi-square distribution with one degree of freedom. Thus, the actual value of p is not likely in the neighborhood of 0.5 but likely closer to 0.3. That is, the estimate $\hat{p} = 0.3$ is not a likely result when $p = 0.5$.

In fact, the comparison of two log-likelihood values produces statistical tests similar to many familiar procedures. Such likelihood comparisons give results similar to chi-square tests, t-tests, and tests based on the normal distribution, such as an approximate tests of a proportion. For example, when, again, $n = 50$ and $x = 15$, a test statistic for the hypothesis of $p = p_0$ is

$$z = \frac{\hat{p} - p_0}{\sqrt{\dfrac{\hat{p}(1 - \hat{p})}{n}}},$$

and $z^2 = X^2$ has an approximate chi-square distribution with one degree of freedom. Specifically, for the thumb tack example and $p_0 = 0.5$

$$z = \frac{0.3 - 0.5}{\sqrt{\dfrac{0.3(1 - 0.3)}{50}}} = -3.086.$$

The test-statistic is then $z^2 = (-3.086)^2 = 9.524$ and is approximately equal to the previous likelihood ratio chi-square value of $X^2 = 8.228$. The difference between these two approaches diminishes as the estimate becomes closer to the hypothesis-generated test value. Such as when $p_0 = 0.4$, then $z^2 = (-1.543)^2 = 2.381$, and the likelihood ratio chi-square test statistic is $X^2 = 2.160$.

Calculating the difference between log-likelihood values is a fundamental statistical tool and provides the opportunity to compare analytic models with any number of parameters. In general, for a model describing the relationship among n observations $x_1, x_2, \cdots, x_n$ using l parameters, the log-likelihood value is represented by

$$log(L_1) = log\text{-}likelihood = log[L(\theta_1, \theta_2, \theta_3, \cdots, \theta_l | x_1, x_2, x_3, \cdots, x_n)].$$

A second log-likelihood value based on creating a nested model by removing m parameters (set equal to zero) is represented by

$$log(L_0) = log\text{-}likelihood = log[L(\theta_1 = 0, \cdots, \theta_m = 0,$$
$$\theta_{m+1}, \cdots, \theta_l | x_1, x_2, x_3, \cdots, x_n)].$$

Or, for a model based on the remaining $l - m$ parameters, the same likelihood value is more simply represented as

$$log(L_0) = log\text{-}likelihood = log[L(\theta_{m+1}, \cdots, \theta_l | x_1, x_2, x_3, \cdots, x_n)].$$

As long as these two log-likelihood values are calculated from the same data, contrast nested models, and differ only because of random variation, the likelihood ratio test statistic $X^2 = -2[log(L_0) - log(L_1)]$ has an approximate chi-square distribution. The degrees of freedom are, as before, m, where m represents the number of parameters deleted from the more complex model to form the simpler and, as required, nested model.

The comparison of two log-likelihood values (almost always calculated with a computer program) reflects the relative difference in "fit" between the two sets of conditions described in term of two nested models. The observed difference indicates the effectiveness of the simpler model (fewer parameters) to summarize the observed data relative to the more complex model. When a parameter value or a set of parameter values is eliminated from a model and the log-likelihood comparison remains essentially unaffected (only a slight difference), the inference is made that the parameters eliminated are unimportant. The log-likelihood difference is said to be likely due to random variation. Conversely, when a parameter value or a set of parameter values is eliminated from a model and the log-likelihood comparison yields a striking difference, the inference is made that the parameters eliminated are important and likely have systematic influences. The comparison of two log-likelihood values, therefore, produces a chi-square test in terms of a significance probability (random or systematic) that allows an evaluation of the difference between two models intentionally created by eliminating selected model parameters.

The following example illustrates a typical contrast of two nested models. Using estimated parameters to generate two log-likelihood values, the linear model $y = a + b_1x_1 + b_2x_2 + b_3x_3$ is compared to the nested model $y = a + b_1x_1$ to evaluate the influence of the variables represented by x_2 and x_3 ($b_2 = b_3 = 0$?). The likelihood ratio chi-square test-statistic

$$X^2 = -2[log(L_0) - log(L_1)] = 6.2 \qquad \text{(last column, Table 3–2)}$$

Table 3–2.   An example evaluation using a likelihood ratio statistic to contrast two nested models (hypothetical)

Nested models	Constraint	d.f.*	Log-likelihood values
$a + b_1 x_1 + b_2 x_2 + b_3 x_3$	–	$n - 4$	$log(L_1) = -145.3$
$a + b_1 x_1$	$b_2 = b_3 = 0$	$n - 2$	$log(L_0) = -148.4$
	–	$m = 2$	$-2[log(L_0) - log(L_1)] = 6.2$

*= Degrees of freedom.

has an approximate chi-square distribution with two degrees of freedom ($m = 2$), producing the p-value $P(X^2 \geq 6.2 | b_2 = b_3 = 0) = 0.045$. The moderately small p-value indicates that the variables x_1 or x_2 or both are likely important components of the more complex model.

The absolute magnitude of a log-likelihood value is primarily determined by the sample size; the larger the sample size, the smaller the log-likelihood statistic. Therefore, a difference between two likelihood values from nested models is not influenced by the sample size (same data for both calculations). However, the difference reflects only a relative change in likelihood values due to differences in the compared models. For example, two models could have similar likelihood values, but neither model is a particularly good representation of the relationships within the sampled data. The worth of a statistical model to summarize the relationships within the sampled data is best measured by directly comparing model-generated values to corresponding observed values. The important issue of the adequacy of the model to represent the relationships within the data cannot always be addressed with likelihood methods.

A sometimes handy rule of thumb states: when the likelihood ratio chi-square test-statistic X^2 is less than m (the number of parameters eliminated), no evidence exists that the eliminated parameters play a systematic role in the model. The rule is an application of the fact that the mean value of a chi-square distribution is its degrees of freedom. The likelihood ratio test statistic has a chi-square distribution with m degrees of freedom when the m eliminated parameters have only random influences. Thus, an observed chi-square value less than its mean value m provides no evidence of a systematic difference between likelihood values. For $X^2 < m$, the smallest possible p-value is always greater than 0.3. Of course, exact probabilities exist in tables or are produced as part of statistical computer programs.

THE STATISTICAL PROPERTIES OF A FUNCTION

Consider a variable denoted x with known or postulated properties, but questions arise concerning a function of x, denoted $f(x)$. Two important statistical questions are: What is the mean, and what is the variance of the distribution of $f(x)$? Or, in symbols,

$$mean \ of \ the \ distribution \ of \ f(x) =? \quad and \quad variance[f(x)] =?$$

Two rules allow the approximate mean and the variance of the distribution of the variable $f(x)$ to be derived from the mean and variance of the distribution of the variable x. They are:

- *Rule 1:* The approximate mean of the distribution of the variable $f(x)$ (denoted μ_f) is the value of the function evaluated at the mean of the distribution of x (denoted μ). That is,

$$\mu_f = mean \ of \ the \ distribution \ of \ f(x) \approx f(\mu)$$

where μ_f represents the approximate mean value of the distribution of the $f(x)$-values and μ represents the mean value of the distribution of the x-values.
- *Rule 2:* The approximate variance of the distribution of the variable $f(x)$ (denoted *variance*$[f(x)]$) is

$$variance \ of \ f(x) = variance[f(x)] \approx \left[\frac{d}{dx} f(\mu) \right]^2 variance(x)$$

where *variance*(x) represents the variance of the distribution of the variable x.

The symbol $\frac{d}{dx} f(\mu)$ represents the derivative of the function $f(x)$ with respect to x evaluated at the mean value μ. Both rules 1 and 2 are an application of a basic mathematical tool called a *Taylor series expansion*, and their application in a statistical context is sometimes referred to as "the delta method" [12].

For example, suppose the variable x has a symmetric distribution (Figure 3–2, left) with a mean value $= \mu = 10$ and a *variance*$(x) = 4$. The distribution of $f(x) = 1/x$ (Figure 3–2, right) then has an approximate mean value $\mu_f \approx 1/\mu = 1/10 = 0.1$ (Rule 1) and an approximate *variance*$[f(x)] \approx \frac{1}{\mu^4} variance(x) = \frac{1}{10^4}(4) = 0.0004$ (Rule 2), because the derivative is $1/x$ is

$$\frac{d}{dx} f(x) = \frac{d}{dx} \left[\frac{1}{x} \right] = -\frac{1}{x^2} \quad and \quad \left[\frac{d}{dx} f(\mu) \right]^2 = \frac{1}{\mu^4} = \frac{1}{10^4}.$$

Application 1: Poisson Distribution

A *Poisson distributed variable* is sometimes transformed by taking the square root to produce a more normal-like distribution. For a Poisson distribution, the mean value (represented by the mean value $\mu = \lambda$) and the variance (represented by

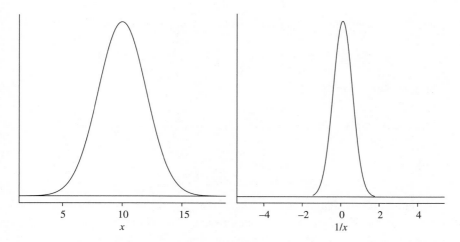

Figure 3–2. The distributions of x and $f(x) = \frac{1}{x}$.

$variance(x) = \lambda$) are equal. The function $f(x) = \sqrt{x}$ produces a more symmetric and approximate normal distribution (if λ is not too small) with mean value = $\mu_f = \sqrt{\lambda}$ and $variance(\sqrt{x}) = 1/4$.

Applying Rules 1 and 2, the approximate mean value of the normal-like distribution of the function $\sqrt{x}$ is

$$\mu_f = \text{mean of the distribution of } \sqrt{x} = \mu_{\sqrt{x}} \approx \sqrt{\mu} = \sqrt{\lambda} \quad \text{(Rule 1)}.$$

The approximate variance is

$$\text{variance of } f(x) = \text{variance}(\sqrt{x}) = \frac{1}{4\lambda} \text{ variance}(x) = \frac{1}{4\lambda}\lambda = \frac{1}{4} \quad \text{(Rule 2)},$$

because the derivative of $\sqrt{x}$ is

$$\frac{d}{dx}f(x) = \frac{d}{dx}\sqrt{x} = \frac{1}{2\sqrt{x}} \quad \text{and} \quad \left[\frac{d}{dx}f(\lambda)\right]^2 \approx \frac{1}{4\lambda}.$$

Application 2: Variance of a Logarithm of a Variable

Applying Rules 1 and 2 to the logarithm of a variable x again yields an expression for the approximate mean value and variance of the distribution of the transformed variable $log(x)$. Thus, when $f(x) = log(x)$, applying Rule 1 yields

$$\mu_f = \text{mean of the distribution of } f(x) = \mu_{log(x)} \approx log(\mu)$$

where μ represents the mean of the distribution of the variable x. The derivative of $log(x)$ is

$$\frac{d}{dx}f(x) = \frac{d}{dx}log(x) = \frac{1}{x}.$$

Applying Rule 2 yields

$$variance\ of\ f(x) = variance[f(x)] = variance[log(x)] \approx \frac{1}{\mu^2}\ variance(x).$$

Corollary:

$$variance(x) \approx \mu^2 variance[log(x)].$$

Statistical summaries and estimates are sometimes transformed to have more symmetric (normal-like) distributions using logarithms (Chapter 1). Such transformations frequently improve the accuracy of confidence intervals and statistical tests. The mean value and variance of the distribution of the logarithm of a variable then become necessary parts of the statistical evaluation.

Application 3: Variance of the Logarithm of a Count

The variance of the logarithm of a count is estimated by the reciprocal of the count. That is, when a count is denoted x, the estimated variance of $log(x)$ is $variance(log[x]) = 1/x$. Such reciprocal values of counts appear in the variance of the logarithm of odds ratios, the variance of the relative risk, the variance of the logarithm of odds, and the variance of the logarithm of rate-ratios.

When the count x has a binomial distribution,

$$the\ mean = \mu = np \quad and \quad variance(x) = np(1 - p).$$

When the count x has a Poisson distribution,

$$the\ mean = \mu = \lambda = np \quad and \quad variance(x) = \lambda = np.$$

Therefore, when p is small ($1 - p \approx 1$) or when x has a Poisson distribution,

$$variance(log[x]) \approx \left[\frac{1}{np}\right]^2 np = \frac{1}{np} \quad (rule\ 2)\ because \quad \left[\frac{d}{dx}f(\mu)\right]^2 = \left[\frac{1}{np}\right]^2.$$

When x events occur among a series of n observations, the probability of the occurrence of x is estimated by $\hat{p} = x/n$. Therefore, a natural estimate of the variance of the logarithm of x is

$$variance(log[x]) = \frac{1}{n\hat{p}} = \frac{1}{x} \quad because\ n\hat{p} = x.$$

4

LINEAR LOGISTIC REGRESSION: DISCRETE DATA

Epidemiologic data frequently consist of discrete variables, such as cases of disease or deaths, or continuous variables made into categorical variables to create a table. Converting continuous variables into categorical variables simplifies their presentation and is usually based on traditional definitions. For example, individuals are considered hypertensive when their systolic blood pressure exceeds 140 mm Hg, or smokers are placed into exposure categories based on the reported number of cigarettes smoked per day. A table is certainly a valuable summary of collected data, but, in addition, it is often important to explore the sometimes complex relationships within a table. Such a table (Table 4–1) describes three risk factors and the likelihood of coronary heart disease (CHD) using data from the Western Collaborative Group Study (WCGS; described in detail at the end of this chapter).

Table 4–1 contains the counts of CHD events and counts of individuals at risk classified into behavior type, systolic blood pressure, and smoking exposure categories. It is apparent that increased likelihood of a CHD event is associated with increasing amounts smoked, high blood pressure, and type-A behavior. A number of questions, however, are not as easily answered. Among them are:

- Does smoking have a nonlinear influence on CHD risk, or does smoking increase risk in a more or less linear pattern?

Table 4–1. Coronary heart disease events classified by behavior type (type-A or type-B), systolic blood pressure (<140 mm Hg or ≥140 mm Hg), and smoking exposure (cigarettes/day, four categories): a summary table

Blood pressure	Behavior type	Smoking frequency, cigarettes per day			
		0	1–20	21–30	≥30
≥140 mm Hg	type-A	29/184 = 0.158	21/97 = 0.216	7/52 = 0.135	12/55 = 0.218
≥140 mm Hg	type-B	8/179 = 0.045	9/71 = 0.127	3/34 = 0.088	7/21 = 0.333
<140 mm Hg	type-A	41/600 = 0.068	24/301 = 0.080	27/167 = 0.162	17/133 = 0.128
<140 mm Hg	type-B	20/689 = 0.029	16/336 = 0.048	13/152 = 0.086	3/83 = 0.036

- What is the magnitude of the combined influences of blood pressure and smoking on the behavior–CHD relationship?
- Is the relationship between the measure of behavior type and CHD risk the same regardless of an individual's blood pressure level?
- What is the relative contribution of each risk factor measure to the description of the likelihood of a coronary event?
- What is the combined influence of the three risk factors on the likelihood of a coronary event?
- Historically, the WCGS data were collected to assess lifestyle behavior as a possible risk factor for a coronary event. Therefore, the primary question was: Does behavior type reflect a systematic and direct influence on the likelihood of a CHD event (an unanswered and even controversial question when the study was undertaken)?

The inability to answer complex or even elementary questions about risk–disease relationships in a satisfactory way results, to a large extent, from lack of data. When large numbers of individuals are classified into a table with numerous categories, most questions can be directly answered about the role of risk factors in the likelihood of a disease. When more than a few variables are investigated, or large numbers of observations are not available, a table alone frequently fails to reveal effectively the relationships between risk and disease. In addition, human disease is almost always a rare event, causing at least a few categories to have low frequencies in most tabulated data. For example, only three coronary events occur in the high blood pressure, moderate smoking (21–30 cigarettes/day), type-B category among the 3154 men studied. Even for this relatively large study, it becomes necessary to apply specialized statistical tools to effectively identify the relationships within a table, primarily because of the presence of substantial sampling variation caused by low frequencies of observations. A statistical model is designed for this situation. A model approach is a highly efficient and frequently provides a coherent description of the relationships within a table. That is, a small number of summary values, each estimated from the entire data set, potentially provide a simple, precise, and sometimes comprehensive description of the relationships within the collected data. A *logistic regression model* is such a model and is a statistical tool designed for identifying and assessing the relationships between a series of risk factors and a binary outcome classified into a multivariable table.

THE SIMPLEST LOGISTIC REGRESSION MODEL: THE 2 × 2 TABLE

A 2 × 2 table produces the simplest possible application of a logistic model. To start, the variables to be studied are again the presence and absence of a disease ($D = 1$, disease present and $D = 0$, disease absent) and a two-level risk factor ($F = 1$, risk factor present and $F = 0$, risk factor absent). The general notation (repeated from Chapters 1 and 2) for a 2 × 2 table applies (Table 4–2).

A baseline statistic calculated as the first step in describing disease risk using a logistic model is an estimate of the log-odds associated with individuals who do not possess the risk factor (risk factor is absent or $F = 0$), then

$$\hat{a} = estimated\ log\text{-}odds = log\left[\frac{n_{01}/(n_{01} + n_{00})}{n_{00}/(n_{01} + n_{00})}\right] = log\left[\frac{n_{01}}{n_{00}}\right]$$

so that

$$\hat{a}\ \text{is an estimate of}\ a\ \text{where}\ a = log(odds) = log\left[\frac{P(D|F = 0)}{P(\overline{D}|F = 0)}\right].$$

One measure of the influence of a risk variable on the likelihood of disease is the change in the log-odds associated with individuals who possess the risk factor ($F = 1$) relative to the log-odds associated with individuals who do not possess the risk factor ($F = 0$). Specifically, this difference in log-odds is

$$\hat{b} = log\left(\frac{n_{11}}{n_{10}}\right) - log\left(\frac{n_{01}}{n_{00}}\right) = log\left[\frac{n_{11}/n_{10}}{n_{01}/n_{00}}\right] = log\left[\frac{n_{11}n_{00}}{n_{10}n_{01}}\right] = log(\hat{or})$$

Table 4–2. Notation for a 2 × 2 table

	Disease: $D = 1$	No disease: $D = 0$	**Total**
Factor present: $F = 1$	n_{11}	n_{10}	$n_{1.}$
Factor absent: $F = 0$	n_{01}	n_{00}	$n_{0.}$
Total	$n_{.1}$	$n_{.0}$	n

so that

$\hat{b}$ is an estimate of b where $b = log\left[\dfrac{P(D|F=1)}{P(\overline{D}|F=1)}\right] - log\left[\dfrac{P(D|F=0)}{P(\overline{D}|F=0)}\right]$

$$= log(or).$$

Furthermore, exponentiating the differences b and $\hat{b}$, then

$$e^b = \frac{P(D|F=1)/P(\overline{D}|F=1)}{P(D|F=0)/P(\overline{D}|F=0)} = or \quad \text{and} \quad e^{\hat{b}} = \frac{n_{11}/n_{10}}{n_{01}/n_{00}} = \hat{or}$$

yield the odds ratio and estimated odds ratio measures of association from a 2×2 table (Chapter 1). This relationship between the log-odds and the odds ratio characterizes the logistic model.

The two quantities (denoted a and b), called *parameters* in the context of a model, form the simplest possible linear logistic model. The model is

$$log\text{-}odds = a + bF$$

where $F = 0$ or $F = 1$ so that,

when $F = 0$, the estimated baseline log-odds is $log\text{-}odds = log\left(\dfrac{n_{01}}{n_{00}}\right) = \hat{a}$

and

when $F = 1$, the estimated log-odds is $log\text{-}odds = log\left(\dfrac{n_{11}}{n_{10}}\right) = \hat{a} + \hat{b}$

and, as before, the difference in log-odds is $(\hat{a} + \hat{b}) - \hat{a} = \hat{b} = log(\hat{or})$.

The estimate $\hat{b}$ measures, on the log-odds scale, the change in likelihood of disease associated with the presence of a risk factor ($F = 1$) relative to the absence of the same risk factor ($F = 0$). A difference in log-odds is not a particularly intuitive description of a risk–disease association, but it has tractable statistical properties and, of most importance, relates directly to the odds ratio measure of association, which is the primary reason for selecting a logistic regression model in the first place. In general, this relationship is

$$odds\ ratio = or = e^{difference\ in\ log\text{-}odds}.$$

Consider a 2×2 table from the WCGS data (Table 4–3) summarizing the relationship between behavior type (a binary risk factor) and a coronary event (a binary disease outcome).

Table 4–3.   CHD by A/B-behavior type

	CHD	No CHD	**Total**
Type-A	178	1411	1589
Type-B	79	1486	1565
Total	257	2897	3154

From these data, the specific parameter estimates are $\hat{a} = log(79/1486) =$ −2.934 (baseline) and $\hat{a} + \hat{b} = log(178/1411) = -2.070$. The difference in the estimated log-odds of a CHD event associated with type-A individuals (risk factor present) relative to type-B individuals (risk factor absent, baseline) is $\hat{b} = (\hat{a} + \hat{b}) - \hat{a} = -2.070 - (-2.934) = 0.864$ (difference in log-odds, Figure 4–1). For the CHD data (Table 4–3), the model estimated odds ratio is then $\hat{or} = e^{\hat{b}} = e^{0.864} = 2.373$. The odds of a coronary event is, therefore, estimated to be 2.373 times greater for a type-A individual than for a type-B individual. The odds ratio calculated directly from the table yields the identical value where $\hat{or} = (178/1411)/(79/1486) = 2.373$.

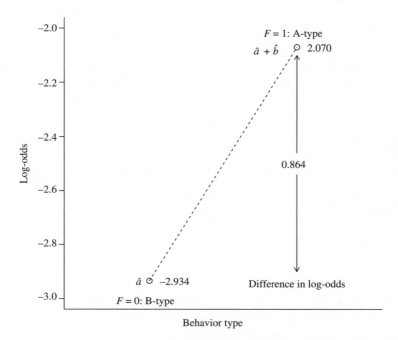

Figure 4–1.   The geometry of the log-odds associated with likelihood of a CHD event and behavior type (A/B).

When the number of model parameters equals the number of observed log-odds values, the results from applying a logistic model to describe associations and making calculations directly from the data are always identical. Such a model is said to be *saturated*. The two-parameter logistic model applied to estimate the two log-odds values generated by a 2×2 table is an example of a saturated model.

The two primary ways to account for the influence of sampling variation on an estimated value, a confidence interval, and a significance test, directly apply to model-generated estimates.

> Note: The relative merits of a confidence interval versus a significance test have been occasionally discussed, sometimes debated (for example, [13], [14] and [15]). For a single estimate, a confidence interval and a two-sided significance test yield essentially the same result. The confidence interval conveys more information, in the sense that the interval width gives some sense of the range of the parameter possibilities (statistical power). A confidence interval is expressed in the same units as the estimated quantity, which is sometimes helpful. A significance test reported in isolation tends to reduce conclusions to two choices ("significant" or "not significant") which, perhaps, characterizes the role of chance variation too simply. For example, an estimate can be "significant" (chance not a plausible explanation) because a large number of observations is involved but does not reflect an important biological or physical association. On the other hand, a confidence interval approach is complicated when more than one estimate is involved. In these situations, several estimates are easily assessed simultaneously with a significance test where the analogous confidence region is complex to construct and difficult to interpret. Of course, a significance test and a confidence interval could both be presented. However, if one approach must be chosen, a confidence interval allows a direct and comprehensive description of the influence of sampling variation on a single estimated quantity, enhancing the description of most estimates.

Sampling variability occurs because the collected data represent a fraction of the population sampled, and this variation must be taken into account to assess realistically the results of a statistical analysis. To evaluate the influence of sampling variation on the estimated log-odds, the calculations of both a significance test and a confidence interval require an estimate of the variance of the distribution of the estimated value $\hat{b}$. An estimate of this variance is

$$variance(\hat{b}) = \frac{1}{n_{11}} + \frac{1}{n_{10}} + \frac{1}{n_{01}} + \frac{1}{n_{00}}$$

where, to repeat, $\hat{b} = $ *difference in log-odds* $= log$ log(*estimated odds-ratio*) $= log(\hat{or})$. This is the same estimate of the variance introduced in Chapters 1 and 2. For the behavior type data (Table 4–3), the estimated variance associated with the distribution of the estimate $\hat{b} = 0.864$ is

$$variance(\hat{b}) = \frac{1}{178} + \frac{1}{1411} + \frac{1}{79} + \frac{1}{1486} = 0.020.$$

To test the hypothesis that a risk factor is unrelated to the disease outcome ($b = 0$), the commonly used test statistic

$$X^2 = \frac{(\hat{b} - 0)^2}{variance(\hat{b})} = \frac{(log(\hat{or}) - 0)^2}{variance(log[\hat{or}])}$$

has an approximate chi-square distribution with one degree of freedom when no risk–disease association exists (Chapters 1 and 3). A statistical test of the hypothesis that $b = 0$ is equivalent to testing the hypothesis that the odds ratio $= or = 1.0$. More concretely, the test statistic X^2 addresses the question: Is the disease outcome and risk factor statistically independent or, in symbols, $P(D|F) = P(D)$?

For the WCGS data, the chi-square distributed test statistic

$$X^2 = \frac{(\hat{b} - 0)^2}{variance(\hat{b})} = \frac{(0.864 - 0)^2}{0.020} = 37.985$$

yields a p-value of $P(X^2 \geq 37.985 | b = 0) < 0.001$, providing substantial evidence that A/B-behavior is associated with the likelihood of a CHD event.

The maximum likelihood estimate $\hat{b}$ has an approximate normal distribution that is particularly accurate for large samples of observations (Chapter 3). Therefore, an approximate 95% confidence interval based on the estimate $\hat{b}$ and its estimated variance has bounds

$$lower\ bound = \hat{A} = \hat{b} - 1.960\ \sqrt{variance(\hat{b})}$$

and

$$upper\ bound = \hat{B} = \hat{b} + 1.960\ \sqrt{variance(\hat{b})}\ .$$

A 95% confidence interval based on the estimated odds ratio $\hat{or} = e^{\hat{b}}$ is then (e^{lower}, e^{upper}).

Specifically, the estimate $\hat{b} = 0.864$ and the normal distribution yield the approximate 95% confidence interval $(0.589, 1.139)$. The approximate 95% confidence interval based on the estimated odds ratio $e^{\hat{b}} = e^{0.864} = 2.373$ is then $(e^{0.589} = 1.803, e^{1.139} = 3.123)$, indicating a likely range of the possible values for the underlying odds ratio.

A linear model representing the log-odds directly describes the probabilities from a 2×2 table with a logistic function; thus, the name *logistic regression model*. The logistic function, which has been historically important in a variety of contexts, is formally

$$f(x) = \frac{1}{1 + e^{-x}}.$$

The logistic function $f(x)$ is an S-shaped curve where large negative values of x yield values of $f(x)$ near but never less than zero, and large positive values of x yield values of $f(x)$ near but never greater than 1. Because the logistic function simply produces values that are always between zero and 1, it is ideal for representing probabilities that are also always between zero and 1.

In symbols, the logistic model probabilities from a 2×2 table are

$$P(D|F = 0) = \frac{1}{1 + e^{-a}} \quad \text{and} \quad P(D|F = 1) = \frac{1}{1 + e^{-(a+b)}}$$

where a and b are the coefficients previously defined in terms of a log-odds linear model. In other words, the same two parameters (a, b) equally describe the relationship between risk factor and disease within a 2×2 table in terms of a difference in log-odds values, odds ratios, or probabilities.

Logistic probabilities from a 2×2 table imply a linear relationship among the log-odds values and vice versa. For example, the log-odds measure of the likelihood of disease when the risk factor is present ($F = 1$) becomes

$$log\text{-}odds = log\left[\frac{P(D|F = 1)}{P(\overline{D}|F = 1)}\right] = log\left[\frac{1/(1 + e^{-(a+b)})}{e^{-(a+b)}/(1 + e^{-(a+b)})}\right]$$

$$= log\left[e^{(a+b)}\right] = a + b.$$

When the risk factor is absent ($F = 0$), then

$$log\text{-}odds = log\left[\frac{P(D|F = 0)}{P(\overline{D}|F = 0)}\right] = log\left[\frac{1/(1 + e^{-a})}{e^{-a}/(1 + e^{-a})}\right] = log(e^a) = a.$$

In general, the relationship between the log-odds and the probability of disease is

$$probability\ of\ disease = \frac{1}{1 + e^{-log\text{-}odds}}$$

and, based on this expression, then

$$odds\text{-}ratio = e^{difference\ in\ log\text{-}odds}.$$

A summary of the logistic regression model applied to evaluate the association between behavior type and coronary heart disease (2×2 table) using the WCGS data is given in Table 4–4.

The estimated probabilities of a CHD event are $\hat{P}(D|F = 0) = 0.050$ and $\hat{P}(D|F = 1) = 0.112$ calculated from either the logistic model using estimates $\hat{a}$ and $\hat{b}$ or directly from the data, indicating again that the logistic model is saturated when applied to a 2×2 table. Specifically, for the type-A individuals ($F = 1$ and

Table 4–4.   CHD by A/B-behavior: a two parameter logistic model
applied to the WCGS data ($n = 3{,}154$)

Variables	Terms	Estimates	Std. errors	p-Values	$\hat{or}$
Constant	a	-2.934	0.115	–	–
A/B	b	0.864	0.140	<0.001	2.373

LogLikelihood $= -870.172$

$log(odds) = \hat{a} + \hat{b} = -2.070$), the probability of a CHD event is

$$\hat{P}(D|F = 1) = \frac{1}{1 + e^{-(\hat{a}+\hat{b})}} = \frac{1}{1 + e^{2.070}} = 0.112 \quad \text{or}$$

$$\hat{P}(D|F = 1) = \frac{178}{1589} = 0.112$$

and for the type-B individuals ($F = 0$ and $log(odds) = \hat{a} = -2.934$), the probability of a CHD event is

$$\hat{P}(D|F = 0) = \frac{1}{1 + e^{-\hat{a}}} = \frac{1}{1 + e^{2.934}} = 0.050 \quad \text{or}$$

$$\hat{P}(D|F = 0) = \frac{79}{1565} = 0.050.$$

The estimated odds ratio necessarily follows the same pattern, and

$$\hat{or} = e^{\hat{b}} = e^{0.864} = 2.373 \quad \text{or} \quad \hat{or} = \frac{0.112/0.888}{0.050/0.950} = 2.373.$$

THE LOGISTIC REGRESSION MODEL: THE 2 × 2 × 2 TABLE

When an association between two variables is identified, the question immediately arises: Is the association influenced by other factors? The answer is almost always yes. The WCGS data show a strong association between behavior type and coronary heart disease, but an important question remains: Is this association, at least in part, due to other risk factors? For example, systolic blood pressure is related to the risk of coronary disease as well as behavior type, and could substantially influence the observed association. It is entirely possible that type-A individuals have on average higher blood pressure levels than do type-B individuals, and this higher level of blood pressure is responsible for much of the observed increased CHD risk associated with type-A behavior. A 2 × 2 × 2 table sheds light on the role of a third binary variable.

To illustrate, the influence of systolic blood pressure on the association between behavior type and coronary disease is explored by creating two separate

Table 4–5.   CHD by A/B-behavior and systolic blood pressure: counts ($n = 3{,}154$ men)

	Blood pressure ≥ 140			Blood pressure < 140		
	CHD	No CHD	**Total**	CHD	No CHD	**Total**
Type-A	69	319	388	109	1092	1201
Type-B	27	278	305	52	1208	1260
Total	96	597	693	161	2300	2461

$$\hat{or}_1 = 2.227 \qquad\qquad\qquad \hat{or}_2 = 2.319$$

Table 4–6.   CHD by A/B-behavior and systolic blood pressure: log-odds measure of risk factor influence ($n = 3{,}154$ men)

Blood pressure	Behavior type	At-risk	CHD	No CHD	Notation	Log-odds
≥ 140	type-A	388	69	319	$\hat{l}_{11}$	−1.531
≥ 140	type-B	305	27	278	$\hat{l}_{10}$	−2.332
< 140	type-A	1201	109	1092	$\hat{l}_{01}$	−2.304
< 140	type-B	1260	52	1208	$\hat{l}_{00}$	−3.145

2×2 tables of counts from the WCGS data (a $2 \times 2 \times 2$ table, Table 4–5). Blood pressure is measured as a binary variable (high ≥ 140 or low < 150). An alternative description of these data in terms of four log-odds values is also useful (Table 4–6).

The influence of behavior type again measured by the difference in log-odds is $\hat{b}_1 = \hat{l}_{11} - \hat{l}_{10} = -1.531 - (-2.332) = 0.801$ for individuals with high blood pressure, and by the difference in log-odds $\hat{b}_2 = \hat{l}_{01} - \hat{l}_{00} = -2.304 - (-3.145) = 0.841$ for individuals with low blood pressure. The estimation and interpretation of these two quantities does not differ from the log-odds measure previously calculated from a single 2×2 table, but they are estimated twice, once for each blood pressure level (each 2×2 table). Also parallel to estimates from a single 2×2 table, the estimated odds ratios are $\hat{or}_1 = e^{0.801} = 2.227$ (blood pressure ≥ 140) and $\hat{or}_2 = e^{0.841}$ (blood pressure < 140) $= 2.319$.

In the case of a $2 \times 2 \times 2$ table, measures of the influence on the risk of a CHD event associated with blood pressure are similarly estimated for each A/B-behavior category. Specifically, for type-A individuals $\hat{c}_1 = \hat{l}_{11} - \hat{l}_{01} = -1.531 - (-2.304) = 0.773$ and for type-B individuals $\hat{c}_2 = \hat{l}_{10} - \hat{l}_{00} = -2.332 - (-3.145) = 0.813$, producing the corresponding estimated odds ratios $e^{0.773} = 2.166$ (type-A) and $e^{0.813} = 2.256$ (type-B), measuring the influence of blood pressure.

The fact that these two measures of association ($\hat{b}_i$-values or $\hat{c}_i$-values) are not equal introduces a fundamental analytic issue. One of two possibilities exists:

1. The underlying measures of the influence of the risk factor in each subtable are the same ($b_1 = b_2$ or $or_1 = or_2$), and the observed difference arises only because of random variation or
2. The underlying measures of the influence of the risk factor in each subtable systematically differ ($b_1 \neq b_2$ or $or_1 \neq or_2$).

The first possibility suggests that the two estimates should be combined to produce a single summary measure of the association between risk factor and disease. A single estimate is more parsimonious and precise than two separate estimates. The second possibility suggests the opposite. When a summary measure behaves differently in each subtable, creating a single estimate likely understates or overstates the extent of association and is occasionally completely misleading (Chapter 1).

In symbolic terms, for a $2 \times 2 \times 2$ table, a simple measure of the difference between subtable estimates (denoted d) is

$$difference(behavior\ type) = d = b_1 - b_2 = (l_{11} - l_{10}) - (l_{01} - l_{00})$$
$$= l_{11} - l_{10} - l_{01} + l_{00}$$

or, similarly,

$$difference(blood\ pressure) = d = c_1 - c_2 = (l_{11} - l_{01}) - (l_{10} - l_{00})$$
$$= l_{11} - l_{10} - l_{01} + l_{00}.$$

The expression $d = l_{11} - l_{10} - l_{01} + l_{00}$ is the difference between two measures of association on the log-odds scale. It is the difference between two differences. Therefore, the estimate of d reflects the magnitude of the interaction associated with behavior type and blood pressure. The specific estimate from the WCGS data (Table 4–5) is $\hat{d} = \hat{b}_1 - \hat{b}_2 = \hat{c}_1 - \hat{c}_2 = \hat{l}_{11} - \hat{l}_{10} - \hat{l}_{01} + \hat{l}_{00} = -1.531 + 2.332 + 2.304 - 3.145 = -0.040$.

The quantity represented by d indicates the extent of the failure of the measures of association (log-odds) between the risk variable and disease outcome to be the same for both levels of the other risk factor. A key issue is whether the data provide substantial evidence that this difference is nonrandom. Testing the hypothesis that no interaction effect exists, or $d = l_{11} - l_{10} - l_{01} + l_{00} = 0$, is equivalent to testing the hypothesis that $b_1 = b_2 = b$ or $c_1 = c_2 = c$ or $or_1 = or_2 = or$.

A statistical test to evaluate the influence of random variation on an estimated interaction effect, estimated by $\hat{d}$, requires an expression for its variance. The variance associated with the distribution that produced the estimated interaction effect ($\hat{d}$) is estimated by

$$variance(\hat{d}) = variance(\hat{l}_{11} - \hat{l}_{10} - \hat{l}_{01} + \hat{l}_{00}) = \sum\sum\sum \frac{1}{n_{ijk}}$$

$$= \frac{1}{n_{111}} + \frac{1}{n_{112}} + \frac{1}{n_{121}} + \cdots + \frac{1}{n_{222}}$$

where n_{ijk} represents one of the eight cell frequencies in the $2 \times 2 \times 2$ table. For the CHD example, the estimated interaction effect associated with blood pressure and behavior type is $\hat{d} = -0.040$, and the estimated variance associated with its distribution is

$$variance(interaction) = \frac{1}{69} + \frac{1}{319} + \frac{1}{27} + \frac{1}{278} + \frac{1}{109} + \frac{1}{1092} + \frac{1}{52} + \frac{1}{1208} = 0.088.$$

The test statistic (a version of Wald's test)

$$X^2 = \frac{(\hat{l}_{11} - \hat{l}_{10} - \hat{l}_{01} + \hat{l}_{00} - 0)^2}{variance(interaction)} = \frac{(\hat{d} - 0)^2}{variance(\hat{d})}$$

has an approximate chi-square distribution with one degree of freedom when no interaction exists. Continuing the WCGS example, the chi-square test statistic

$$X^2 = \frac{(-0.040 - 0)^2}{0.088} = 0.018$$

yields a p-value of $P(X^2 \geq 0.018 | d = 0) = 0.892$. Such a large significance probability formally provides no evidence of an interaction. That is, it appears that the measures of the relationship between behavior type and a CHD event are likely estimates of the same underlying odds ratio from each blood pressure group. More simply, the odds ratio estimates $\hat{or}_1 = 2.227$ and $\hat{or}_2 = 2.319$ likely differ only because of sampling variation (Table 4–5).

Another view of the interaction parameter d is

$$d = b_1 - b_2 \quad \text{and} \quad e^d = e^{b_1 - b_2} = \frac{e^{b_1}}{e^{b_2}} = \frac{or_1}{or_2}$$

where or_1 is the odds ratio from the first 2×2 subtable and or_2 is the odds ratio from the second 2×2 subtable. For the blood pressure and behavior type data, $\hat{or}_1 = 2.227$ (blood pressure ≥ 140) and $\hat{or}_2 = 2.319$ (blood pressure <140) yield $e^{\hat{d}} = e^{-0.040} = 2.227/2.319 = 0.960$. When $d = 0$ ($e^0 = 1.0$), the odds ratios are identical in both subtables; otherwise the magnitude of $e^{\hat{d}}$ measures the extent of interaction as the ratio of two odds ratios. It should be expected that differences measured on a ratio scale are necessarily expressed in terms of a ratio (Chapter 1).

The linear regression model underlying the log-odds approach describing an interaction in a $2 \times 2 \times 2$ table is

$$l_{11} = a + b_2 + c_2 + d,$$
$$l_{10} = a + c_2,$$
$$l_{01} = a + b_2, \text{ and}$$
$$l_{00} = a$$

where, as before, d represents the magnitude of the interaction effect. The parameters b_2 and c_2 represent the influences of behavior type and blood pressure as defined earlier. The parameters b_1 and c_1 are unnecessary because $b_1 = b_2 + d$ and $c_1 = c_2 + d$. The parameter a represents the log-odds measure of the baseline level of risk, sometimes called the *referent category*. The four parameters a, b_2, c_2, and d are directly estimated by the four log-odds values from the $2 \times 2 \times 2$ table because this model is saturated (four log-odds values = four parameters).

For the $2 \times 2 \times 2$ table, the saturated logistic regression model is typically represented by the expression

$$log\text{-}odds = a + b_2 F + c_2 C + d(F \times C)$$

where $F = 1$ (type-A) or $F = 0$ (type-B) and $C = 1$ (blood pressure ≥ 140) or $C = 0$ (blood pressure <140). Table 4–7 summarizes the model and presents the four estimated model parameters that describe the likelihood of coronary disease associated with the binary risk variables blood pressure and behavior type in terms of the saturated logistic regression model. As noted, saturated model parameter estimates can be directly calculated from the data.

For example, from Table 4–6, the direct estimate $\hat{b}_2 = log(109/1092) - log(52/1208) = -2.304 - (-3.145) = 0.841$. As with all saturated models, the parametric model exactly reproduces the data. For example, for a type-A individual with high blood pressure

$$log\text{-}odds = \hat{a} + \hat{b}_2 F + \hat{c}_2 C + \hat{d}(F \times C)$$
$$= -3.145 + 0.841(1) + 0.814(1) - 0.040(1 \times 1) = -1.531$$

and $log(69/319) = -1.531$.

The application of the logistic regression model to a $2 \times 2 \times 2$ table is geometrically described as two lines on a log-odds scale, each depicting the influence of one risk variable at the two levels of the other variable. This representation is the same as the 2×2 case (Figure 4–1), but repeated twice, one

Table 4–7. CHD by A/B-behavior by systolic blood pressure: four-parameter logistic model and estimated coefficients

Blood pressure	Behavior type	C	F	$F \times C$	Model
≥ 140	type-A	1	1	1	$a + b_2 + c_2 + d$
≥ 140	type-B	1	0	0	$a + c_2$
<140	type-A	0	1	0	$a + b_2$
<140	type-B	0	0	0	a

Variables	Terms	Estimates	Std. errors	p-Values	Odds ratios
Constant	a	–3.145	0.142	–	–
A/B	b_2	0.841	0.174	<0.001	2.319
Blood pressure	c_2	0.814	0.246	0.001	2.256
Interaction	d	–0.040	0.297	0.892	0.960

LogLikelihood $= -854.967$

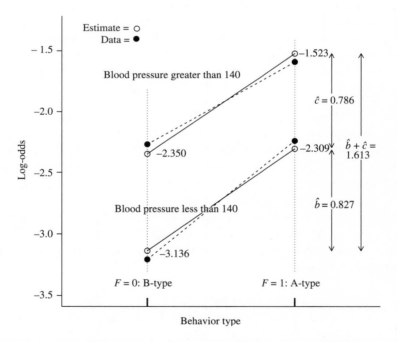

Figure 4–2. Log-odds associated with CHD risk and behavior types (A/B-behavior) and systolic blood pressure (<140 and $\geq$140).

line displaying risk for each 2×2 table (dashed lines, Figure 4.2). The parameter d indicates the degree to which these two lines are not parallel. Because the four-parameter model is saturated, a plot of the model values is identical to a plot of the four observed log-odds values (Figure 4–2, dots).

ADDITIVE LOGISTIC REGRESSION MODEL

When no interaction exists ($d = 0$; that is, $or_1 = or_2$), a logistic regression model (not saturated) represents the relationships in a $2 \times 2 \times 2$ table and is called an *additive logistic model*. Again, in terms of the log-odds, the three-parameter additive logistic regression model is

$$l_{11} = a + b + c,$$
$$l_{10} = a + c,$$
$$l_{01} = a + b, \quad and$$
$$l_{00} = a.$$

A compact expression for this model is

$$log\text{-}odds = a + bF + cC \qquad \text{(details in Table 4–8)}$$

where, again, $F = 1$ (type-A) or $F = 0$ (type-B) and $C = 1$ (blood pressure ≥ 140) or $C = 0$ (blood pressure < 140).

This statistical model is called *additive* because the log-odds associated with possessing both risk factors (l_{11}) relative to possessing neither risk factor (l_{00}) is exactly the sum of the log-odds values from each risk factor, namely parameters b and c. In symbols, $l_{11} - l_{00} = (a + b + c) - a = b + c$. The central property of this additive model is that $d = 0$ or $d = l_{11} - l_{10} - l_{01} + l_{00} = (a + b + c) - (a + c) - (a + b) + a = 0$. The values b and c take the place of the previous pairs of values b_1, b_2, and c_1, c_2 from the saturated model because $b_1 = b_2 = b$ and $c_1 = c_2 = c$,

Table 4–8.   CHD by A/B-behavior by systolic blood pressure: three-parameter additive logistic model

Blood pressure	Behavior type	C	F	Model
≥ 140	type-A	1	1	$a+b+c$
≥ 140	type-B	1	0	$a+c$
< 140	type-A	0	1	$a+b$
< 140	type-B	0	0	a

Variables	Terms	Estimates	Std. errors	p-Values	$\hat{or}$
Constant	a	−3.136	0.124	–	–
A/B	b	0.827	0.141	<0.001	2.287
Blood pressure	c	0.786	0.138	<0.001	2.194

LogLikelihood $= -854.976$

or $d = b_1 - b_2 = c_1 - c_2 = 0$. An iterative procedure or a computer program is necessary to calculate the maximum likelihood estimates of the model parameters a, b, and c from data contained in a $2 \times 2 \times 2$ table.

The maximum likelihood estimated coefficients from the WCGS data are $\hat{a} = -3.136$, $\hat{b} = 0.827$, and $\hat{c} = 0.786$ (Table 4–8). Using these estimates, Figure 4–2 displays the four log-odd values from the additive model estimated from the CHD data (circles, solid lines).

Based on the additive model and its estimated coefficients, the model-generated log-odds and probabilities of a CHD event can be calculated (Table 4–9).

For example, the log-odds associated with type-A individuals with high blood pressure (≥ 140) is $\hat{l}_{11} = \hat{a} + \hat{b} + \hat{c} = -3.136 + 0.827 + 0.786 = -1.523$, and the probability of a CHD event is then

$$\hat{P}(CHD \mid type\text{-}A \ and \ blood \ pressure \geq 140) = \hat{P} = \frac{1}{1 + e^{-log\text{-}odds}}$$

$$= \frac{1}{1 + e^{-l_{11}}} = \frac{1}{1 + e^{1.523}} = 0.179.$$

Using the model-estimated probability, the number of model-generated cases of CHD is $n\hat{P} = 388/(1 + e^{1.523}) = 388(0.179) = 69.46$ among the $n = 388$ type-A individuals with high blood pressure. The model-estimated number of type-A study participants with high blood pressure without a coronary event is directly $388 - 69.46 = n(1 - \hat{P}) = 0.388(0.821) = 318.54$. The other seven model frequencies are similarly estimated (Table 4–9). All estimates conform exactly to the additive model (Figure 4–2).

The additive (no-interaction) model requires that the measure of association of each risk factor be exactly the same at both levels of the other risk factor. A single estimated odds ratio $\hat{or}_{A/B} = e^{\hat{b}} = e^{0.827} = 2.286$, therefore, reflects the CHD risk associated with behavior type for both levels of blood pressure. In other words, a type-A individual has odds of a coronary event 2.286 times greater than a type-B individual regardless of blood pressure group (≥ 140 or < 140). Similarly, the estimated odds ratio $\hat{or}_{bp} = e^{\hat{c}} = e^{0.786} = 2.195$ reflects the likelihood of a CHD

Table 4–9. CHD by A/B-behavior and systolic blood pressure: theoretical values based on the additive model parameter estimates

Blood pressure	Behavior type	At risk	CHD	No CHD	Notation	Log-odds
≥ 140	type-A	388	69.46	318.54	$\hat{l}_{11}$	–1.523
≥ 140	type-B	305	26.54	278.46	$\hat{l}_{10}$	–2.350
< 140	type-A	1201	108.54	1092.46	$\hat{l}_{01}$	–2.309
< 140	type-B	1260	52.46	1207.55	$\hat{l}_{00}$	–3.136

event associated with blood pressure levels equal to or exceeding 140 relative to individuals with levels less than 140 for both behavior types. In addition, the product of these odds ratios $\hat{or}_{A/B} \times \hat{or}_{bp} = (e^{0.827})(e^{0.786}) = (2.286)(2.195) = 5.019$ indicates the CHD risk associated with possessing both risk factors (type-A with blood pressure ≥ 140) relative to possessing neither risk factor (type-B with blood pressure <140). In terms of the additive logistic model, the estimated difference in log-odds associated with possessing both risk factors ($F = C = 1$) relative to possessing neither factor ($F = C = 0$) is $l_{11} - l_{00} = \hat{a} + \hat{b} + \hat{c} - \hat{a} = \hat{b} + \hat{c} = 0.827 + 0.786 = 1.613$. Therefore, the estimated odds ratio is again

$$odds\ ratio = e^{difference\ in\ log\text{-}odds} = e^{l_{11}-l_{00}} = e^{\hat{b}+\hat{c}}$$
$$= e^{0.827+0.786} = (e^{0.827})(e^{0.786}) = e^{1.613} = 5.019.$$

Factors influencing the outcome that act additively on the log-odds scale act multiplicatively on the odds ratio scale. Additivity requires each risk factor to contribute to the likelihood of disease separately, and the overall odds ratio (or) becomes a product of these separate variable-specific odds ratios (or_i). In symbols, $or = \prod or_i$. The risk factors of an additive regression model are said to have "independent" influences on the likelihood of disease—independent in the sense that the influence on the outcome variable from a specific variable is not affected by the value of any other variable in the model. Estimated measures of association derived from an additive model are also referred to as "statistically adjusted."

A comparison of the model-estimated values from the additive model to the corresponding observed values (Figure 4–2) shows that no important differences occur when the interaction term is excluded from the model. Or, more simply, when the coefficient d is set to zero, the model-estimated values are essentially unaffected.

For the WCGS data, the estimation of the additive and interaction models generates two log-likelihood statistics. These values are

$$log(L_{d \neq 0}) = -854.967\ from\ the\ saturated\ model\ \text{(Table 4–7)}$$

and

$$log(L_{d=0}) = -854.976\ from\ additive\ model\ \text{(Table 4–8).}$$

A formal likelihood ratio chi-square test verifies that setting $d{=}0$ in the logistic model has only a small and likely random influence on the description of CHD risk. The chi-square distributed likelihood ratio test statistic

$$X^2 = log(L_{d=0}) - log(L_{d \neq 0}) = -2[-854.976 - (-854.967)] = 0.018,$$

with one degree of freedom produces a p-value of $P(X^2 \geq 0.018 | d = 0) = 0.892$.

To evaluate the influence of systolic blood pressure on the likelihood of a CHD event, a single-variable logistic regression model with blood pressure variable excluded from the model ($log\text{-}odds = a + b$ or $c = 0$) can be contrasted to the two-variable additive model with the blood pressure variable included ($log\text{-}odds = a + b + c$ or $c \neq 0$). The model with the parameter c set to zero is summarized in Table 4–4. The difference in the log-likelihood statistics between these two nested models indicates the importance of blood pressure in the description of CHD risk. The log-likelihood values

$$log(L_{c=0}) = -870.172 \text{ (blood pressure variable excluded, Table 4–4)}$$

and

$$log(L_{c \neq 0}) = -854.976 \text{ (blood pressure variable included, Table 4–8)}$$

produce the test statistic

$$X^2 = -2[log(L_{c=0}) - log(L_{c \neq 0})] = -2[-870.172 - (-854.976)] = 30.392.$$

The value X^2 has a chi-square distribution with one degree of freedom when $c = 0$. The associated p-value $P(X^2 \geq 30.392 | c = 0) < 0.001$ shows that the influence of systolic blood pressure is a vital part of the description of CHD risk. The log-likelihood comparison is not affected by behavior type. Its separate influence (additive) is accounted for in both regression models.

Comparing log-likelihood values to assess a single parameter is not basically different from the statistical test of the hypothesis that the parameter is zero (Chapter 3). As indicated earlier, a squared estimated coefficient divided by its estimated variance has an approximate chi-square distribution with one degree of freedom when the underlying value of the coefficient is zero. Specifically, the blood pressure test statistic (Wald's test, $c = 0$)

$$X^2 = \frac{(\hat{c} - 0)^2}{variance(\hat{c})} = \frac{(0.786 - 0)^2}{0.019} = 32.436$$

is, as expected, not substantially different from the likelihood ratio test statistic (30.392).

A NOTE ON THE STATISTICAL POWER TO IDENTIFY INTERACTION EFFECTS

The power of a statistical test to detect an interaction is relatively low compared to tests to detect additive effects. In terms of the WCGS data, the probability of identifying a blood pressure–behavior type interaction is less than the probability that variables such as blood pressure or behavior type will be identified as significant factors in an additive model (lower statistical power).

The reason for this lower power is directly seen in the analysis of a $2 \times 2 \times 2$ table. Recall that the expression for the variance of the estimated measure of interaction $(\hat{d})$ is

$$variance(interaction) = variance(\hat{d}) = \frac{1}{n_{111}} + \frac{1}{n_{112}} + \frac{1}{n_{121}} + \cdots + \frac{1}{n_{222}}$$

where n_{ijk} represents a cell frequency in the $2 \times 2 \times 2$ table. From the CHD example, the estimated variance of the distribution of the estimated coefficient $\hat{d}$ is

$$variance(\hat{d}) = \frac{1}{69} + \frac{1}{319} + \frac{1}{27} + \frac{1}{278} + \frac{1}{109} + \frac{1}{1092} + \frac{1}{52} + \frac{1}{1208} = 0.088.$$

Because this estimate is the sum of the reciprocal values of each of the eight cell frequencies in the table, its magnitude is primarily determined by the cell with the lowest frequency; in this case, 27. Therefore, the variance of the estimate of d cannot be less than $1/27 = 0.037$ regardless of the numbers of observations in the other seven cells. Because the variance of an interaction is largely determined by the cells with the fewest observations, estimates of the interaction effects usually have large variances yielding low statistical power. Effectively, the "sample size" is determined by the cell or cells with the smallest number of observations. Tabulations of even large data sets typically produce a few categories containing a small number of observations. On the other hand, the additive model parameters are estimated from combined cell frequencies and, therefore, based on these larger numbers of observations, produce more precise estimates. These smaller variances yield increased power. The estimated variances of the estimates $\hat{b}$ and $\hat{c}$ from the additive CHD model, for example, are close to 0.02 (Table 4–8).

In more complex situations, the investigation of interactions often suffers from similar problems of low power for much the same reason as illustrated by the case of a $2 \times 2 \times 2$ table. Failure of a statistical test to reject the hypothesis of no interaction provides some justification for relying on an additive model, but the power of this test is frequently low and sometimes extremely low.

Another concern when assessing the influence of an interaction term in a model is the typically high correlation between the interaction variable and its components. An interaction term $x \times y$ is, not surprisingly, highly correlated with the single variables x and y that are required to be included in the regression model. This high correlation increases the variance associated with the estimated interaction coefficient, further lowering the statistical power to detect the presence of an interaction.

It is essential to detect interaction effects when they exist. It is not as critical to eliminate interaction terms when the data support an additive model. In terms of assessing the hypothesis of no interaction (H_0), a type I error (rejecting H_0 when H_0 is true) is not as important as a type II error (accepting H_0 when H_0 is not true) when it comes to testing for the presence of an interaction. Therefore, it is a good idea to increase the level of significance (the probability of a type I error) to increase the statistical power. Increasing the probability of the type I error to attain more statistical power (decreasing the type II error) is a conservative strategy in the sense that relatively minor losses occur, such as some loss of efficiency and increased complexity of the model, if interaction terms are unnecessarily included in the model (type I error). Erroneously eliminating interaction effects (type II error), however, can substantially disrupt the validity of any conclusions ("wrong model bias").

THE LOGISTIC REGRESSION MODEL: THE 2 × k TABLE

Central to the previous approach to analyzing a $2 \times k$ table is the use of a straight line to summarize a sequence of proportions (Chapter 2), implying a linear relationship between levels of risk and the likelihood of disease. A $2 \times k$ table is also effectively analyzed using a log-odds summary measure of association. Underlying a log-odds approach (logistic model) is the representation the risk factors as if they act in a multiplicative fashion on the likelihood of disease. That is, the log-odds are accurately represented by a straight line. The WCGS data (Table 4–10) classified into a 2×4 table relating CHD occurrence to the amount smoked ($k = 4$ levels) illustrate the logistic regression model approach.

A logistic regression model that exactly duplicates the information contained in a $2 \times k$ table (a saturated model) in terms of log-odds (denoted l_i; $i = 0, 1, 2, \cdots$, $k - 1$) is, for $k = 4$,

$$l_0 = baseline, \quad l_1 = l_0 + b_1, \quad l_2 = l_0 + b_2 \quad \text{and} \quad l_3 = l_0 + b_3$$

Table 4–10.   CHD by smoking: a $2 \times k$ table

	Cigarettes per day				
	0	1 to 20	21 to 30	>30	**Total**
CHD	98	70	50	39	257
No CHD	1554	735	355	253	2897
Total	1652	805	405	292	3154

or, as a single expression,

$$log\text{-}odds = l_0 + b_1 x_1 + b_2 x_2 + b_3 x_3$$

where x_1, x_2, and x_3 are three components of a specially constructed variable that identifies each level of the categorical risk factor. For example, the values $x_1 = 0$, $x_2 = 1$, and $x_3 = 0$ produce a model value $log\text{-}odds = l_2 = l_0 + b_2$, which reflects the risk from smoking 21 to 30 cigarettes per day. The values $x_1 = x_2 = x_3 = 0$ establish a baseline or referent group ($log\text{-}odds = l_0$), namely the CHD log-odds among nonsmokers (Table 4–11 and Figure 4–3).

The logistic model describing four categories of smoking exposure and CHD risk is not restricted in any way, because a saturated model can produce any pattern of log-odds values. As with all saturated models, the pattern of response is entirely determined by the data. In fact, the data are reproduced exactly. Estimates of the saturated model parameters (calculated directly from the data) are:

$$\hat{l}_0 = log(n_{11}/n_{21}), \quad \hat{b}_1 = log(n_{12}/n_{22}) - \hat{l}_0,$$

$$\hat{b}_2 = log(n_{13}/n_{23}) - \hat{l}_0 \text{ and } \hat{b}_3 = log(n_{14}/n_{24}) - \hat{l}_0.$$

These estimates from the WCGS smoking exposure data are displayed in Table 4–11.

The odds ratios (denoted or_{0i} and estimated by $e^{\hat{b}_i}$) measure the multiplicative risk for each smoking category relative to nonsmokers (baseline = nonsmokers).

Table 4–11. CHD logistic regression model: smoking exposure saturated* model and estimates

Smoking exposure	x_1	x_2	x_3	Model
Nonsmoker	0	0	0	l_0
Smoker (1–20)	1	0	0	$l_0 + b_1$
Smoker (21–30)	0	1	0	$l_0 + b_2$
Smoker (>30)	0	0	1	$l_0 + b_3$

Variables	Terms	Estimates	Std. errors	p-Values	$\hat{o}r$
Constant	l_0	−2.764	0.104	–	1.000
Smoker (1–20)	b_1	0.412	0.163	<0.001	1.510
Smoker (21–30)	b_2	0.804	0.183	<0.001	2.233
Smoker (>30)	b_3	0.894	0.201	<0.001	2.444

LogLikelihood = −875.847

* Four parameters estimated from four log-odds (saturated)

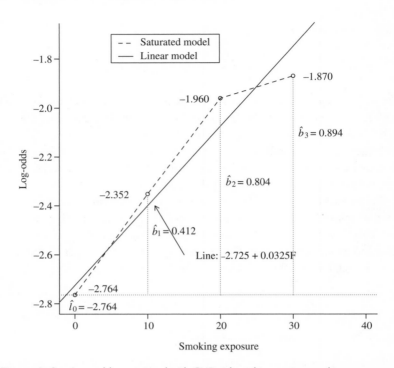

Figure 4–3. Log-odds associated with CHD risk and increasing smoking exposure.

For example, smoking more than 30 cigarettes a day produces an estimated odds ratio of $\hat{or}_{03} = e^{\hat{b}_3} = e^{0.894} = 2.444$. That is, the odds of a CHD event among heavy smokers is an estimated 2.444 times greater than the odds associated with nonsmokers. Because the model is saturated, the identical odds ratio is also directly calculated from the data $[\hat{or}_{03} = (39/253)/(98/1554) = 2.444]$. The odds ratios associated with increasing levels of smoking show an increasing likelihood of a CHD event (increasing from 1.0 to 1.5 to 2.2 to 2.4, Table 4–11). The log-odds values that generate these odds ratios are displayed in Figure 4–3. This increasing pattern is entirely a property of the data and not the model. Any pattern, as mentioned, could emerge from a saturated model.

One reason to construct a $2 \times k$ table is to provide the opportunity to explore the question: Does the likelihood of a coronary event increase in a specific pattern with increasing levels of smoking? A frequently used and certainly simple representation of a dose–response relationship is a straight line. In terms of a logistic regression model, the log-odds described by a straight line are

$$log\text{-}odds = l_i = l_0 + bF_i$$

where F_i represents one of k numeric levels of the risk factor and l_i again represents the log-odds for the ith level of that risk variable. For example, the model parameter l_0 represents the log-odds among the nonsmokers ($F_0 = 0$).

For the WCGS example, the values $F_0 = 0$, $F_1 = 10$, $F_2 = 20$, and $F_3 = 30$ cigarettes per day are chosen to reflect numerically the four smoking categories. As noted (Chapter 2), other equally spaced F_i-values give the same analysis (same p-values and log-likelihood statistics but different values of the model parameters, l_i, a, and b). For example, selecting the values of 0, 0.5, 1.0, and 1.5 packs of cigarettes per day would not change the analytic results ($F_{new} = F_{old}/20$).

This straight-line model constrains the log-odds to follow a linearly increasing or decreasing pattern. That is, a straight line summarizes the risk–outcome relationship, and the data are used to determine the "best" straight line. Such a constrained model no longer reproduces the data perfectly but summarizes the underlying relationships in a simpler and frequently useful way.

Computer-generated maximum likelihood estimates of the linear logistic model parameters from the smoking data are $\hat{l}_0 = -2.725$ and $\hat{b} = 0.0325$, and the estimated model becomes

$$log\text{-}odds = \hat{l}_i = -2.725 + 0.0325 F_i.$$

The model log-odds increase by an amount of 0.325 between each of the four smoking levels (Figure 4–3, solid line).

The log-likelihood statistic reflecting the relative effectiveness of the logistic regression linear model is $log(L_0) = -876.522$ (parameters $= 2$). The previous saturated model yields the log-likelihood value of $log(L_1) = -875.847$ (parameters $= 4$). The primary reason to estimate the parameters of a saturated model is that the log-likelihood value provides a baseline value to assess the consequences of simplifying the model (sometimes called a "reduced" model). The likelihood ratio test statistic applied to the smoking–CHD data has an approximate chi-square distribution with two degrees of freedom when the saturated and nested linear models differ strictly because of sampling variation. Specifically, the chi-square likelihood ratio test statistic (degrees of freedom $= 4 - 2 = 2$) is

$$X^2 = -2[log(L_0) - log(L_1)] = -2[-876.522 - (-875.847)] = 1.350,$$

producing a p-value$=P(X^2 \geq 1.350|$ *no systematic difference*$) = 0.509$. The likelihood ratio comparison suggests that the values estimated from a single straight line accurately predict the smoking–CHD log-odds values. Consequently, the influence from each smoking exposure category is effectively represented as if the increasing likelihood of a CHD event follows a simple multiplicative pattern.

In symbols, the pattern is

$$estimated\ log\text{-}odds = \hat{l}_i = \hat{l}_0 + \hat{b}F_i, \ \ implies\ \ \hat{l}_i - \hat{l}_0 = \hat{b}F_i$$

and

$$\hat{o}r_{0i} = e^{difference\ in\ log\text{-}odds} = e^{\hat{l}_i - \hat{l}_0} = e^{\hat{b}F_i}$$

where, again, $\hat{o}r_{0i}$ represents the model estimated odds ratio associated with the ith level of the risk factor relative to the baseline $\hat{l}_0$. For the smoking data, the model-estimated odds ratios are

$$\hat{o}r_{0i} = (e^{\hat{b}})^{F_i} = (e^{0.0325})^{F_i} = (1.033)^{F_i},$$

relative to the nonsmoking study participants (baseline, $F = 0$). The model dictates that the estimated log-odds increase linearly, causing the estimated odds ratio to increase multiplicatively (Table 4–12).

The linear logistic regression model translated into estimated probabilities

$$\hat{p}_i = \frac{1}{1 + e^{-(log\text{-}odds_i)}} = \frac{1}{1 + e^{-(\hat{l}_0 + \hat{b}F_i)}} = \frac{1}{1 + e^{-(-2.725 + 0.0325F_i)}}$$

provides an alternative description of the relationship between smoking exposure and the likelihood of a CHD event. For the example, based on the estimated linear logistic model, smoking 30 or more cigarettes a day ($F_3 = 30$) produces an odds of a CHD event 2.651 times greater than the odds for nonsmokers and a probability of a CHD event of 0.148. As required by the model, these two model-estimated values are related. Specifically, the model-estimated odds ratio is

$$\hat{o}r_{03} = \frac{\hat{p}_3/(1 - \hat{p}_3)}{\hat{p}_0/(1 - \hat{p}_0)} = \frac{0.148/0.852}{0.062/0.938} = 2.651.$$

Table 4–12. Summary of the CHD risk from smoking exposure: straight line logistic regression model

	Smoking exposures			
	$F = 0$	$F = 10$	$F = 20$	$F = 30$
Odds ratio ($\hat{o}r_{0i}$)	$(1.033)^0$	$(1.033)^{10}$	$(1.033)^{20}$	$(1.033)^{30}$
	1.000	1.384	1.915	2.651
$\hat{p}_i$	0.062	0.083	0.112	0.148
CHD events: $n\hat{p}_i$	101.63	66.96	45.18	43.23
Observed values	98	70	50	39
No CHD events: $n(1 - \hat{p}_i)$	1550.37	738.04	359.82	248.77
Observed values	1554	735	355	253

The model-estimated frequencies of CHD events ($n\hat{p}_i$, CHD events and $n(1 - \hat{p}_i)$, no CHD events) compared to the corresponding observed frequencies (Table 4–12) directly reflect the accuracy of the postulated linear logistic model. For example, the model-estimated number of CHD events among the heaviest smokers is $292(0.148) = 43.228$ and the observed number is 39. A Pearson summary chi-square assessment yields the summary test statistic

$$X^2 = \sum \frac{(observed_i - expected_i)^2}{expected_i}$$
$$= \frac{(98 - 101.635)^2}{101.635} + \cdots + \frac{(253 - 248.772)^2}{248.772} = 1.354.$$

The comparison of eight pairs of values (Table 14–12), summarized by a chi-square statistic (two degrees of freedom), produces a p-value of $P(X^2 \geq 1.354|linear) = 0.508$. The degrees of freedom are the number of model parameters (two) subtracted from the number of log-odds values in the data set (four). The degrees of freedom generated by the chi-square analysis are always identical to those used in the comparison of log-likelihood values. The previous log-likelihood comparison yields almost the same result (p-value $= 0.509$). The likelihood ratio test and the chi-square comparison of observed and estimated values generally produce similar results.

THE LOGISTIC REGRESSION MODEL: MULTIVARIABLE TABLE

Applying a logistic regression model to identify the relationships among three categorical risk variables and a binary disease outcome follows the pattern of the two-variable analysis. Using the WCGS data, interest is again focused on evaluating the influence of behavior type (two levels) on the likelihood of a coronary event while accounting for the confounding influences from smoking (four levels) and blood pressure (two levels). The important question is: After accounting for the influences of blood pressure and smoking, what is the role of behavior type in the likelihood of a coronary event? These three risk variables produce a $2 \times 4 \times 4$ table (Table 4–13). The same data, in a different format, are presented at the beginning of the chapter (Table 4–1).

A 16-parameter saturated model again provides a point of comparison for evaluating simpler models. The maximum log-likelihood statistic associated with the saturated model is $log(L_1) = -833.567$ with 16 degrees of freedom. No other model possibly "fits" the data better. A perfect correspondence between data and estimates makes a chi-square goodness-of-fit test statistic exactly zero. The perfect fit serves as a reminder that the accuracy of the model is an analytic issue,

Table 4–13. WCGS participants ($n = 3154$) by CHD, smoking, behavior type and blood pressure status ($2 \times 4 \times 4$ table)

	Type-A and blood pressure ≥ 140				
Cigs/day	0	1–20	21–30	>30	**Total**
CHD	29	21	7	12	69
No CHD	155	76	45	43	319
Total	184	97	52	55	388

	Type-A and blood pressure <140				
Cigs/day	0	1–20	21–30	≥ 30	**Total**
CHD	41	24	27	17	109
No CHD	559	277	140	116	1092
Total	600	301	167	133	1201

	Type-B and blood pressure ≥ 140				
Cigs/day	0	1–20	21–30	≥ 30	**Total**
CHD	8	9	3	7	27
No CHD	171	62	31	14	278
Total	179	71	34	21	305

	Type-B and blood pressure <140				
Cigs/day	0	1–20	21–30	≥ 30	**Total**
CHD	20	16	13	3	52
No CHD	669	320	139	80	1208
Total	689	336	152	83	1260

and statistical models do not indicate specific biologic or physical relationships among the variables studied. That is, any saturated model perfectly predicts the observations regardless of the form of the model or underlying relationships within the data.

An analytic question becomes: To what extent can the 16-parameter saturated model be simplified (fewer parameters), yet still maintain a useful description of the relationships among the risk variables (behavior type, smoking, and blood pressure) and the likelihood of a CHD event? The minimum model that accounts for the simultaneous influences of the three risk variables requires four parameters. In addition, smoking exposure is postulated to have the same linear influence on CHD risk within each of the four levels of the other two binary risk variables. The expression for this four-parameter additive logistic model is

$$log\text{-}odds = a + bF_i + cC + dD$$

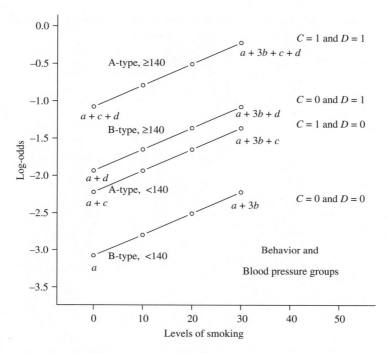

Figure 4–4. A graphic representation of the four-parameter additive CHD/risk logistic model applied to a 2 × 4 × 4 table of WCGS data.

where, again, the variable F_i incorporates the four levels of smoking into the model (coded again F_i for 0, 10, 20, and 30 cigarettes per day), the variable $C = 0$ or 1 indicates the behavior types (B, A), and the variable $D = 0$ or 1 indicates systolic blood pressure levels (<140, ≥ 140).

Geometrically, the model represents the influence of smoking as four parallel straight lines on a log-odds scale. The distances between these lines indicate the extent of the influences of the four combinations of the binary blood pressure and behavior type variables on the likelihood of a coronary event (Figure 4–4).

The maximum likelihood estimates of the four parameters of this additive model (Table 4–14) yield a log-likelihood statistic of $log(L) = -844.211$. The utility of this four-parameter logistic model evaluated by a chi-square statistic contrasting the log-likelihood statistics $log(L_0)$ [minimum model] to $log(L)$ [saturated model] is

$$X^2 = -2[log(L) - log(L_0)] = -2[-844.211 - (-833.569)] = 21.284.$$

The resulting p-value is $P(X^2 \geq 21.284 | model\ fits) = 0.046$, based on 12 degrees of freedom. The degrees of freedom again are the number of model

Table 4–14. Additive logistic model: A/B-behavior, smoking exposure, and blood pressure

Variables	Terms	Estimates	Std. errors	p-Values	or
Constant	a	−3.365	0.136	–	–
Smoking	b	0.029	0.006	<0.001	1.029
A/B	c	0.769	0.142	<0.001	2.157
Blood pressure	d	0.779	0.139	<0.001	2.179

LogLikelihood = −844.211

Table 4–15. CHD by A/B-behavior by systolic blood pressure by smoking: model estimated odds ratios

Blood pressure	Behavior type	$F = 0$	$F = 10$	$F = 20$	$F = 30$
≥140	type-A	4.701	6.256	8.324	11.077
≥140	type-B	2.179	2.900	3.859	5.135
<140	type-A	2.157	2.871	3.820	5.083
<140	type-B	1.000	1.331	1.771	2.356

parameters subtracted from the total number of log-odds values ($16 - 4 = 12$). The considerably simpler logistic model (16 vs. 4 parameters) does not appear to be an extremely accurate reflection of the relationships among the three risk variables and the likelihood of a coronary event. The decrease in the log-likelihood statistic reflects the magnitude of the inevitable trade-off between accuracy (goodness-of-fit) and simplicity of the model. Simpler models always fit less well. Although the four-parameter model is not ideal, a strictly additive model produces an extremely parsimonious description of the three risk variables (Table 4–15 and Figure 4–4).

The additive model-estimated odds ratios (Table 4–15) are calculated from combinations of the parameter estimates $\hat{b}$, $\hat{c}$, and $\hat{d}$ using the relationship

$$\hat{or} = e^{\hat{b}F_i + \hat{c}C + \hat{d}D} = (1.029)^{F_i}(2.157)^C(2.179)^D.$$

The estimated odds ratios associated with the 15 different levels of the risk factors are relative to the baseline category [nonsmokers ($F = 0$), type-B ($C = 0$) with blood pressure < 140 ($D = 0$), $or = 1$].

GOODNESS-OF-FIT: MULTIVARIABLE TABLE

For tabulated data, the goodness-of-fit of a model is directly assessed by generating a series of model-dictated counts (denoted e_k) and comparing these theoretical values to the corresponding observed counts (denoted o_k). For the WCGS data, the four estimated logistic model parameters generate 16 logistic probabilities that produce 32 estimated numbers of individuals with and without CHD events (Table 4–16). The logistic model probabilities are estimated from the relationship

$$\hat{p}_{chd} = \frac{1}{1 + e^{-(log\text{-}odds)}}$$

$$= \frac{1}{1 + e^{-(\hat{a}+\hat{b}F_i+\hat{c}C+\hat{d}D)}} = \frac{1}{1 + e^{-(-3.365+0.029F_i+0.769C+0.779D)}},$$

and e_k represents either $n\hat{p}_{chd}$, the number of individuals with CHD events, or $n(1 - \hat{p}_{chd})$, the number of individuals without CHD events when n represents the total number of individuals in the category, namely the sum of the CHD and no CHD individuals (Table 4–16). For example, when $C = 1$, $D = 1$, and $F = 30$ ($n = 55$), the probability of a CHD event is

$$\hat{p}_{chd} = \frac{1}{1 + e^{-[-3.365+0.029(30)+0.769(1)+0.779(1)]}} = \frac{1}{1 + e^{0.959}} = 0.277,$$

then $e_4 = n\hat{p}_{chd} = 55(0.277) = 15.230$ is the number of model-estimated individuals with a CHD event, and $e_8 = 55 - 15.230 = 55(0.923) = 39.770$ is the number of model-estimated individuals without a CHD event among $n = 55$ study subjects who are type-A ($D = 1$) with blood pressures greater than or equal to 140 ($C = 1$) who smoke more than 30 cigarettes per day ($F = 30$). The corresponding observed numbers of individuals are $o_4 = 12$ and $o_8 = 43$. The remaining 31 model-generated values are directly calculated and compared to the corresponding observed values (Table 4–16). A chi-square goodness-of-fit statistic (the sum of the last column, Table 4–16) yields $X^2 = \sum(o_k - e_k)^2/e_k = 22.107$ with 12 degrees of freedom ($k = 1, 2, \cdots, 32$). The p-value is $P(X^2 \geq 22.107 | differ\ by\ chance) = 0.036$. The model estimates compared to the observed values based on the less intuitive likelihood ratio chi-square test statistic

$$G^2 = -2[log(L) - log(L_0)] = -2\sum o_i log\left(\frac{e_i}{o_i}\right)$$

is the previously calculated likelihood ratio test statistic, $G^2 = 21.284$. This likelihood expression is no more than an explicit form of the more general likelihood ratio test statistic (Chapter 3) when applied to categorical data.

The values estimated from the four-parameter logistic model, as seen in Table 4–16 (columns 8 or 9), are good or reasonable estimates of the observed frequencies in almost all categories. That is, these contributions to the chi-square test statistic are small. Only three categories are seriously misrepresented by the

Table 4–16. Goodness-of-fit, data and various summaries

Outcome	Type	B.P.	F_i	o_k	e_k	$o_k - e_k$	$(o_k - e_k)/\sqrt{e_k}$	$(o_k - e_k)^2/e_k$
Behavior type A								
CHD	A	≥ 140	0	29	25.723	3.277	0.646	0.417
CHD	A	≥ 140	10	21	17.248	3.752	0.903	0.816
CHD	A	≥ 140	20	7	11.621	-4.621	-1.355	1.837
CHD	A	≥ 140	30	12	15.230	-3.230	-0.828	0.685
No CHD	A	≥ 140	0	155	158.277	-3.277	-0.260	0.068
No CHD	A	≥ 140	10	76	79.752	-3.752	-0.420	0.177
No CHD	A	≥ 140	20	45	40.379	4.621	0.727	0.529
No CHD	A	≥ 140	30	43	39.770	3.230	0.512	0.262
CHD	A	< 140	0	41	41.642	-0.642	-0.099	0.010
CHD	A	< 140	10	24	27.175	-3.175	-0.609	0.371
CHD	A	< 140	20	27	19.482	7.518	1.703	2.901
CHD	A	< 140	30	17	19.880	-2.880	-0.646	0.488
No CHD	A	< 140	0	559	558.358	0.642	0.027	0.001
No CHD	A	< 140	10	277	273.825	3.175	0.192	0.037
No CHD	A	< 140	20	140	147.518	-7.518	-0.619	0.383
No CHD	A	< 140	30	116	113.120	2.880	0.271	0.073

Table 4–16. (Continued)

Outcome	Type	B.P.	F_i	o_k	e_k	$o_k - e_k$	$(o_k - e_k)/\sqrt{e_k}$	$(o_k - e_k)^2/e_k$
Behavior type B								
CHD	B	≥140	0	8	12.541	-4.541	-1.282	1.644
CHD	B	≥140	10	9	6.469	2.531	0.995	0.996
CHD	B	≥140	20	3	4.002	-0.002	-0.501	0.251
CHD	B	≥140	30	7	3.166	3.834	2.155	4.643
No CHD	B	≥140	0	171	166.459	4.541	0.352	0.124
No CHD	B	≥140	10	62	64.531	-2.531	-0.315	0.099
No CHD	B	≥140	20	31	29.998	1.002	0.183	0.033
No CHD	B	≥140	30	14	17.834	-3.834	-0.908	0.824
CHD	B	<140	0	20	23.024	-3.024	-0.630	0.457
CHD	B	<140	10	16	14.778	1.222	0.318	0.101
CHD	B	<140	20	13	8.768	4.232	1.429	1.377
CHD	B	<140	30	3	6.252	-3.252	-1.301	3.526
No CHD	B	<140	0	669	665.976	3.024	0.117	0.014
No CHD	B	<140	10	320	321.222	-1.222	-0.068	0.005
No CHD	B	<140	20	139	143.232	-4.232	-0.354	0.125
No CHD	B	<140	30	80	76.748	3.252	0.371	0.138
Total	–	–	–	3154	3154	0.0	0.0	22.107

additive four-parameter linear model. Particularly, the number of individuals who are type-B, with high blood pressure, and who smoke more than 30 cigarettes per day ($C = 0$, $D = 1$, and $F = 30$) is predicted least accurately ($e_{20} = 3.166$ and $o_{20} = 7$ and $(o_{20} - e_{20})^2/e_{20} = 4.643$, 21% of the total chi-square test-statistic).

Although the four-parameter logistic regression model is not ideal, it simply and unambiguously addresses the role of behavior type in CHD risk (Table 4–1). As always, the simplicity of the model must be balanced against its accuracy. When the risk factors behavior type, blood pressure, and smoking are assessed as additive influences on the likelihood of a CHD event, they allow separate evaluations. Statistical tests demonstrate that each risk variable represents a substantial and independent (dictated by the model) influence that is not likely due to chance alone (p-values < 0.001). The separate contributions to the likelihood of a CHD event expressed in terms of odds ratios are: $\hat{o}r_{A/B} = 2.157$ (behavior type), $or_{bp} = 2.179$ (blood pressure type), and $\hat{o}r_{30+} = (1.029)^{30} = 2.358$ (smoking more than 30 cigarettes per day). The three variables have about equal influence on CHD risk. The risk of individuals with high blood pressure (≥ 140), type-A behavior who smoke more than 30 cigarettes per day ($F = 30$, $C = 1$, and $D = 1$) is 11 times the risk of individuals with low blood pressure (<140), type-B behavior who do not smoke (referent group, $F = 0$, $C = 0$, and $D = 0$, $or = 1$). Specifically, the joint influences produce a model-estimated odds ratio of $(2.157)(2.179)(2.358) = 11.083$. The log-odds measure of CHD risk increases linearly and again independently as the level of smoking increases (as required by the model). The joint confounding influences of blood pressure and smoking on the behavior–CHD association, measured in terms of odds ratios, are $\hat{o}r = e^{0.846} = 2.373$ (behavior type only, Table 4–4) compared to $\hat{o}r = e^{0.827} = 2.287$ (all three risk variables, Table 4–8).

This description of the influence of the three risk factors on the likelihood of a CHD event is unequivocally a function of the additive logistic regression model and its estimated parameters. However, as illustrated by the CHD data, the correspondence between the model and the data can be a difficult issue.

LOGISTIC REGRESSION MODEL: THE SUMMARY ODDS RATIO

A summary odds ratio estimated from a series of k-independent 2×2 tables is simply accomplished with a weighted average (Chapter 2). The same task is also simply accomplished with a logistic regression model. In addition, with minor modifications, the model approach is an effective statistical tool to combine and summarize relationships within a variety of kinds of tables.

Table 4–17. Data: Mother/infant observations classified by smoking exposure, birth weight, and race/ethnicity (four 2 × 2 tables or a 2 × 2× 4 table)

White	< 2500g	≥ 2500g	**Total**
Smokers	98	832	930
Nonsmokers	169	3520	3689
Total	267	4352	4619

African-American	< 2500g	≥ 2500g	**Total**
Smokers	54	227	281
Nonsmokers	55	686	741
Total	109	913	1022

Hispanic	< 2500g	≥ 2500g	**Total**
Smokers	11	85	96
Nonsmokers	61	926	987
Total	72	1011	1083

Asian	< 2500g	≥ 2500g	**Total**
Smokers	7	102	109
Nonsmokers	90	1936	2026
Total	97	2038	2135

Maternal smoking and infant birth weight data (Chapter 2) illustrate the logistic model approach applied to four 2 × 2 tables. The data are repeated in Table 4–17. In addition, the geometry of the log-odds analysis of the likelihood of a low-birth-weight infant is displayed in Figure 4–5. Each dashed line represents the change in log-odds associated with smoking relative to nonsmoking mothers within each of the four 2 × 2 tables (one line for each race/ethnicity group).

The relationship between a logistic model generated probability (denoted p_{ij}) and the corresponding log-odds, as before, is

$$probability = p_{ij} = \frac{1}{1 + e^{-(log\text{-}odds_{ij})}} \quad or \quad log\text{-}odds_{ij} = log\left[\frac{p_{ij}}{1 - p_{ij}}\right].$$

The likelihood of a low-birth-weight infant associated with smoking exposure and race/ethnicity in terms of the log-odds described by the additive logistic

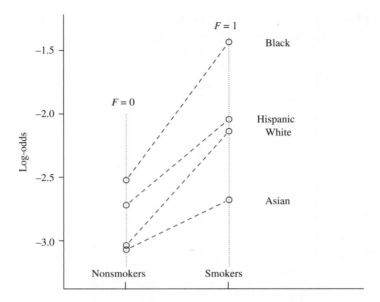

Figure 4–5. The-low-birth weight log-odds from the mother/infant data in Table 4–15 (four 2 × 2 tables or a 2 × 2 × 4 table).

regression model is

$$log\text{-}odds_{ij} = log\left[\frac{p_{ij}}{1 - p_{ij}}\right] = a + bF_j + c_1x_{i1} + c_2x_{i2} + c_3x_{i3}.$$

The variable F_j is a binary indicator that equals 0 for nonsmokers and 1 for smokers ($j = 1$ and 2). The three x_{ij}-components are indicator variables (sometimes called *dummy variables*) that make up a design variable used to include influences of four race/ethnicity groups in a regression model ($i = 0, 1, 2,$ and 3).

Note: Variables characterized numerically are typically entered directly into a regression analysis, as reported. Frequently, categorical variables do not have specific numeric values or even an ordering. Nevertheless, these nominal variables can also be entered into a regression model using specifically designed indicator variables. For example, when two races are considered, say white and African-American, and the member of one group is coded 0 and the other 1, the associated logistic model coefficient and corresponding odds ratio are then relative to the influence of the group coded zero. If the model-estimated odds ratio is 2.0, and whites are coded as 0 and African-Americans as 1, then the odds are two times greater among African-Americans than whites.

The principle of using a binary indicator variable extends to any number of categories. When more than two categories are considered (for example, Whites, African-American, Hispanics, and Asians), indicator variables are again used. For k categories,

$k - 1$ indicator variables, each taking on the values 0 or 1, allow a nominal variable to play a role in a regression model. Such a variable is typically called a *design variable*. Again, a baseline category is established by setting the $k - 1$ components of the design variable to zero. The members of other groups are then identified by a single component of the design variable that takes on the value one while the remaining components are zero. For example, if African-Americans, Hispanics, and Asian are to be compared to the whites in a regression model, then for these $k = 4$ nominal categories, the design variable is

baseline or referent category:

   Whites: $x_1 = 0$, $x_2 = 0$, and $x_3 = 0$;

other categories:

   African-Americans: $x_1 = 1$, $x_2 = 0$, and $x_3 = 0$;

   Hispanics: $x_1 = 0$, $x_2 = 1$, and $x_3 = 0$;

   Asians: $x_1 = 0$, $x_2 = 0$, and $x_3 = 1$.

Parallel to the binary case, the resulting odds ratios (regression coefficients) reflect the influence of each categorical variable relative to the category with all components set equal to zero. Categories identified with a design variable allow the assessment of their influence using a regression model without requiring a numeric value or even requiring that the categories be ordered. Some computer statistical analysis systems create design variables automatically.

A design variable to identify four race/ethnicity categories is illustrated (Table 4–18). Twelve individuals (three Whites, four African-Americans, two Hispanics, and three Asians) make up the "data."

Table 4–18. Illustration of a design variable used to establish membership in four Race/ethnicity categories

Race/ethnicity	i	x_{i1}	x_{i2}	x_{i3}
African–American	1	1	0	0
White	2	0	0	0
Asian	3	0	0	1
White	4	0	0	0
African–American	5	1	0	0
African–American	6	1	0	0
Hispanic	7	0	1	0
Asian	8	0	0	1
White	9	0	0	0
Asian	10	0	0	1
African–American	11	1	0	0
Hispanic	12	0	1	0

Table 4–19. The details of an additive model describing the probability of a low-birth-weight infant associated with maternal smoking exposure among four race/ethnicity groups ($2 \times 2 \times 4$ table)

| Race/ethnicity | Design variable | | | Nonsmokers ($F_j = 0$) | Smokers ($F_j = 1$) |
	x_{i1}	x_{i2}	x_{i3}	log-odds$_{i0}$	log-odds$_{i1}$
White	0	0	0	a	$a + b$
African-American	1	0	0	$a + c_1$	$a + b + c_1$
Hispanic	0	1	0	$a + c_2$	$a + b + c_2$
Asian	0	0	1	$a + c_3$	$a + b + c_3$

The details of an additive model representing the log-odds in each of the eight smoking/race categories are presented in Table 4–19. The parameter b reflects the summary influence of smoking exposure on the log-odds of a low-birth-weight infant, and the three parameters c_1, c_2, and c_3 identify the influence of race/ethnicity. As noted previously, additivity means that the model is constructed so that the influence on risk associated with one variable is unaffected by the values of other variables in the model. For the example, the influence on the log-odds of a low-birth-weight infant associated with smoking exposure (b or e^b) is the same regardless of race/ethnicity (Figure 4–6). The postulated additive logistic regression model dictates that the influence of smoking exposure is constant for the four race/ethnicity categories because

$$[log\text{-}odds\ (smokers)] - [log\text{-}odds\ (nonsmokers)]$$
$$= [a + b(1) + c_i] - [a + b(0) + c_i] = b.$$

Thus, the geometry of an additive logistic model requires the log-odds (nonsmoking vs. smoking) to differ by the same constant distance, b, within each race/ethnicity category (perfect homogeneity or perfect independence or perfect additivity or exactly no interaction). A visual evaluation of a model, particularly the additive influence of smoking exposure ($b =$ constant), becomes again a question of the similarity between observed and model-generated values. In geometric terms, the specific question becomes: Do the lines (Figure 4–5, dashed lines) randomly deviate from the parallel lines (Figure 4–6, solid lines)?

Since an additive model requires the same change in log-odds between smoking exposures for all race/ethnicity groups, an important issue concerns the accuracy of this simple and theoretical relationship. Two possibilities exist; the underlying influence from smoking measured by the odds ratio is the same within the four race/ethnicity groups and observed differences occur only because of random variation (additive relationships), or systematic differences exist among the odds ratios (interaction) in one or more of the four groups. The maximum

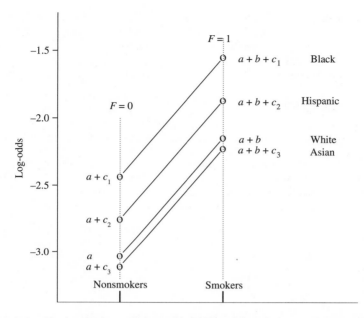

Figure 4–6. The low-birth-weight log-odds for the additive logistic model describing the mother/infant data in Table 4–16.

Table 4–20. Additive logistic regression model: coefficients estimated from the birth weight data, an analysis of a $2 \times 2 \times 4$ table (Table 4–17)

Variables	Symbols	Estimates	Std. errors
Intercept	a	−3.032	0.073
Smoking exposure	b	0.885	0.101
African-American	c_1	0.598	0.121
Hispanic	c_2	0.279	0.139
Asian	c_3	−0.080	0.124

LogLikelihood $= -1.521$

likelihood estimated coefficients for the additive model (Table 4–20) provide estimates of the eight log-odds values producing eight estimates of the probabilities of a low or "normal" birth weight infant. These eight probabilities (denoted $\tilde{p}_{ij}$) produce 16 model-generated counts of infants (denoted e_{ij}) that exactly correspond to the additive model (Table 4–21).

For the example data, the model-estimated log-odds of a low-birth-weight infant associated with an Asian mother who smokes is

$$estimated\ log\text{-}odds = \hat{a} + \hat{b} + \hat{c}_3 = -3.032 + 0.885 - 0.080 = -2.227$$

Table 4–21.   Observed (o_{ij}) and model (e_{ij}) estimated cell frequencies for the 16 birth weight, smoking exposure, and race/ethnicity categories, a $2 \times 2 \times 4$ table

Weight	Race/ethnicity	Exposure	Total	$\tilde{p}^*_{ij}$	o_{ij}	e_{ij}
$< 2500g$	White	Smoker	930	0.105	98	97.3
$\geq 2500g$	White	Smoker	930	0.895	832	832.7
$< 2500g$	White	Nonsmoker	3689	0.046	169	169.7
$\geq 2500g$	White	Nonsmoker	3689	0.954	3520	3519.3
$< 2500g$	African-American	Smoker	281	0.175	54	49.2
$\geq 2500g$	African-American	Smoker	281	0.825	227	231.8
$< 2500g$	African-American	Nonsmoker	741	0.081	55	59.8
$\geq 2500g$	African-American	Nonsmoker	741	0.919	686	681.2
$< 2500g$	Hispanic	Smoker	96	0.134	11	12.8
$\geq 2500g$	Hispanic	Smoker	96	0.866	85	83.2
$< 2500g$	Hispanic	Nonsmoker	987	0.060	61	59.2
$\geq 2500g$	Hispanic	Nonsmoker	987	0.940	926	927.8
$< 2500g$	Asian	Smoker	109	0.097	7	10.6
$\geq 2500g$	Asian	Smoker	109	0.903	102	98.4
$< 2500g$	Asian	Nonsmoker	2029	0.043	90	86.4
$\geq 2500g$	Asian	Nonsmoker	2029	0.957	1936	1939.6

*= Estimated from the additive logistic model (for example, Asian and smoker – $\tilde{p}_{13} = 0.097$).

giving the estimated probability of a low-birth-weight infant as

$$\tilde{p}_{13} = P(low\ birth\ weight \mid Asian,\ smoking\ mother) = \frac{1}{1 + e^{2.227}} = 0.097.$$

Because $\tilde{p}_{13} = 0.097$ and there are 109 Asian smokers, the number of model-estimated low-birth-weight infants is $109(0.097) = 10.616$ among smokers compared to the seven observed. The model-estimated number of "normal" weight infants is $109 - 10.616 = 109(0.903) = 98.384$ among nonsmokers compared to the 102 observed. Similarly, the other 14 logistic model-generated values are estimated and compared to the corresponding observed values (Table 4–21, last two columns), directly measuring the accuracy of the additive logistic model. As usual, the classic Pearson chi-square goodness-of-fit statistic effectively summarizes these differences, providing a statistical evaluation of the correspondence between the additive model-estimated counts and the observed data. For the smoking exposure data

$$X^2 = \frac{(98 - 97.291)^2}{97.291} + \cdots + \frac{(1936 - 1939.616)^2}{1939.616} = 2.866.$$

The chi-square test statistic (degrees of freedom $= 8 - 5 = 3$) generates the p-value $= P(X^2 \geq 2.866|additive\ model) = 0.413$ and is a formal assessment of the clearly close correspondence between the 16-model estimated and the observed counts (Table 4–21). The degrees of freedom are the number of parameters in the model (five) subtracted from the number of log-odds values in the table (eight).

To evaluate the always-present influence of random variation on the estimated relationship between smoking exposure and the likelihood of a low-birth-weight infant as measured by the single estimated coefficient $\hat{b} = 0.885$, the usual statistical test (Wald's test) is appropriate. Thus, the test statistic

$$X^2 = \frac{(\hat{b} - 0)^2}{S_{\hat{b}}^2} = \frac{(0.885 - 0)^2}{0.010} = 76.627$$

has an approximate chi-square distribution with one degree of freedom when no association exists ($b = 0$) and yields a p-value of $P(X^2 \geq 76.627|b = 0) < 0.001$. The statistical assessment shows clear evidence of an association between smoking exposure and probability of a low-birth-weight infant. Not unexpectedly, similar results are obtained using Woolf's model-free estimate $\overline{log(or)} = 0.892$, where $z^2 = (8.683)^2 = 75.394 \approx 76.627$ (Chapter 2).

Again, behaving as if the influence of maternal smoking exposure is the same in all four race/ethnicity groups (b is constant), the focus becomes the estimated coefficients from the additive logistic regression model (Table 4–20), specifically the coefficient $\hat{b} = 0.885$. The maximum likelihood estimated odds ratio is $\hat{or}_{mlk} = e^{\hat{b}} = e^{0.885} = 2.423$ and, as dictated by the model, is an estimate of the constant influence of smoking/nonsmoking on the likelihood of a low-birth-weight infant for all four race/ethnicities. The estimated coefficient $\hat{b} = 0.885$ and its standard error, generated as part of the maximum likelihood estimation, produce the approximate 95% confidence interval (0.687, 1.083). Therefore, the confidence interval based on the estimated common odds ratio $\hat{or} = 2.423$ is $(e^{0.687}, e^{1.083}) = (1.987, 2.954)$. Using a weighted average estimate (Chapter 2) yields almost the same summary odds ratio, 2.441, and confidence interval (1.996, 2.986).

The logistic model provides two advantages over the weighted average approach to estimating a summary odds ratio. First, the goodness-of-fit evaluation provides statistical evidence to justify an additive model ($b = $ constant). Second, similar logistic models apply to the analysis of tables that are far more complex than a series of 2×2 tables.

DESCRIPTION OF THE WCGS DATA SET

The WCGS data consist of middle-aged men (ages 39–59) recruited from ten California companies during the years 1960–61 resulting in 3,154 participating individuals. High-risk subjects were deliberately selected to study the relationship between lifestyle behavior and the risk of coronary disease. A number of other risk variables were also measured to provide the best possible assessment of the likelihood of a CHD event associated with a specific measure of lifestyle behavior. The data analyzed in this chapter are three of these risk factors (blood pressure, behavior type, and smoking exposure), and more extensive data are explored in the following chapters, particularly Chapter 11.

A binary behavior classification, called *type-A* or *type-B*, was created from tape-recorded interviews administered by specifically trained personal. A precise definition of type-A and type-B behavior is complicated and equivocal. In general terms, type-A behavior is characterized by a sense of time urgency, aggressiveness, and ambition. A type-A individual is typically thought to have a competitive personality. A type-B individual is essentially the opposite and is characterized by a relaxed, noncompetitive, less hurried personality. A total of 1589 type-A and 1565 type-B individuals were identified.

The outcome variable is the occurrence of a CHD event determined by an independent medical referee. Clinical coronary disease occurred in 257 subjects during about 7 years of follow-up, producing a crude incidence rate of CHD events of 11.1 per 1000 person-years. The study subjects lost to follow-up (504) were considered to be non-CHD cases and were close to evenly divided between type-A and type-B individuals. A total of 92.5% of all possible person-years of follow-up was accomplished.

The WCGS data are completely described in a number of places ([16], [17] and [18]) and a report on the mortality experience 22 years later has been published [19]. This long-term follow-up of WCGS participants indicates that the relationship between behavior type and CHD is not simple. Behavior type originally showed a strong association with the incidence of a CHD event (Chapters 4 and 11). However, no similar association was found when the same WCGS subjects were studied 22 years later using mortality data. The predictive association between behavior and CHD incidence, as well as the absence of the same association with mortality, are not likely explained by artifact or bias. An explanation may lie in the possibility that behavior type is related to recovery from a nonfatal heart attack. This conjecture, the WCGS data, and the associations originally observed are discussed in detail elsewhere [19].

5

LOGISTIC REGRESSION: CONTINUOUS DATA

An expression for a general linear multivariable regression model describing an observed outcome represented by y_i ($i = 1, 2, \cdots, n =$ number of observations) predicted from the k observed values represented by $x_{i1}, x_{i2}, \cdots, x_{ik}$ is

$$f(y_i) = a + s_1(x_{i1}) + s_2(x_{i2}) + \cdots + s_k(x_{ik}) + \varepsilon_i.$$

The value represented by y_i is called the *dependent variable* and $f(y_i)$ represents a function of the observation y_i. The value represented by x_{ij} is called the *independent variable*, and $s_j(x_{ij})$ represents one of k possible functions of the independent variable x_{ij} ($j = 1, 2, \cdots, k =$ number of variables). Regression equations have a sense of direction indicated by these two names. The independent variables in some sense "cause" the dependent variable. At the very least, the independent variable is antecedent to the dependent variables. For example, a variable such as exposure to intense sound (independent variable) is possibly associated with increased likelihood of hypertension (dependent variable). The converse makes no sense. The most commonly used form of the functions s_j is linear or, in symbols, $s_j(x_{ij}) = b_j x_{ij}$. The value denoted b_j, called a *regression coefficient*, then reflects the linear influence of the jth-independent variable x_{ij} on the ith-dependent variable y_i or a function of y_i. Other forms of the function s_j characterize more sophisticated relationships between an independent and a dependent variable, potentially enhancing the correspondence between the mode-predicted values and the observed outcomes. For example, the function $s_j(x_{ij})$

could represent a polynomial function such as

$$s_j(x_{ij}) = c_1 x_{ij} + c_2 x_{ij}^2 + c_3 x_{ij}^3$$

or, s_j could represent a spline function (more details to follow in this chapter and Chapter 10). The constant term a and the $s(x)$-functions make up the *deterministic* part of the linear model—the part of the model that is not subject to random variation—sometimes called the *fixed effects*. The remaining term (denoted ε_i) represents the *stochastic* part of the model and incorporates the influences of random variation into the description of the dependent variable.

The most fundamental and common multivariable regression model (k-variable) is

$$y_i = a + b_1 x_{i1} + b_2 x_{i2} + \cdots + b_k x_{ik} + \varepsilon_i$$

where $f(y_i) = y_i$, $s_j(x_{ij}) = b_j x_{ij}$ and ε_i is assumed to have a normal distribution, with a mean value of zero and a variance that is the same for the relevant sets of x_{ij}-values. This multivariable model is called somewhat ambiguously a linear *regression model*. Perhaps it should be called a "linear-linear regression model," because it is a sum of regression model terms and these terms, themselves have a linear influence ($b_j x_{ij}$). Another and less ambiguous name is an *additive linear regression model*.

Specific functions of the dependent variable are associated with specific statistical distributions (distributions of the stochastic term ε_i). Three frequently used regression models and their associated statistical distributions are:

Models	$f(y)$	Distributions of ε
Linear	y	Normal
Logistic	$log[y/(1-y)]$	Binomial
Poisson	$log(y)$	Poisson

The function $f(y)$ is chosen to create a linear model, so that the regression coefficient b directly relates to a chosen measure of association, sometimes called a *link function*. It is the "link" between the dependent variable and a measure of association describing its influence on the independent variable. Table 5–1 displays the relationship between three of the most commonly used link functions $f(y)$, the regression coefficients (b), and their corresponding measure of association.

Therefore, the estimates and the analysis are in terms of a linear model but the end results are described in terms of a chosen measure of association. For example, when $f(y) = log(y)$ is the selected link function of the dependent variable, the regression coefficient (b) measures the influence of the independent variables (x) in terms of the logarithm of a ratio, making e^b a ratio measure of association between each independent variable x and the dependent variable y. Selecting a

Table 5–1. Three examples of link functions and their corresponding measures of association

Link function $= f(y)$	Coefficient $= b = f(y') - f(y)$	Interpretation
$f(y) = y$	$b = y' - y$	linear difference
$f(p) = log\left[\dfrac{p}{1-p}\right]$	$b = log(p'/[1-p']) - log(p/[1-p])$ $= \left[\dfrac{p'/[1-p']}{p/[1-p]}\right]$	log(odds ratio)
$f(y) = log(y)$	$b = log(y') - log(y) = log\left[\dfrac{y'}{y}\right]$	log(ratio)

model determines the measure of association or selecting a measure of association determines the model.

FOUR BASIC PROPERTIES OF MULTIVARIABLE REGRESSION MODEL ANALYSIS

The following presents four examples of generally important issues that arise frequently in the analysis and interpretation of many statistical results. In the context of a multivariable regression model, their description is clearly and unambiguously illustrated. The intent of these examples is primarily a clear and simple explanation. The same issues are revisited in more realistic applications of the logistic (this chapter and Chapter 7), the Poisson (Chapter 6), and the log-linear (Chapter 13) regression models.

Additivity

In nontechnical terms, additivity means that each independent variable included in a multivariable regression model adds it own contribution to the prediction of the dependent variable, unaffected by the values of the other variables in the model. In the bivariate case ($k = 2$), for example, the expression for an additive linear regression model is

$$y_i = a + b_1 x_{i1} + b_2 x_{i2} + \varepsilon_i.$$

Geometrically, this model describes observations that randomly deviate from a plane. The regression coefficients b_1 and b_2 represent the slopes of the plane in the x_1-direction and x_2-direction, respectively. Because of the geometry of a plane, the slope in the x_1-direction is the same for all slopes in the x_2-direction and vice versa. The model influence of x_1 on the variable y is $b_1 x_1$, and stays $b_1 x_1$ for any value of b_2 or x_2. Each dependent variable, therefore, influences the outcome, unaffected by the other variable in the additive model.

When more than two variables are included in an additive regression model, the geometry is considerably more complicated, but the principle remains the same. The regression coefficients (the "slopes") reflect the degree of influence of each variable, and this influence is not affected by the values of other variables in model. Thus, the influence of a specific variable x_i on the variable y, measured by the regression coefficient b_i, again remains $b_i x_i$, regardless of the values of the other variables, as long as the model is additive. The statistical consequence of additivity is a clear separation of the influences from each dependent variable on the outcome under study. Confusingly, the independent variables are then frequently said to have "independent" influences.

To algebraically describe the property of additivity, consider two additive k-variable linear regression models:

Model 1

$$y_i = a + b_1 x_{i1} + b_2 x_{i2} + \cdots + b_m x_{im} + \cdots + b_k x_{ik} + \varepsilon_i$$

and Model 2, where a single dependent variable x_m is increased by one unit

$$y_i' = a + b_1 x_{i1} + b_2 x_{i2} + \cdots + b_m(x_{im} + 1) + \cdots + b_k x_{ik} + \varepsilon_i,$$

yielding

$$y_i' - y_i = b_m.$$

Therefore, the regression coefficient, b_m, measures the degree of influence of a one-unit increase in the dependent variable, x_m, in terms of the response of the independent variable y, unaffected by the other $k-1$ values of the variables in the model. When the model is not additive, the regression coefficients are not so simply interpreted because the multivariable influences are not simply separated into individual contributions.

For an additive regression model, it is said that x-variables are independent, the x-variables do not interact, the x-variables make separate contributions, the x-variables are adjusted for the influence of other model variables, or the other x-variables are held constant. Regardless of the language, additivity means one thing. An additive model represents the influence from each independent variable on the outcome variable as a simply interpreted and separate measure of association derived from a single model regression coefficient (b). Of course, it is the model that is additive and not necessarily the relationships within the data. Therefore, the correspondence between an additive model and the data analyzed is always a critical issue.

Confounding Influence

An additive regression model provides a clear and unequivocal example of the concept frequently called *confounding* (Chapter 1). In general terms, confounding occurs when a variable or variables influence the relationship between another variable and the outcome being studied. The following discussion applies to k-variate regression models, but the bivariate linear model ($k = 2$) provides an easily understood special case of the general principle.

A confounding influence of a specific variable is directly illustrated by comparing the coefficients estimated from two regression models. For the two-variable case, the two additive models are:

$$a \text{ single variable model}: \quad y_i = A + B_1 x_{i1} + \varepsilon_i \quad \text{and}$$
$$a \text{ bivariate model}: \quad y_i = a + b_1 x_{i1} + b_2 x_{i2} + \varepsilon_i.$$

The extent of the confounding bias caused by variable x_2 is defined as $\hat{B}_1 - \hat{b}_1$, where $\hat{B}_1$ represents the estimate of the coefficient B_1 in the single-variable model and $\hat{b}_1$ represents the estimate of the coefficient b_1 in the bivariate model, estimated from the same set of observations. That is, the relationship of the variable x_1 to the dependent variable y depends on the presence of the variable x_2 to the extent that the estimated regression coefficient $\hat{B}_1$ differs from $\hat{b}_1$. Thus, when $\hat{B}_1 \neq \hat{b}_1$, the variable x_2 is said to have a confounding influence on the relationship between x_1 and y. Conversely, when $\hat{B}_1 = \hat{b}_1$, then the variable x_2 does not influence the relationship between x_1 and y, sometimes called a "nonconfounder."

Expressions for the estimates of the two regression coefficients, B_1 and b_1, identify the basic properties of a confounding bias. For the single-variable model, the estimate of $\hat{B}_1$ is

$$\hat{B}_1 = \frac{S_{y1}}{S_1^2}.$$

and for the bivariate model the estimate of $\hat{b}_1$ is

$$\hat{b}_1 = \frac{S_{y1} S_2^2 - S_{y2} S_{12}}{S_1^2 S_2^2 - S_{12}^2}$$

where S_1^2 and S_2^2 represent the estimated variances of the variables x_1 and x_2, and S_{ij} represents the estimated covariance between two variables. The difference between estimates $\hat{B}_1$ and $\hat{b}_1$ produces the expression

$$extent \text{ of confounding bias from } x_2 = \hat{B}_1 - \hat{b}_1 = \frac{S_{12}\hat{b}_2}{S_1^2} = \frac{r_{12}\hat{b}_2 S_2}{S_1}$$

where r_{12} represents the estimated correlation coefficient between x_1 and x_2.

Two properties of confounding become apparent:

1. If correlation coefficient $r_{12} = 0$, then $\hat{B}_1 - \hat{b}_1 = 0$, and
2. If $\hat{b}_2 = 0$, then $\hat{B}_1 - \hat{b}_1 = 0$.

Thus, the variable x_2 does not have a confounding influence when x_2 is linearly unrelated to x_1 ($r_{12} = 0$) or when y is independently unrelated to x_2 ($\hat{b}_2 = 0$). It is also important to note that the variable x_2 can have a confounding influence when the dependent variable y is linearly unrelated to the independent variable x_2 ($r_{y2} = 0$). In symbols, when $r_{y2} = 0$, then $\hat{B}_1 - \hat{b}_1 = \hat{B}_1 r_{12}^2/(r_{12}^2 - 1)$. The confounding influence of x_2 results entirely from the relationship of x_2 to x_1 and the relationship of variable x_1 to y. Thus, the variable x_2 has a confounding influence only when it is related to both x_1 ($r_{12} \neq 0$) and the dependent variable y ($b_2 \neq 0$).

Confounding is a property of the sample and not the population sampled. It is defined and measured as the difference between estimated values. In other words, when a substantial confounding influence exists, the difference remains important even if it is largely a result of random variation. Furthermore, the extent of confounding depends on the choice of the analytic model (measure of association). Therefore, the determination of whether a confounding variable or variables are important contributors to understanding the outcome variable is primarily a subject matter decision. Other than estimating the magnitude of the confounding influence, further statistical analysis is not much help.

To be specific, consider an example. For a sample of 754 newborn infants, their birth weights (y) and gestational ages (x_2) were recorded. Also, it was determined whether the infant's mother smoked cigarettes during the year prior to her pregnancy (x_1). Two linear regression models (a two-variable and a one-variable model) produce the estimates given in Tables 5–2 and 5–3. When gestational age (x_2) is excluded from the model, the coefficient $\hat{b}_1$ remains equal to –0.190 because the estimated correlation between gestational age and smoking status is essentially zero ($r_{12} = 0$). Therefore, gestational age does not have a confounding influence on the relationship between smoking and birth weight because $\hat{B}_1$ and $\hat{b}_1$ equal –0.190 in both analyses ($\hat{B}_1 - \hat{b}_1 = 0$). That is, age ($x_2$) has no influence on the relationship between smoking and birth weight.

Although gestational age (x_2) does not have a confounding influence, deleting gestational age from the bivariate model increases the standard error of the estimated regression coefficient associated with smoking from $S_{\hat{b}_1} = 0.046$ to $S_{\hat{B}_1} = 0.050$.

These two properties of a nonconfounding variable ($r_{12} = 0$ causes $\hat{B}_1 = \hat{b}_1$ and a reduction of variance) occur for the linear model ($f(y) = y$) but are not properties of regression models in general. For example, when using the same data ($n = 754$) and defining birth weight as a binary variable (<2500 grams and

Table 5–2. Birth weight (y) analyzed using a bivariate linear regression model (x_1 = smoking status and x_2 = gestational age)

Variables	Terms	Estimates	Std errors	z-Values
Constant	$\hat{a}$	1.007	0.235	–
Smoking	$\hat{b}_1$	−0.190	0.046	−4.108
Gestation	$\hat{b}_2$	0.009	0.001	10.792

Table 5–3. Birth weight (y) analyzed using a single-variable linear regression model (x_1 = smoking status)

Variables	Terms	Estimates	Std. errors	z-Values
Constant	$\hat{A}$	3.532	0.020	–
Smoking	$\hat{B}_1$	−0.190	0.050	−3.825

Table 5–4. Birth weight (y) analyzed using a bivariate logistic regression model (x_1 = smoking status and x_2 = gestational age)

Variables	Terms	Estimates	Std. errors	z-Values
Constant	$\hat{a}$	−36.705	5.672	–
Smoking	$\hat{b}_1$	−1.032	0.693	−1.489
Gestation	$\hat{b}_2$	0.152	0.022	6.895

Table 5–5. Birth weight (y) analyzed using a single-variable logistic regression model (x_1 = smoking status)

Variables	Terms	Estimates	Std. errors	z-Values
Constant	$\hat{A}$	3.709	0.261	–
Smoking	$\hat{B}_1$	−0.705	0.493	−1.430

$\geq$2500 grams), applying a logistic regression analysis shows that the two properties observed in the linear models (Tables 5–2 and 5–3) are not observed in the logistic model (Tables 5–4 and 5–5). The correlation between smoking and gestational age remains essentially zero ($r_{12} = 0$); however, the one- and two-variable regression models produce different coefficients $\hat{B}_1 = -0.705$ and $\hat{b}_1 = -1.032$ with estimated standard errors $S_{\hat{B}_1} = 0.493$ and $S_{\hat{b}_1} = 0.693$ ($S_{\hat{B}_1} < S_{\hat{b}_1}$). For the logistic model analysis, gestational age (x_2) has a substantial confounding influence on the relationship between smoking and birth weight ($\hat{B}_1 - \hat{b}_1 = -0.705 - (-1.032) = 0.327$).

The Geometry of Interaction and Confounding

Much of statistical analysis can be viewed as the art of creating and evaluating summary values calculated from collected data. Such summary values become the focus of the analysis, frequently producing coherent, accurate, and intuitive descriptions of relationships among the variables under study, particularly when accompanied by rigorous statistical inferences. The concepts of interaction and confounding are central to creating summary values and are readily illustrated in the context of a linear regression model.

To be concrete, consider two variables, denoted X and C, that are potentially related to an outcome variable denoted Y. Variables X and C could be the blood pressure and sex of a study subject, and the outcome Y the probability of CHD. Or, the variable X could be the age of a mother and C indicates whether she smokes or not, and the outcome Y might be the birth weight of her newborn infant. Regardless of the kinds of variables, two important questions are key to creating a single statistical summary of the X/Y-relationship (discussion continued from Chapter 1).

First question: Is the measure of the relationship between X and Y the same for the relevant values of C? If the answer is no, a single summary is not useful. Different relationships cannot be summarized by a single value. Figure 5–1A illustrates three straight lines with different slopes. No single line (slope) or any other summary measure accurately captures the relationship between X and Y, because no single relationship exists. As before, such a situation is called an *interaction* or sometimes *effect statistical measure modification*.

If the answer to the question is yes, it is usually possible to create an easily interpreted summary line reflecting the X/Y-relationship. Figure 5–1B illustrates a linear relationship between X and Y that is identical for three levels of C (exactly no interaction) that is effectively summarized by a single value, namely the X/Y-slope of the lines.

Only in the absence of an interaction, a second question arises: What is the role of variable C in creating a summary slope? There are two obvious possibilities. The variable C influences the measurement of the relationship between X and Y (Figure 5–1C) or has little or no influence on the measurement of the X/Y-relationship (Figure 5–1D). In epidemiologic terms, the same question becomes: Does the variable C have a confounding influence? If the answer is yes, then taking C into account, a useful summary statistic can be created that reflects the relationship between X and Y. The resulting summary estimate is said to be *adjusted* for the influence of variable C. If the answer to the question is no, then the variable C can be ignored, and a useful summary estimate can be created directly from the variables X and Y (Figure 5–1D). The X/Y-relationship is said to be independent of the variable C.

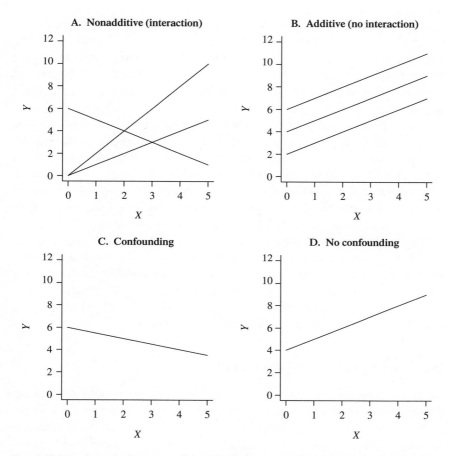

Figure 5–1. A simple illustration of the role of interaction and confounding in the creation of a statistical summary of the relationship between X and Y.

The process of creating a statistical summary described schematically is

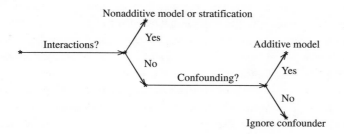

The considerations of interaction and confounding in creating a summary of the X/Y-relationship are sequential. If interactions exists, confounding is not an issue because summarization is not possible, and confounding concerns a choice among kinds of summaries. When no interaction exits, the role of C becomes of fundamental importance. The choice of the kind of summary then depends on the presence or absence of an influence of the variable C.

This discussion of interaction and confounding in the context of a simple regression model is presented for the purpose of a clear and concise description. In reality, the issues are rarely clear cut and require sometimes sophisticated statistical tools to identify and evaluate interaction and confounding influences. More realistic situations typically involve a number of variables producing a large number of possible interactions. The influence of sampling variation produces added complications. Confounding influences are also not always obvious. For example, in a regression analysis context, confounding influences cannot be investigated until a useful additive model is chosen—not always a simple task. Considerable statistical analysis is frequently necessary to determine the extent of confounding and to make realistic decisions about the role of specific variables in the study of an outcome. The fact remains, however, that confounding is a consideration only when interaction influences are absent.

The Geometry of Statistical Adjustment

Direct comparisons of human mortality rates between time periods is frequently not simply accomplished because of changes in the age distributions between the periods. Age can a have a substantial confounding influence on the comparison. Similarly, direct comparison of mortality risk between white and African-American newborn infants is not useful because differences in birth weight distributions complicate the interpretation summary of any pattern. The same issues are encountered in comparing CHD incidence between type-A and type-B individuals, because these individuals differ in a number of ways, such as different distributions of blood pressure levels, different distributions of cholesterol levels, and different levels of smoking exposure (Chapters 4 and 11). That is, a direct comparison of a specific variable between behavior types is influenced by differences among other variables not equally distributed (not balanced) between the compared groups. Groups that are balanced for all relevant variables rarely occur in observational data. However, comparisons of summary values from unbalanced groups are frequently improved by statistical adjustment strategies. Although a variety of strategies exist, the underlying geometry of a typical adjustment technique is illustrated by the following elementary regression analysis.

Consider comparing a variable labeled y between two groups (denoted group I and group II) that differ with respect to the distribution of a variable labeled x. That

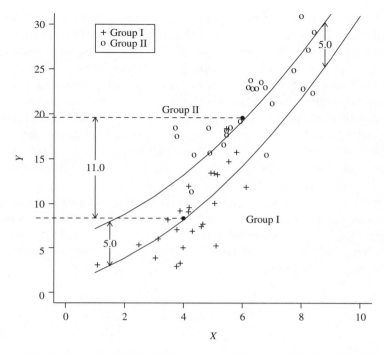

Figure 5–2. The adjusted difference between two groups based on a nonlinear relationship between the variables X and Y.

is, the variable x is not balanced between the two groups. Furthermore, these two variables (x and y) are related. Fictional data ($+$ = group I and o = group II) and mean values of these two groups (solid dots) are displayed in Figure 5–2. The mean value of the y-values in group I is $\bar{y}_1 = 8.5$, and in group II, the mean value is $\bar{y}_2 = 19.5$ (dashed lines). These two mean values occur at the mean values of the x-variable, $\bar{x}_1 = 4.0$ and $\bar{x}_2 = 6.0$, respectively. That is, the two groups are unbalanced with respect to the distribution of x ($\bar{x}_1 \neq \bar{x}_2$). The difference between the mean values $\bar{y}_1$ and $\bar{y}_2$ ($\bar{y}_2 - \bar{y}_1 = 11.0$, dashed lines), therefore, has two components. First, the mean values differ because the two groups differ with respect to the values of y. Second, the mean values differ because the y-values are related to the x-values, and the x-values in group II, by and large, are greater than those in group I. Consequently, the difference between the group mean values $\bar{y}_1$ and $\bar{y}_2$ is increased to some extent by the differences between the variable x. This lack of balance produces a confounding influence. It is this influence that complicates the interpretation of the directly observed difference between groups, namely the difference $\bar{y}_2 - \bar{y}_1 = 11.0$.

A statistical adjustment is one way to produce a summary value that behaves as if the distributions of other relevant variables (such as the x-values in the example) are the same between the compared groups. Specifically, the difference in mean values $\bar{y}_2 - \bar{y}_1 = 11.0$ is adjusted so that the difference between groups I and II can be estimated as if the groups were balanced for the distribution of x. The adjusted mean difference is then said to be "free" of the confounding influence of the x-variable. For example, the adjusted difference in mortality rates (y) between white and African-American newborn infants would be "free" of the confounding influence of the difference in the birth-weight distributions (x). The adjusted mortality rates then behave as if the compared groups have the same birth-weight distributions (Chapter 6).

A typical and perhaps the easiest way to create a summary value adjusted for another variable starts with a postulated model that describes the relationship between x and y. In addition, this model relationship is required to be the same for the compared groups (additivity or no interaction). For the example data (Figure 5–2), such a model is

$$y = a + dF + bx + cx^2$$

where $F = 0$ indicates observations from group I and $F = 1$ indicates observations from group II. The proposed model describes the x/y-relationship within both groups with the same curve (Figure 5–2). Furthermore, the model separates the influence of the variable x from the comparison between groups. In symbols, for group I ($F = 0$), $y = a + bx + cx^2$, and for group II ($F = 1$), $y' = a + d + bx + cx^2$. The distance between the two curves ($y' - y = d$) is constant (*distance* $= d = 5.0$, in the example) and is, therefore, not influenced by the value of x. The value remains $d = 5$ for any value of x. The difference $d = 5$ is then said to be the adjusted difference between the groups I and II.

Implicit in this example, and for model-based adjustment procedures in general, is that a useful model can be found to adequately characterize the relationship between the variables x and y. The adequacy of the model is typically part of a complete analysis. The contexts change, the models differ, and the complexity is generally greater than this example but the geometry of underlying adjustment strategies frequently follows a similar pattern. A model is constructed so that the influence of one variable can be studied as if the influences of another variable or several other variables are the same between the compared groups (statistically balanced). Geometrically, an adjusted estimate then becomes the distance between the two curves at any point.

LOGISTIC REGRESSION ANALYSIS

To study the relationship between the likelihood of hypertension and exposure to high levels of noise, data were collected from 1101 women working in a textile factory in Beijing, China (only women make up the workforce). All study participants were employed for at least 5 years and worked at essentially the same task during their period of employment. Workers were assigned to these tasks at "random." That is, when a current worker retired or quit (a rare event), a new worker (about age 19) was assigned to the vacated job and typically continued to do the same task until her retirement. The textile factory environment was chosen for study because of the stable work force and the spatial uniformity of each worker's exposure to elevated noise levels measured by sound pressure level (SPL, in decibels). An SPL measure is a time-weighted average producing a continuous measurement of exposure. Hypertension was defined as systolic blood pressure over 160 mm Hg or diastolic blood pressure greater than 95 mm Hg. In addition, workers taking antihypertension drugs were classified as hypertensive regardless of their blood pressure levels. This definition produced 44 hypertensive women (4.0%). Along with the measurement of each worker's noise exposure, an interview determined the worker's age, the number of years employed, her salt consumption (self-reported), and whether or not she had a family history of hypertension (medical records). In this exceptionally homogeneous cohort, one worker reported smoking, no women had more than one child, and only seven reported drinking alcohol regularly. Furthermore, all workers lived in the same industrial commune [20]. These data constitute what is sometimes called a "natural experiment."

A linear logistic regression model is an ideal statistical tool to analyze and describe the association between workplace exposure to elevated noise levels and a binary outcome variable such as the presence/absence of hypertension, while accounting for the potentially confounding influences of age, years-worked, salt consumption, and family history of high blood pressure.

An additive multivariable logistic model relating k risk variables (denoted x_{ij}, risk factor j measured on individual i) to the probability of disease (denoted p_i) is

$$P(disease|x_{i1}, x_{i2}, \cdots, x_{ik}) = p_i = \frac{1}{1 + e^{-(b_0 + b_1 x_{i1} + b_2 x_{i2} + \cdots + b_k x_{ik})}}.$$

The link function $log[p_i/(1 - p_i)]$ transforms the logistic probability into an additive linear regression model where

$$f(p_i) = log\text{-}odds_i = log\left[\frac{p_i}{1 - p_i}\right] = b_0 + b_1 x_{i1} + b_2 x_{i2} + \cdots + b_k x_{ik}.$$

More simply, as before, the relationship is expressed as

$$p_i = \frac{1}{1 + e^{-log\text{-}odds_i}} \quad \text{or} \quad log\text{-}odds_i = log\left[\frac{p_i}{1 - p_i}\right].$$

The transformed regression model is additive, and its components are estimated and interpreted, in terms of the log-odds, in the same way as all linear regression models. For the hypertension data, two variables are continuous (age and years worked), one variable is also continuous but classified into seven numeric categories (SPL), and two variables are binary (family history and salt consumption). Brief descriptions of these five independent variables are presented in Table 5–6. The relationship between the likelihood of hypertension and SPL is summarized in Table 5–7.

The estimated log-odds measure of hypertension risk based on SPL measures alone (denoted x) is

$$log\text{-}odds_x = \hat{a} + \hat{b}x = -10.400 + 0.077x.$$

Table 5–6. Summary of the five risk factors (independent variables) relevant to the study of likelihood of hypertension (binary dependent variable) in Chinese textile workers ($n = 1{,}101$ women)

Continuous variables

Variables	Symbols	Means	Medians	Std. dev.	Minimums	Maximums
Sound pressure level	*spl*	90.8	90.0	8.83	75.0	104.0
Age	*age*	35.5	33.9	8.43	22.1	53.0
Years-worked	*work*	16.2	16.3	9.64	5.0	38.4

Binary variables

	Symbol	Yes	No	**Total**
Family history	*history*	604	497	1101
Salt consumption	*salt*	554	557	1101

Table 5–7. Frequency and proportion of hypertension by SPL observed in the Chinese textile factory workers ($n = 1{,}101$ women)

SPL levels	<77	77–80	80–87	87–90	90–96	96–104	>104	**Total**
Hypertensive	4	1	0	1	5	17	16	44
Non-hypertensive	149	38	23	47	375	277	148	1057
Total	153	39	23	48	380	294	164	1101
Proportion ($\hat{p}_i$)	0.026	0.026	0.000	0.021	0.013	0.058	0.098	0.040
Estimated ($\hat{p}_x$)	0.010	0.012	0.015	0.025	0.031	0.049	0.087	0.040

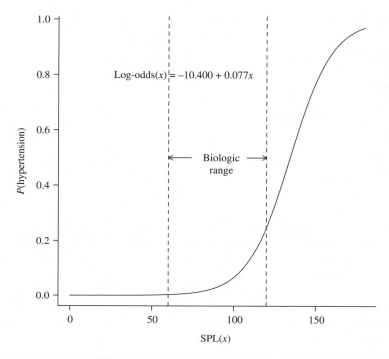

Figure 5–3. Estimated logistic curve displaying the probability of hypertension associated with sound pressure levels (x = SPL), Chinese textile workers data (n = 1101).

The parameter estimates $\hat{a} = -10.400$ and $\hat{b} = 0.077$ are maximum likelihood estimates from the 1101 textile factory workers data. The log-odds values can be directly transformed to estimate the probability that an individual is hypertensive for any selected SPL level. Specifically, the probabilities

$$\hat{P}(hypertension|x) = \hat{p}_x = \frac{1}{1 + e^{-log\text{-}odds_x}} = \frac{1}{1 + e^{-(\hat{a} + \hat{b}x)}}$$

$$= \frac{1}{1 + e^{-(-10.400 + 0.077x)}}$$

are displayed in Figure 5–3. These model-estimated probabilities of hypertension $\hat{p}_x$ are between zero and 1 for all SPL levels, which is a property of the logistic model in general. However, realistic probabilities are between 0.0 and 0.1. (Table 5–7, last line).

The relationship between the likelihood of hypertension and SPL summarized by a more comprehensive additive logistic model, in terms of the log-odds, is

$$log\text{-}odds_i = b_0 + b_1 spl_i + b_2 age_i + b_3 work_i + b_4 history_i + b_5 salt_i$$

Table 5–8. Estimated regression coefficients for the five-variable logistic regression model, Chinese textile workers data ($n = 1101$)

Variables	Coefficients	Estimates	Std. errors	z-Values	p-Values	Odds ratios
Intercept	b_0	−14.719	2.770	–	–	–
SPL	b_1	0.056	0.021	2.595	0.009	1.057
Age	b_2	0.150	0.075	1.990	0.047	1.162
Years-worked	b_3	−0.012	0.065	−0.183	0.855	0.988
Family history	b_4	0.326	0.330	0.986	0.324	1.385
Salt consumption	b_5	0.800	0.335	2.387	0.017	2.226

LogLikelihood $= -153.093$

again, $i = 1, 2, \cdots, n = 1101$ workers. As with all regression models, the form of the independent variables in a logistic model is unrestricted. For the hypertension data, the observed values of these five independent variables are entered into the estimation process as reported (Table 5–8).

A notable property of the Beijing textile factory workers data is the high correlation between a worker's age and years-worked. Each sampled worker was hired at about the same age. Therefore, the correlation between these two variables is almost collinear ($correlation = 0.97$) because $age \approx years\text{-}worked + 19$. As expected, almost no change in the log-likelihood value occurs when either variable is excluded from the model. For the full model (all five risk factors included), the log-likelihood value is −153.093 and, when years-worked is removed, the log-likelihood value decreases slightly to −153.109 (Table 5–9).

The extremely high correlation between age and years worked, however, dramatically affects the precision of the estimated regression coefficients associated with these two nearly collinear variables. The estimated standard error associated with the age coefficient ($\hat{b}_2$) is $S_{\hat{b}_2} = 0.075$ when years-worked is included in the five-variable model (Table 5–8). When years-worked is not included in the model, the standard error of the estimate associated with the worker's age, $\hat{b}_2$, falls sharply to 0.025. The three-fold decrease in variability increases the z-statistic

Table 5–9. Summary of the roles of highly correlated (nearly collinear) variables in a logistic model of the hypertension data, age and years-worked

Model	Age		Yrs-wrk		log-likelihood
	$\hat{b}_2$	$S_{\hat{b}_2}$	$\hat{b}_3$	$S_{\hat{b}_3}$	
All five variables	0.150	0.075	−0.012	0.065	−153.09
Years worked removed	0.137	0.025	–	–	−153.11
Age removed	–	–	0.113	0.021	−154.91

associated with evaluating the influence of age from 1.990 to 5.530. The p-value correspondingly decreases from 0.047 (Table 5–8) to less than 0.001. However, the price paid for the increased precision is a biased estimate of the age–hypertension regression coefficient. The estimated coefficient measuring the influence of age is $\hat{b}_2 = 0.150$ when years-worked is included in the regression model and becomes 0.137 when years-worked is excluded from the model. The difference (0.150 vs. 0.137) is the bias incurred by not accounting for the confounding influence of years-worked.

Excluding age from the logistic model has a similar but more pronounced influence on the analysis. When the variable age is removed, the estimated standard error of the estimated coefficient associated with years-worked, $\hat{b}_3$, is sharply reduced, again by a factor of three (0.113 to 0.021). For the full model (Table 5–8), the coefficient associated with years-worked is $\hat{b}_3 = -0.012$, but when the age variable is removed from the regression model, the estimated coefficient becomes 0.113. This considerable difference (−0.012 vs. 0.113) is the bias incurred by not accounting for the important confounding influence of age. A summary of the roles of the variables measuring the influences of age and years-worked is given in Table 5–9.

Occasionally, a statistical analysis presents a trade-off between bias and precision. A decision then must be made between two alternatives: a biased estimate with relatively higher precision or an unbiased estimate with lower precision. The choice is typically made on the basis of subject-matter considerations. For the textile workers analysis, it is undoubtedly better to trade a decrease in precision for a less biased estimate. Because the SPL influence is the focus of the analysis, the precision of the estimated regression coefficients associated with age and years-worked are a minor concern. The reduction of bias in the measure of the SPL–hypertension relationship is the primary reason age and years-worked were included in the sampled data.

Goodness-of-fit is always an issue in the interpretation of the results from a postulated model, particularly an additive model. For a logistic regression model with continuous independent variables, evaluating the goodness-of-fit is not a straightforward comparison of observed to model-estimated values. The observed outcomes are binary (hypertensive or not), and the values estimated from a logistic model are either log-odds or probabilities. The observed binary outcome cannot be directly estimated from a logistic model, causing a lack of correspondence between the observed and estimated values, regardless of the accuracy of the model.

To produce a goodness-of-fit procedure, the estimated logistic model is used to create an artificial table based on model-generated probabilities of hypertension. Once the table is constructed, observed cell frequencies based strictly on the data are compared to model-estimated cell frequencies. The degree of correspondence, evaluated with a chi-square statistic in the usual way, reflects the goodness-of-fit of the proposed model.

To create a "goodness-of-fit table," the first step is to estimate the probability of hypertension from the estimated logistic model. Using each participant's five measured risk factors produces 1101 estimated probabilities ($\hat{p}_i$-values), one from each study subject. These model-estimated probabilities of hypertension are then used to classify study subjects into "risk" categories. Typically, the 10% of the sampled individuals with the lowest estimated probabilities form the first category, the next lowest 10% form the second category, and so forth, until the last category is made up of the 10% of sampled individuals with the highest estimated probabilities of hypertension. These ten categories are sometimes referred to as *deciles of risk*. For most data sets, all the deciles of risk will not contain exactly 10% of the observations. In this case, the table is constructed so that each decile contains 10% or as close as possible to 10% of the data. Ten mean probabilities (denoted $\bar{p}_k$) are then calculated, one from each decile. In symbols, for the kth decile, the model-generated mean probability is

$$\bar{p}_k = \frac{1}{n_k} \sum \hat{p}_j$$

where $j = 1, 2, \cdots, n_k$, $n_k \approx n/10$ and $k = 1, 2, \cdots, 10$.

For the textile factory workers, these ten model-generated mean probabilities are given in Table 5–10 (column 3). Furthermore, these probabilities allow 20 model-generated frequencies to be calculated. For the kth decile, these frequencies are $n_k \bar{p}_k$ cases and $n_k(1 - \bar{p}_k)$ non-cases generated from the model-estimated mean probabilities. From the hypertension data, for example, the eighth decile ($k = 8$) yields $\bar{p}_8 = 0.052$. The model-estimated frequency of cases of hypertension becomes $n_8 \bar{p}_8 = 110(0.052) = 5.74$ and non-cases $n_8(1 - \bar{p}_8) = 110(0.948) = 104.26$, since $n_8 = 110$. The corresponding observed frequencies are 5 and 105, respectively. The 20 model-generated frequencies (denoted e_k) compared to the 20 frequencies observed from the data tabulated into the same deciles (denoted o_k, Table 5–10) reflect the goodness-of-fit of the estimated logistic model.

The Pearson chi-square goodness-of-fit test statistic for the textile factory data is $X^2 = \sum(o_k - e_k)^2/e_k = 11.181$. The observed test statistic X^2 has an approximate chi-square distribution with eight degrees of freedom when the model is "correct." The term "correct" means that the only reason the 20 model-generated frequencies differ from the 20 observed frequencies is random variation. The justification of the degrees of freedom is not simple nor intuitive, and the explanation is left to more detailed descriptions of the logistic model goodness-of-fit procedure [21]. The p-value is $P(X^2 \geq 11.181 \mid model\ is\ "correct") = 0.192$. A p-value in the neighborhood of 0.2 provides no strong evidence that the logistic regression

Table 5–10. The components of the goodness-of-fit procedure for the Chinese textile factory worker's logistic regression analysis

Decile	n_k	Cases $\bar{p}_k$	e_k	o_k	Non-cases $1 - \bar{p}_k$	e_k	o_k
1	111	0.002	0.25	1	0.998	110.75	110
2	110	0.004	0.46	0	0.996	109.54	110
3	110	0.006	0.68	0	0.994	109.32	110
4	110	0.009	0.97	0	0.991	109.03	110
5	110	0.013	1.44	0	0.987	108.56	110
6	110	0.020	2.17	4	0.980	107.83	106
7	110	0.031	3.44	3	0.969	106.56	107
8	110	0.052	5.74	5	0.948	104.26	105
9	110	0.089	9.81	15	0.911	100.19	95
10	110	0.173	19.06	16	0.827	90.94	94
Total	1101	0.040	44.00	44	0.960	1057.00	1.057

model based on the additive influences of the five risk factors is an adequate or an inadequate description of the risk–hypertension relationship.

The "table approach" to assessing the fit of the logistic model is not ideal for several reasons. First, classifying a large number of estimated and observed values into 20 categories incurs some loss of information, causing an associated loss in statistical efficiency. Second, the Pearson chi-square approximation is least accurate when the cell frequencies are small. Small cell frequencies are common when data are distributed into deciles based on logistic model-estimated probabilities. For the hypertension data, seven of the ten model-estimated frequencies are less than five. Third, small inconsequential changes in the estimated parameters lead to small changes in the model-estimated values. As expected, slightly redefining the decile boundaries can shift the numbers of observed values found in the newly defined categories. These small shifts, however, occasionally produce deceptively large changes in the contributions to the chi-square statistic from decile categories containing small numbers of observations. Perhaps of most importance, the chi-square assessment of the goodness-of-fit table does not produce a rigorous comparison of nested models. A simpler model (fewer parameters) can produce a chi-square summary statistic that is smaller than the same summary value calculated from a more complex model. If variables are deleted from a regression model, the simpler model always "fits" the data less well. Comparison of the log-likelihood values always reflects this fact. However, a chi-square statistic calculated from the decile-of-risk approach can decrease when a variable or variables are deleted from the model, thus yielding a comparison between models that has no rigorous interpretation. Such a procedure is certainly useless as a guide to the selection of an appropriate model to represent the relationships within the data.

The following example emphasizes a failure of the goodness-of-fit strategy derived from a chi-square statistic as a tool for model selection. A variable (denoted x) was created by selecting $n = 1101$ random values between 0 and 100. Using these values and the hypertension outcome, the model $log\text{-}odds = a + bx$ produced the estimated regression coefficient $\hat{b} = 0.005$ ($\hat{or} = 1.005$). However, the decile-at-risk table yields a goodness-of-fit chi-square statistic of $X^2 = 6.950$, with the corresponding p-value of 0.542 (degrees of freedom = 8). A value with no relationship to the outcome ($b = 0$) should produce a large chi-square value (a small p-value) because it is clearly not predictive in any way of the hypertension outcome. Chapter 11 continues the goodness-of-fit discussion for logistic regression analysis.

The primary purpose of applying a logistic model to the Chinese textile factory data is to describe the influence of elevated noise exposure on the likelihood of hypertensive disease. The first model based on the SPL measurements alone (Table 5–7) produces a measure of influence in terms of the estimated regression coefficient $\hat{b} = 0.077$. The second analysis based on the same SPL measurements but including four additional variables (age, years-worked, history, and salt) produces the adjusted estimate $\hat{b}_1 = 0.056$ (Table 5–8). The difference occurs because the second model accounts for the joint confounding bias incurred by not including four relevant variables. It is to reduce this bias that these four variables were collected and included in the analysis.

Similar to the coefficients from additive regression models in general, the coefficients from a logistic regression model measure the amount of change in the log-odds for each unit increase in a specific independent variable. That is, a one-unit increase in the ith independent variable yields a b_i-unit change in the log-odds. The estimated coefficient associated with SPL is $\hat{b}_1 = 0.056$. A one-unit increase in SPL then increases the log-odds associated with the likelihood of hypertension by an estimated 0.056 per decibel, while accounting for the influence of the other four variables in the regression equation ("held constant"). An increase of 0.056 in the log-odds translates into an estimated increase in the odds by a factor of $e^{\hat{b}} = e^{0.056} = 1.057$ per decibel increase in SPL, also reflecting the influence of noise exposure on the likelihood of hypertension. For an additive logistic model, the influence of a variable measured by an odds ratio is multiplicative and, for the SPL logistic regression model, this multiplicative increase is an estimated 1.057 per unit increase in SPL. Thus, a 20-decibel increase in SPL produces an estimated odds ratio of

$$\hat{or} = (1.057)(1.057)\cdots(1.057) = (1.057)^{20} = 3.060.$$

In general, an increase of x units of a variable with an estimated coefficient $\hat{b}$ produces the estimated odds ratio

$$\hat{or}_x = e^{[\hat{b}_i \times x]} = [e^{\hat{b}_i}]^x, \quad \text{and for the hypertension data} \quad \hat{or}_x = [1.057]^x$$

where x represents SPL-levels. Because the model is additive, this change in the odds ratio is unaffected by the values of the other variables in the model.

The estimated logistic regression model (Table 5–8 and Figure 5–4) dictates a linear relationship between each of three continuous independent variables (SPL, age, and years-worked) and the log-odds associated with the likelihood of hypertension. No reason exists to assume that these variables are so simply related to the log-odds. The variables family history and salt consumption, however, consist of two values and necessarily have binary influences.

A model postulating a nonlinear relationship between a risk factor and a binary outcome is easily created. Using polynomial expressions to describe the influence of each of the three continuous independent variables, the logistic regression model becomes

$$log\text{-}odds_i = a_0 + s_1(spl_i) + s_2(age_i) + s_3(work_i) + a_1 history_i + a_2 salt_i.$$

When a cubic polynomial representation is chosen, then

$$s_j(x) = b_j x + c_j x^2 + d_j x^3.$$

A cubic polynomial possibly improves the description of the influence of an independent variable on the log-odds measure of association. The individual regression coefficients estimated from this more extensive but additive model are not simply interpreted but are usually not of great interest. The focus is not on each coefficient but on each polynomial expression, defined by three coefficients. Using a polynomial function $s(x)$ rather than a single linear term x adds flexibility to the description of the independent variable and provides a potentially more accurate nonlinear characterization of the relationship between an independent and outcome variable. It is certainly not necessary that the patterns of risk influence be simple (perhaps, simplistic) straight lines (Figure 5–4). Estimated nonlinear patterns are displayed in Figure 5–5 for the variables years-worked, age, and SPL, each adjusted for the influence of the other four variables because the logistic regression model remains additive. For example, the polynomial representation of the nonlinear relationship between SPL and the likelihood of hypertension is not influenced by the kind of representation or the specific values of the other four variables in the model.

Two choices exist with regard to the interpretation of nonlinear influences— the measure of the relationship is essentially linear, and the apparent nonlinearity

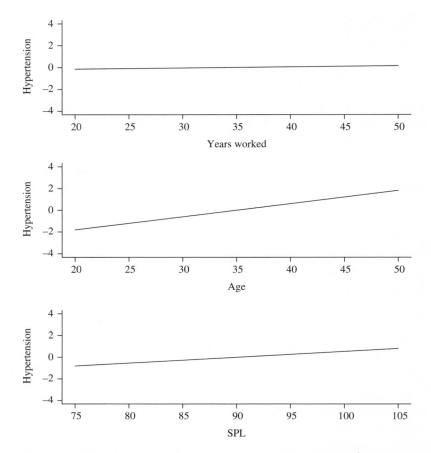

Figure 5–4. Estimated linear influences on the likelihood of hypertension for each of the three continuous risk variables (years-worked, age, and SPL).

results from the estimation process capitalizing on the inherent random variation of the observations, or the measure of the relationship has an underlying systematic nonlinear influence on the outcome variable. To formally evaluate these two possibilities, a model consisting of nonlinear influences for all continuous variables is compared to a model with a strictly linear influence assigned to a single independent variable. In symbols, the linear term $b_j x_i$ replaces the polynomial $s_j(x_i)$. For example, the polynomial hypertension model

$$log\text{-}odds_i = a_0 + s_1(spl_i) + s_2(age_i) + s_3(work_i) + a_1 history_i + a_2 salt_i$$

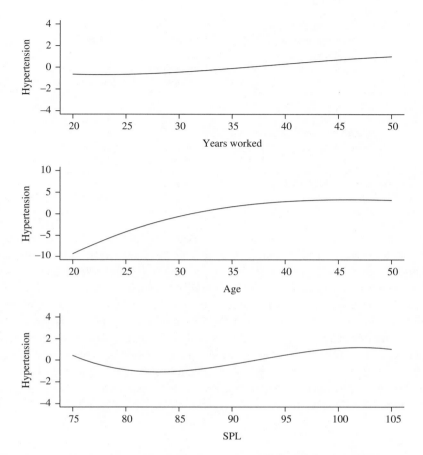

Figure 5–5. Estimated polynomial influences on the likelihood of hypertension for each of the three continuous risk variables (years-worked, age, and SPL).

is compared to the same model with the influence of the SPL variable represented as a linear influence where

$$log\text{-}odds_i = a_0 + b_1 spl_i + s_2(age_i) + s_3(work_i) + a_1 history_i + a_2 salt_i.$$

The difference in log-likelihood values measures the increased influence of a nonlinear representation of the SPL variable. The extent of the influence of a polynomial representation of each of the three continuous risk variables is evaluated by a series of likelihood ratio comparisons (Table 5–11, column 4).

No convincing evidence of a nonlinear association with years-worked emerges from the textile factory workers data ($X^2 = -2[-147.361 - (-146.589)] = 1.547$, p-value $= 0.461$). However, some evidence exists that the likelihood

Table 5–11. Comparison of a polynomial representation $[s(x) = bx + cx^2 + dx^3]$ to a linear representation $[s(x) = bx]$ for each continuous risk factor

Models	Log-likelihoods	Degrees of freedom	$-2 \times$ Differences	p-Values
$s_1(spl) + s_2(age) +$ $s_3(work)*$	−146.589	1089	–	–
$s_1(work)$ replaced by $work$	−147.361	1091	1.547	0.461
$s_2(age)$ replaced by age	−149.382	1091	5.589	0.061
$s_3(spl)$ replaced by spl	−149.821	1091	6.464	0.039

* Full five-variable model (including *history* and *salt* variables).

of hypertension linearly increases as a worker's age increases until about ages 35 or 40. Then, further increases appear to have relatively little additional influence ($X^2 = -2[-149.382 - (-146.589)] = 5.589$, p-value = 0.061). As noise exposure increases, initially the log-odds decreases at the lower SPL levels and then increases for exposures greater than about 85 decibels. The statistical analysis (Table 5–11) provides evidence that the observed pattern is not likely an artifact of random variation and potentially represents a systematic nonlinear relationship between the SPL exposure and the likelihood of hypertension ($X^2 = -2[-149.821 - (-146.589)] = 6.466$, p-value = 0.039). The discussion of nonlinear representations of independent variables as part of a regression analysis is continued in Chapter 10.

6

ANALYSIS OF COUNT DATA: POISSON REGRESSION MODEL

Counts come in a variety of forms. They are the numerators of rates, the numerators of proportions, and values directly entered into tables. Regression model tools provide effective and efficient analyses of counts when they are sampled from Poisson probability distributions (another application of the Poisson distribution is presented in Chapter 7). Clearly, not all counts have Poisson distributions, and other probability distributions potentially improve the description of their variation. A regression approach based on the assumption or knowledge that sampled counts have Poisson distributions, however, is a good place to start.

Three properties of a model relevant to regression analysis are: (1) a dependent variable that is a function of an outcome observation, (2) a specific summary measure of association, and (3) a probability distribution that describes the population sampled (Chapter 5). For the additive linear regression case, the function of the dependent variable is the variable itself, the natural measure of association is the difference between model-estimated values, and the observations are typically assumed to be sampled from normal probability distributions. For the logistic regression case, the function of the dependent variable is the log-odds, the measure of association is the odds ratio, and the observations are assumed to be sampled from binomial probability distributions. For the Poisson case, the function of the dependent variable is the logarithm of a rate, the logarithm of a probability, or the logarithm of a count, and the measure of association is a rate-ratio, a relative risk, or a ratio. The counts, as the name indicates, are assumed to be sampled from Poison probability distributions.

POISSON MULTIVARIABLE REGRESSION MODEL: TECHNICAL DESCRIPTION

The influence on a rate, a probability, or a count from k independent variables is frequently expressed in terms of a multiplicative model. In symbols, to describe a rate, one such a model is

$$rate = A \times B_1^{x_1} \times B_2^{x_2} \times B_3^{x_3} \times \cdots \times B_k^{x_k}.$$

The choice of multiplicative influences of the independent variables, represented by $x_1, x_2, x_3, \cdots, x_k$, is a continuation of a pattern established in the early studies of mortality risk. Rate-ratios have long been a traditional measure of association used to describe mortality and disease data.

The logarithm of a rate then yields an additive model that is a linear function of the k independent variables or

$$log(rate) = log(A) + log(B_1)x_1 + log(B_2)x_2 + log(B_3)x_3 + \cdots + log(B_k)x_k$$

and, expressed more simply, is

$$log(rate) = a + b_1x_1 + b_2x_2 + b_3x_3 + \cdots + b_kx_k \quad log(B_j) = b_j.$$

In yet another form, this additive regression model is

$$log(d) = a + b_1x_1 + b_2x_2 + b_3x_3 + \cdots + b_kx_k + log(P) \quad (rate = \frac{d}{P})$$

where d represents the number of deaths or cases of disease in the numerator of a *rate* and P represents the person-time-at-risk or the number of individuals at risk in the denominator. The value represented by $log(P)$ is a nonrandom quantity technically called an *offset* in a regression context.

As with most regression models, it is necessary to know or assume that the dependent variable has a specific probability distribution. For a Poisson regression model, the observed counts (d) are required to be sampled from Poisson distributions. Under this condition, the model coefficients and their variances are estimated with maximum likelihood techniques. As usual, the variance estimates are essential for evaluating the influence of sampling variation on the model-estimated parameters (statistical tests and confidence intervals). Of greater importance, the estimated model frequently becomes a statistical tool to identify and assess important features of the sampled data.

The measure of association, as noted, generated by a Poisson regression model, is a ratio. For the analysis of rates, the measure of association is a rate-ratio. Consider a specific independent variable denoted x_m; then the additive Poisson models

$$log(rate) = a + b_1x_1 + b_2x_2 + b_3x_3 + \cdots + b_mx_m + \cdots + b_kx_k$$

and

$$log(rate)' = a + b_1x_1 + b_2x_2 + b_3x_3 + \cdots + b_m(x_m + 1) + \cdots + b_kx_k,$$

differ by

$$log(rate)' - log(rate) = b_m \quad or \quad log\left(\frac{rate'}{rate}\right) = b_m.$$

Therefore, the coefficient b_m directly indicates the amount of change in the log-rate associated with a one-unit increase in the mth variable, while the other $k - 1$ variables are "held constant." The same change is more commonly reported in terms of multiplicative change in the rate-ratio, where $e^{b_m} = rate'/rate$ per unit increase.

ILLUSTRATION OF THE POISSON REGRESSION MODEL

Before exploring the Poisson regression model in detail, the basic properties are illustrated by a small artificial example. Artificial data consisting of the counts of deaths and the person-time-at-risk from two populations classified into four age strata are contained in Table 6–1.

A traditional summary value used to compare two sets of mortality rates is the *standard mortality ratio (SMR)*. This statistical summary, calculated from the hypothetical data using population 1 as a standard and applying these age-specific rates to the age-specific counts in population 2, produces an expected number of deaths and a standard mortality ratio comparison of

$$
\begin{aligned}
SMR &= \frac{observed\ deaths\ population\ 2}{expected\ deaths\ population\ 2} \\
&= \frac{0.001(10000) + 0.00083(12000) + 0.002(20000) + 0.008(10000)}{0.002(10000) + 0.0017(12000) + 0.004(20000) + 0.016(10000)} \\
&= \frac{10 + 10 + 40 + 80}{20 + 20 + 80 + 160} = \frac{140}{280} = 0.5.
\end{aligned}
$$

Table 6–1. Artificial age-specific mortality rates per 100,000 person-years created to have exactly constant rate-ratios (exactly homogeneous)

Age	Population 1			Population 2			Ratios
	Deaths	At-risk	Rates*	Deaths	At-risk	Rates*	
40–50	400	200,000	200.0	10	10,000	100.0	0.5
50–60	600	360,000	166.7	10	12,000	83.3	0.5
60–70	2000	500,000	400.0	40	20,000	200.0	0.5
70–80	3200	200,000	1600.0	80	10,000	800.0	0.5

* Per 100,000 person-years

A SMR is a single-value summary of the strata-specific rate-ratios and, in this artificial example, perfectly reflects the common rate-ratio (0.5). The SMR is "adjusted" in the sense that the compared observed and expected counts of deaths have the same age distributions, namely the age distribution of population 2.

Using a Poisson model to estimate a parallel summary mortality rate-ratio serves as an introduction to the application of Poisson regression tools. An additive model defined in terms of the logarithms of the strata-specific rates is given by

$$log\text{-}rate = a + bF + c_1z_1 + c_2z_2 + c_3z_3$$

and exactly represents the theoretical relationships described in detail in Table 6–2. The variable $F = 0$ indicates population 1 and $F = 1$ indicates population 2. The values z_1, z_2, and z_3 are components of a design variable used to identify each of the four age strata. The model produces values for the log-rates constructed from the five parameters (a, b, c_1, c_2, and c_3). This additive regression model dictates perfect homogeneity among the rate-ratios. That is, the parameter b is the constant difference between the logarithms of the rates within each of the four age strata. The quantity e^b then becomes the summary rate-ratio ratio and is necessarily also constant (exactly no interaction). The parameters c_i reflect the influences of the age strata, and e^{c_i} is the ratio of age-specific rates within each population relative the referent age stratum (age 40–50). The model coefficients can be directly calculated from the data (Table 6–3) because of the perfect correspondence between "data" and model (no random variation).

For the example, the value $\hat{c}_3 = log(3200/400) = log(80/10) = 2.079$, or the rate in the last age category is eight times the rate in first age category ($e^{2.079} = 8$) within both populations. The model-produced summary rate-ratio is $e^{\hat{b}} = e^{-0.693} = 0.5$, and this ratio is identical to the model-free SMR because the four age-specific rate-ratio are exactly 0.5.

Table 6–2. Additive Poisson model: theoretical
relationships between the log-rate and age for two populations
with a constant age-specific mortality ratio

Age	Population 1 Log-rate	Population 2 Log-rate	Difference
40–50	a	$a + b$	b
50–60	$a + c_1$	$a + b + c_1$	b
60–70	$a + c_2$	$a + b + c_2$	b
70–80	$a + c_3$	$a + b + c_3$	b

Table 6–3. The coefficients from the hypothetical data,
two sampled populations classified into four age strata

Variables	Terms	Estimates
Constant	a	−6.215
Population	b	−0.693
Age 50–60	c_1	−0.182
Age 60–70	c_2	0.693
Age 70–80	c_3	2.079

POISSON REGRESSION MODEL: HODGKIN DISEASE MORTALITY

The Poisson regression model and a sample of Hodgkin disease mortality data illustrate the comparison of risk between two groups (males and females) while accounting for influences of another variable (age). More traditional methods that account for the influence of differing age distributions on the comparison of mortality or disease rates employ model-free direct-adjustment or indirect-adjustment techniques, such as an SMR. Regardless of the analytic approach, the underlying rate-ratios are required to be the same for all age strata (differ by chance alone) to create a single accurate summary of the difference in risk. However, model-free methods give no indication whether the requirement is realistic. In addition, traditional approaches provide summaries of mortality risk as if the influences of differing age distributions were eliminated, but it is frequently useful to understand the role of age in creating and interpreting the summary rate or rate-ratio.

A Poisson regression model allows a statistical assessment of the requirement of constant age-specific rate-ratios. A model approach also provides a variety of ways to identify and adjust for the influences from differing age distributions. Furthermore, when the rate-ratios are constant, a model approach yields a simple and easily interpreted age-adjusted summary of the difference in risk between the

Table 6–4. Hodgkin disease deaths, mortality rates (per 1,000,000 person-years), and rate-ratios for males and females, California, 1989

Age	Males			Females			Ratios
	Deaths	At-risk	Rates	Deaths	At-risk	Rates	
30–34	50	1,299,868	38.5	37	1,300,402	28.5	1.352
35–39	49	1,240,595	39.5	29	1,217,896	23.8	1.659
40–44	38	1,045,453	36.3	23	1,045,801	22.0	1.653
45–49	26	795,776	32.7	12	810,260	14.8	2.206
50–54	19	645,991	29.4	7	665,612	10.5	2.797
55–59	17	599,729	28.3	12	633,646	18.9	1.497
60–64	22	568,109	38.7	9	650,686	13.8	2.800
65–69	21	506,475	41.5	19	600,455	31.6	1.310
70–74	18	368,751	48.8	13	474,609	27.4	1.782
75–79	11	252,581	43.6	14	376,781	37.2	1.172
80–84	10	140,053	71.4	5	255,412	19.6	3.647
>85	4	81,850	48.9	3	313,603	9.6	5.109
Total	285	7,545,231	37.8	183	8,345,163	21.9	1.772

compared groups, as well as providing natural assessments of the influence of sampling variation (primarily, statistical tests or confidence intervals).

Hodgkin disease mortality data (Table 6–4) illustrate the application of the Poisson model to the classic problem of providing an age-adjusted comparison of mortality risk between populations with differing age distributions.

Three choices of possible additive Poisson models are:

$$log\text{-}rate = log(R) = a + bF + c_1 z_1 + c_2 z_2 + c_3 z_3 + \cdots + c_{11} z_{11},$$

$$log\text{-}rate = log(R) = a + bF + c(age), \quad and$$

$$log\text{-}rate = log(R) = a + bF + c_1(age) + c_2(age)^2 + c_3(age)^3.$$

The symbol F represents a binary variable ($F = 0 =$ female or $F = 1 =$ male) indicating group membership and R represents an age-specific mortality rate.

The first model characterizes the influences from age with a design variable made up of 11 components. This design variable accounts for the influences of age on the Hodgkin disease log-rate, allowing an age-adjusted estimate of the difference between two groups in terms of a single model parameter b. That is, the difference between male and female model-generated log-rates is the same in all age-specific stratum, making e^b a single summary age-adjusted male–female rate-ratio. Geometrically, the pattern of mortality is represented by two lines separated by the constant distance, b, at each of the 12 age-specific categories (Figure 6–1,

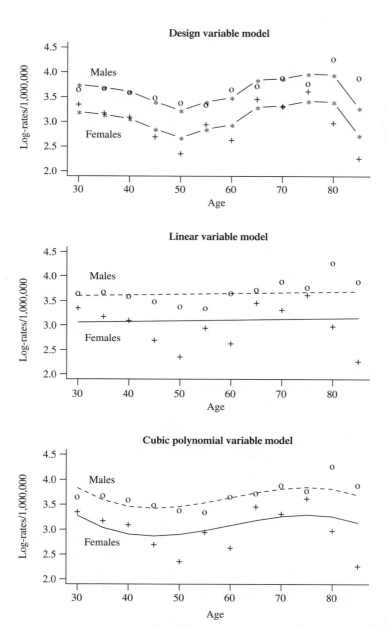

Figure 6–1. Three additive Poisson models for describing sex-specific Hodgkin disease mortality by age, California, 1989.

top). When the number of age strata is large, a multilevel design variable leads to a cumbersome summary of the role of age in terms of an unconstrained categorical variable.

A second model requires the variable age to have a direct and linear influence on the log-rates. This model also provides a single summary male–female rate-ratio accounting for influences from differing age distributions. Specifically, the additive regression models

$$log\text{-}rate(F = 1) = log(R_1) = a + b(1) + c(age)$$

and

$$log\text{-}rate(F = 0) = log(R_0) = a + b(0) + c(age)$$

produce the constant rate-ratio because

$$log(R_1) - log(R_0) = b$$
$$\text{or} \quad log\left[\frac{R_1}{R_0}\right] = b \quad \text{giving a } rate\ ratio = \frac{R_1}{R_0} = e^b$$

for all age strata. The coefficient b represents the geometric distance between two parallel straight lines with slopes c (Figure 6–1, middle). Accounting for the influence age by a simple linear term ($c \times age$), however, is likely an inadequate description of the sometimes complex relationship between age and mortality/disease risk.

The influence of age can be incorporated into a regression model that is a compromise between using an extensive unconstrained design variable with 11 components and a highly constrained linear function. A third model characterizes the influences of age using the cubic polynomial $c_1 age + c_2 age^2 + c_3 age^3$. This more sophisticated but relatively simple expression provides substantial flexibility to describe the relationship between age and mortality/disease rates. In fact, this polynomial representation includes a linear influence as a special case ($c_2 = c_3 = 0$). As with the other two additive models, an age-adjusted summary of the difference in mortality/disease rates continues to be measured by the single coefficient b or by the rate-ratio e^b. That is, the additive model requires the pattern of mortality rates to be described by two curves separated by the constant distance b (Figures 6–1 and 6–2) for all age strata.

Small numbers of deaths, particularly in the older age groups, cause considerable sampling variation in the observed log-rates (Figure 6–2). Despite this variation, the influence of age appears nonlinear. The log-rates sightly decrease up to about age 50 and then increase for the older ages. The coefficients generated

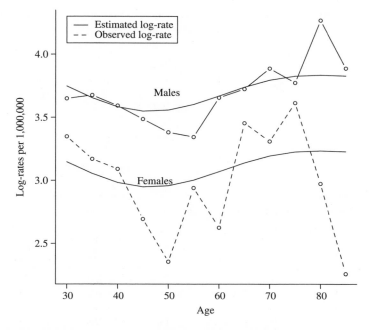

Figure 6–2.   Cubic polynomial model generated sex-specific Hodgkin disease mortality log-rates (solid lines) and observed log-rates by age, California, 1989.

by the cubic polynomial terms in the Poisson model provide an estimate of this nonlinear relationship and, because the model is additive, it is the same nonlinear relationship for both males and females. In other words, regardless of the age–risk relationship, the model estimated male–female rate-ratio is same for all ages.

A cubic polynomial representation of the influence of age and an additive Poisson model allow estimates of male and female age-specific mortality rates, and simply describes the role of age, and produces a single age-adjusted summary, namely the male–female rate-ratio. Of most importance, the model-estimated rates provide an evaluation of the key assumption that the underlying rate-ratios are the same among all age strata.

As with all model-based analyses, it is important to assess the accuracy of the postulated Poisson model as a representation of the pattern of mortality. The maximum likelihood estimated coefficients (Table 6–5), as usual, allow maximum likelihood estimates of Hodgkin disease sex and age-specific mortality rates that conform exactly to the additive model, producing exactly the same rate-ratio for all ages (Table 6–6, rate-ratio = 1.742). The log-rates, the rates, and the numbers of deaths in each of the 12 age strata directly follow from the model and the five model-estimated regression coefficients. For example, for males ($F = 1$) ages

Table 6–5. Poisson model: estimated model coefficients from Hodgkin disease mortality data by age and sex (Table 6–4)

Variables	Terms	Estimates	Std. errors
Constant	a	−5.409	1.881
Sex	b	0.555	0.095
Age-linear	c_1	−0.308	0.114
Age-quadratic	c_2	0.00547	0.00216
Age-cubic	c_3	−0.0000303	0.000013

LogLikelihood = −9.256

Table 6–6. Model estimated Hodgkin disease deaths, mortality rates (per 1,000,000 person-years), and rate-ratios for males and females, California, 1989

Age	Males Deaths	At-risk	Rates	Females Deaths	At-risk	Rates	Ratios
30–34	60.1	1,299,868	46.2	34.5	1,300,402	26.5	1.742
35–39	45.0	1,240,595	36.3	25.4	1,217,896	20.8	1.742
40–44	33.3	1,045,453	31.9	19.2	1,045,801	18.3	1.742
45–49	24.5	795,776	30.7	14.3	810,260	17.6	1.742
50–54	20.5	645,991	31.7	12.1	665,612	18.2	1.742
55–59	20.6	599,729	34.3	12.5	633,646	19.7	1.742
60–64	21.6	568,109	37.9	14.2	650,686	21.8	1.742
65–69	21.3	506,475	42.0	14.5	600,455	24.1	1.742
70–74	16.8	368,751	45.4	12.4	474,609	26.1	1.742
75–79	11.9	252,581	47.0	10.2	376,781	27.0	1.742
80–84	6.4	140,053	45.4	6.7	255412	26.1	1.742
85+	3.3	81,850	40.1	7.2	313,603	23.0	1.742
Total	285	7,545,231	37.8	183	8,345,163	21.9	1.772

60–64, the model estimated log-rate is

$$log\text{-}rate = \hat{a} + \hat{b}(1) + \hat{c}_1(60) + \hat{c}_2(60)^2 + \hat{c}_3(60)^3$$
$$= -5.409 + 0.555 - 18.464 + 19.696 - 6.555 = -10.179.$$

The estimated mortality rate becomes $e^{log\text{-}rate}$, or $rate = e^{-10.179} \times 1,000,000 = 37.937$ deaths per 1,000,000. To estimate the number of deaths for this age category, the estimated rate applied to the number of males at risk gives the model estimated number of deaths as $deaths = (37.937/1,000,000) \times 568,109 = 21.552$ (observed frequency = 22).

The same pattern, for females ($F = 0$) ages 60–64, produces the corresponding estimates. The estimated log-rate is

$$log\text{-}rate = \hat{a} + \hat{b}(0) + \hat{c}_1(60) + \hat{c}_2(60)^2 + \hat{c}_3(60)^3$$
$$= -5.409 - 18.464 + 19.696 - 6.555 = -10.734$$

and the model estimated mortality rate becomes $rate = e^{-10.734} \times 1,000,000 = 21.784$ deaths per 1,000,000. Applying this estimated rate to the number of females at risk gives the estimated number of deaths as $deaths = (21.784/1,000,000) \times 650,686 = 14.174$ (observed frequency $= 9$).

The model-estimated rate-ratio is $37.937/21.784 = 1.742$. Because the male–female rate-ratio is not influenced by age (additive model), all 12 age-specific model-estimated rate-ratio are identical and equal 1.742 (Table 6–6). From another perspective, the difference in male–female log-rates is $\hat{b} = 0.555$ regardless of the value of the polynomial representation of age. In more detail, additivity requires that every age stratum produce exactly the same male–female ratio and, for ages 60–64,

$$log\text{-}rate(males) - log\text{-}rate(females) = -10.179 - (-10.734) = 0.555 = \hat{b},$$

and the estimate rate-ratio is then $e^{\hat{b}} = e^{0.555} = 1.742$ for all age-strata (Table 6–6).

The usefulness of this single estimated rate-ratio as a summary of the male–female Hodgkin disease mortality pattern depends on the accuracy (goodness-of-fit) of the postulated additive Poisson regression model. Specifically, if the rate-ratio is not constant (the additive model fails), then a single summary rate-ratio is likely misleading. The usual Pearson goodness-of-fit chi-square analysis supplies a test statistic to evaluate the correspondence between the observed and model-estimated sex- and age-specific counts of deaths. The strata-specific numbers of deaths (Table 6–4) compared directly to the corresponding model-generated estimates (Table 6–6) produce the chi-square test statistic

$$X^2 = \sum \frac{(o_i - e_i)^2}{e_i} = \frac{(50 - 60.1)^2}{60.1} + \frac{(49 - 45.0)^2}{45.0} + \cdots + \frac{(3 - 7.2)^2}{7.2} = 17.625$$

where the symbol o_i represents the 24 observed numbers of deaths and e_i represents the 24 theoretical numbers of deaths estimated from the additive model. The test statistic $X^2 = 17.625$ is an observation from a chi-square distribution with 19 degrees of freedom when all observed and model-estimated values differ by chance alone. The degrees of freedom are the number of observations (24) minus the number of model parameters (5). A p-value of $P(X^2 \geq 17.625|$ $random\ differences\ only) = 0.548$ supports the use of the estimated additive model as a simple and effective description of the influences of sex and age on the pattern of Hodgkin disease mortality. Therefore, the estimated rate-ratio 1.742 is likely a useful and credible summary.

The model is additive even though it contains nonlinear terms. Additivity refers to the relationship among the variables in the model and does not refer to how the variables themselves are represented. Thus, the theoretical influence of sex on the rate of Hodgkin disease mortality is separate and constant, regardless of the postulated pattern of the influence of age, as long as the model is additive. The curves in Figures 6–1 and 6–2 are the geometric consequence of this additivity, as noted earlier. For all ages, the distance between the age-specific male and female curves (solid line, Figure 6–2) is the same ($\hat{b} = 0.555$), making the rate-ratio of males to females the constant value 1.742 ($e^{\hat{b}} = e^{0.555} = 1.742$). For contrast, the classic standard mortality ratio comparing male-to-female Hodgkin mortality experience is SMR = 1.713.

This Poisson model-estimated ratio is said to be adjusted for the influences of any differences in the male–female age distributions. The estimated and necessarily constant summary rate-ratio of 1.742 (male–female) shows substantially greater mortality among males. Although the precision of this estimate is not much of an issue because the data set contains millions of observations, the 95% confidence interval based on the estimate $\hat{b} = 0.555$ ($S_{\hat{b}} = 0.095$) is

$$lower\ bound = \hat{A} = 0.555 - 1.960(0.095) = 0.368 \quad and$$
$$upper\ bound = \hat{B} = 0.555 + 1.960(0.095) = 0.742.$$

The approximate 95% confidence interval based on the estimated rate-ratio of $e^{0.555} = 1.742$ is then ($e^{0.368}$, $e^{0.742}$) = (1.445, 2.099).

The direct comparison of the "crude" rate-ratio (Table 6–4, 1.772; ignoring the age influences) and the age-adjusted rate-ratio (Table 6–6, 1.742; accounting for the age influences) clearly shows that differences in the male–female age distributions have almost no confounding influence on the comparison of male and female Hodgkin disease mortality risk. That is, essentially the same estimated rate-ratio is directly calculated, ignoring the variable age (*rate-ratio* = 37.777/21.928 = 1.722, Table 6–4).

THE SIMPLEST POISSON REGRESSION MODEL: THE 2 × 2 TABLE

An estimate of the relative risk from a 2 × 2 table (Chapter 1) based on a Poisson model follows essentially the same pattern as the estimation of an odds ratio based on a logistic model (Chapter 4). The Poisson model link function is the logarithm of the dependent variable, in this case the logarithm of a probability.

When the risk factor and disease are binary variables, the regression model is

$$log(p_F) = a + bF$$

where, once again, $F = 0$ indicates that the risk factor is absent, $F = 1$ indicates that the risk factor is present, and p_F represents the probability of disease. Therefore, the two log-probabilities associated with the absence and presence of the risk factor in terms of the model parameters are

$$risk\ factor\ absent\ or\ F = 0: \ \ log(p_0) = a$$

and

$$risk\ factor\ present\ or\ F = 1: \ \ log(p_1) = a + b.$$

These two log-probabilities of disease then produce the following estimate of the relative risk where

$$log(p_1) - log(p_0) = (a + b) - a = b = log\left[\frac{p_1}{p_0}\right] = log(rr)$$

and, therefore,

$$relative\ risk = rr = e^b.$$

The 2×2 table generated from the WCGS data (Table 4–3 or Table 6–7) describing behavior type and coronary heart disease (CHD) illustrate. The model parameter $F = \{0, 1\}$ indicates type-B and type-A individuals, respectively.

For the behavior–CHD data, the probability of a CHD event among type-B individuals is denoted p_B and among type-A individuals as p_A, making the relative risk

$$relative\ risk = rr = \frac{P(CHD|type\text{-}A\ individual)}{P(CHD|type\text{-}B\ individual)} = \frac{p_A}{p_B}.$$

The maximum likelihood estimates of the two model parameters produce the estimates of the relative risk and its variance (Table 6–8).

Table 6–7. CHD by A/B behavior type (repeated from Chapter 4)

	CHD	No CHD	Total
Type-A	178	1411	1589
Type-B	79	1486	1565
Total	257	2897	3154

Table 6–8. CHD by A/B-behavior type: a two parameter Poisson model
applied to the WCGS data

Variables	Terms	Estimates	Std. errors	p-Values	$\hat{rr}$
Constant	a	−2.986	0.113	–	–
A/B	b	0.797	0.135	<0.001	2.219

Directly from the model estimate $\hat{b}$,

$$estimated\ relative\ risk = \hat{rr} = e^{\hat{b}} = e^{0.797} = 2.219,$$

and the estimated probabilities of a CHD event for type-B (p_B) and type-A (p_A) individuals are

$$F = 0: \quad \hat{p}_B = e^{\hat{a}} = e^{-2.986} = 0.051 \quad \text{and}$$
$$F = 1: \quad \hat{p}_A = e^{\hat{a} + \hat{b}} = e^{-2.986 + 0.797} = 0.112.$$

These estimated probabilities are identical to the values calculated directly from the data ($\hat{p}_B = 179/1565 = 0.051$ and $\hat{p}_A = 178/1589 = 0.112$) because the model is saturated. There are two observed probabilities, and the model contains two parameters. Necessarily, the same estimated relative risk also follows directly from the 2×2 table ($\hat{rr} = \hat{p}_A/\hat{p}_B = 0.112/0.051 = 2.219$).

The approximate 95% confidence interval based on the estimate $\hat{b}$ and the normal distribution is $\hat{b} \pm 1.960 S_{\hat{b}}$ and $0.797 \pm 1.960(0.135)$ or (0.532, 1.062). The approximate 95% confidence interval for the relative risk based on the estimate $\hat{rr} = 2.219$ becomes ($e^{0.532}$, $e^{1.062}$) or (1.703, 2.892).

Along the same lines, the usual Wald chi-square test statistic

$$X^2 = \left[\frac{\hat{b} - 0}{0.135} \right]^2 = 34.766$$

leaves little doubt that the observed relative risk ($\hat{rr} = 2.219$) is not a random deviation from 1.0 (p-value <0.001). Because the frequency of a CHD event is relatively rare, the estimated odds ratio is expectedly greater but similar to the estimated relative risk ($\hat{or} = 2.373$ and $\hat{rr} = 2.219$, Chapter 1).

APPLICATION OF THE POISSON REGRESSION MODEL: CATEGORICAL DATA

Consider again the relationship between smoking exposure, behavior type, and the risk of a coronary disease event. The WCGS data described earlier (Chapter 4) are again used to illustrate (Table 6–9).

A Poisson regression model that postulates additive influences of behavior type and smoking exposure on the log-probability of a coronary event is

$$log\text{-}probability = a + bF + c_1z_1 + c_2z_2 + c_3z_3$$

where F represents behavior type ($F = 1 = $ type-A and $F = 0 = $ type-B) and the values z_1, z_2, and z_3 are the components of a design variable incorporating the four levels of smoking exposure into the regression model as an unconstrained categorical variable. Furthermore, the model requires that the number of coronary events in each of the eight smoking categories ($70, 45, 34, \cdots, 94$) result from sampling Poisson distributions. The maximum likelihood estimates of the five model coefficients ($a, b, c_1, c_2,$ and c_3) provide a succinct summary description of the influence of behavior type and smoking on the likelihood of a CHD event (Table 6–10).

As with the analysis of rates, the model-generated probabilities are directly calculated from the estimated model parameters. For example, the log-probability associated with a heavy smoker (>30 cigarettes per day) who is a type-A individual is estimated by

$$log\text{-}probability = \hat{a} + \hat{b} + \hat{c}_3 = -3.248 + 0.747 + 0.695 = -1.806$$

Table 6–9. WCGS data: probability of a CHD event by smoking exposure and A/B-behavior type

Type-A	Nonsmoker	1–20	21–30	>30
		Cigarettes smoked per day		
CHD	70	45	34	29
No CHD	714	353	185	159
Probability	0.089	0.113	0.155	0.154

Type-B	Nonsmoker	1–20	21–30	>30
CHD	28	25	16	10
No CHD	840	382	170	94
Probability	0.032	0.061	0.086	0.096

Table 6–10.   CHD data classified by behavior and smoking exposure: coefficients estimated from an additive Poisson model

Variables	Terms	Estimates	Std. errors	Relative risks
Constant	a	−3.248	0.135	–
A/B	b	0.747	0.136	2.111
Smoking (1–20)	c_1	0.368	0.157	1.445
Smoking (21–30)	c_2	0.686	0.174	1.986
Smoking (>30)	c_3	0.695	0.190	2.005

Table 6–11.   Observed and estimated counts and probabilities of CHD events by behavior type and smoking exposure (WCGS data, Chapter 4)

	Data				Model		
	At-risk	Probability	CHD	No CHD	Probability	CHD	No CHD
Type-A, nonsmoker	784	0.089	70	714	0.082	64.3	719.7
Type-A, 1–20	398	0.113	45	353	0.118	47.2	350.8
Type-A, 21–30	219	0.155	34	185	0.163	35.7	183.3
Type-A, >30	188	0.154	29	159	0.164	30.9	157.1
Type-B, nonsmoker	868	0.032	28	840	0.039	33.7	834.3
Type-B, 1–20	407	0.061	25	382	0.056	22.8	384.2
Type-B, 21–30	186	0.086	16	170	0.077	14.3	171.7
Type-B, >30	104	0.096	10	94	0.078	8.1	95.9

yielding an estimated probability of a CHD event of $\hat{P}(CHD|type\text{-}A \ and > 30$ cigarettes$) = e^{-1.806} = 0.164$. This estimated probability produces $0.164(188) = 30.9$ CHD events theoretically occurring among type-A heavy smokers. The corresponding observed number is 29. Observed and model-estimated counts (numbers of CHD cases and non-cases) for all eight behavior–smoking categories are displayed in Table 6–11.

A comparison of the 16 observed and model-estimated values provides evidence that the proposed additive Poisson model is a faithful representation of the relationships within the observed data. Once again, a formal comparison using the Pearson chi-square test statistic yields a statistically rigorous contrast (Table 6–11) where

$$X^2 = \frac{(70 - 64.286)^2}{64.286} + \frac{(45 - 47.156)^2}{47.156} + \cdots + \frac{(94 - 95.902)^2}{95.902} = 2.812.$$

The test-statistic X^2 has an approximate chi-square distribution with three degrees of freedom, yielding a p-value of $P(X^2 \geq 2.812|no \ association) = 0.421$ (*degrees of freedom* = number of probabilities – number of model parameters = $8 - 5 = 3$).

An additive Poisson model provides estimates of the separate influences of behavior type (b) and cigarette exposure (c_i). The influence of behavior type is summarized by the estimated relative risk ratio

$$\frac{\hat{P}(CHD|A)}{\hat{P}(CHD|B)} = \frac{e^{\hat{a} + \hat{b}(1) + \hat{c}_i}}{e^{\hat{a} + \hat{b}(0) + \hat{c}_i}} = e^{\hat{b}} = e^{0.747} = 2.111$$

and is 2.111 regardless of the level of smoking exposure. For example, for heavy smokers, the model estimated A/B-relative risk ratio is 0.164/0.078 = 2.111, and for nonsmokers the relative risk ratio is identically 0.082/0.039 = 2.111 (Table 6–11).

The smoking exposure risks are similarly independent of behavior type. For example, the model-generated relative risk ratio reflecting the influence from smoking more than 30 cigarettes per day compared to a nonsmoker is

$$\frac{\hat{P}(CHD| > 30 \; cigarettes)}{\hat{P}(CHD|nonsmoker)} = \frac{e^{\hat{a} + \hat{b}F + \hat{c}_3}}{e^{\hat{a} + \hat{b}F}} = e^{\hat{c}_3} = e^{0.695} = 2.005.$$

More technically, because the model is additive, values of the regression model term bF do not influence the comparison of the CHD probabilities between smokers and nonsmokers. These relative risk ratios are, therefore, 0.164/0.082 = 0.078/0.039 = 2.005 (Table 6–11) for both type-A and type-B individuals. Furthermore, the joint estimated relative risk for type-A behavior and heavy smokers (>30) relative to type-B and nonsmokers is the product of the two individual risk ratios, where (2.111)(2.005) = 4.232 or 0.164/0.039 = 4.232, or

$$\frac{\hat{P}(CHD| > 30 \; cigarettes \; and \; type\text{-}A)}{\hat{P}(CHD|nonsmoker \; and \; type\text{-}B)} = \frac{e^{\hat{a} + b + \hat{c}_3}}{e^{\hat{a}}} = e^{\hat{b} + \hat{c}_3} = e^{\hat{b}}e^{\hat{c}_3}$$

$$= 2.111(2.005) = 4.232.$$

The estimated relative risk accurately summarizes the separate influences of behavior type and smoking exposure on the probability of a CHD event, as long as the additive model accurately represents the data. The analysis gives some evidence that additivity is the case.

APPLICATION OF THE POISSON REGRESSION MODEL: COUNT DATA

A table containing the counts (denoted n_i) of children under the age of 8 diagnosed with autism in California during the years 1987–1994 (Table 6–12 and Figure 6–3) illustrates another application of Poisson regression tools.

Table 6–12. Frequencies and log-frequencies of cases of autism in California by year (1987–1994)

	1987	1988	1989	1990	1991	1992	1993	1994
Counts (n_i)	192	248	293	382	559	623	633	599
Log-counts	5.257	5.513	5.680	5.945	6.326	6.435	6.450	6.395

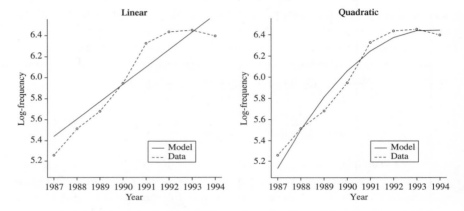

Figure 6–3. Autism data: linear and quadratic Poisson regression models.

A linear log-frequency regression model potentially summarizing the trend in the cases of autism data is

$$log\text{-}frequency = log(n_i) = a + b\ year_i$$

where the variable $year_i$ takes on the values $1987 = 1, 1988 = 2, 1989 = 3, \ldots, 1994 = 8$. The years-variable is analyzed as the difference ($years - 1986$) to improve the computational accuracy and, as noted earlier, does not affect the analytic results (Chapter 2). The maximum likelihood estimated parameters that describe this linear model are given in Table 6–13.

Using the estimated model $log(\hat{n}_i) = 5.276 + 0.165\ year_i$ produces estimated counts of autistic children for each year (Table 6–14 and Figure 6–3). The estimated log-frequencies increase 0.165 cases per year and, because the model requires a linear increase, the increase is 0.165 every year. The model-generated log-frequencies, therefore, produce model-generated counts that increase by a factor of $e^{0.165} = 1.179$ cases per year. That is, over an 8-year period, the log-linear

Table 6–13. Two-parameter Poisson linear model: autism by year of diagnosis

Variables	Terms	Estimates*	Std. errors	p-Values
Constant	a	5.276	0.044	–
Year	b	0.165	0.008	<0.001

LogLikelihood = –40.371

* = Years coded 1, 2, ... , 8 for computation accuracy

Table 6–14. Cases of autistic children during the period 1987–1994 predicted by a linear Poisson model

	1987	1988	1989	1990	1991	1992	1993	1994
Observed (n_i)	192	248	293	382	559	623	633	599
Predicted ($\log[\hat{n}_i]$)	5.441	5.606	5.771	5.936	6.101	6.266	6.431	6.596
Predicted ($\hat{n}_i$)	230.8	272.2	321.0	378.6	446.5	526.6	621.0	732.5

model predicts that the number of affected children would increase by a factor of $(1.179)^8 = 3.733$. The observed increase is $599/192 = 3.120$.

A comparison of the model-estimated and the observed counts (Table 6–12 or Figure 6–3) suggests that the straight line representing the estimated log-frequencies does not accurately characterize the observed pattern over the 8-year period. The log-frequency increase appears roughly constant from 1991 to 1994, after a striking linear increase during the period 1987 to 1991 (Figure 6–3).

Inspection of the apparent lack of fit suggests that adding a quadratic term to the linear model will improve the representation of the trend in the log-frequency of cases of autism. Such a log-frequency model is

$$log\text{-}frequency = log(n_i) = a + b\,year_i + c\,year_i^2$$

where the variable $year_i$ again takes on the values 1987 = 1, 1988 = 2, ..., 1994 = 8. The maximum likelihood parameter estimates for this quadratic model are given in Table 6–15. The estimated quadratic model $log(\hat{n}_i) = 4.700 + 0.462$ $year_i - 0.031$ $year_i^2$ considerably improves the correspondence of the observed and estimated counts of autistic children (Table 6–16 and Figure 6–3).

The assumption that Poisson distributions describe the number of observed autism cases per year is not critically important. The goal of the analysis is a clear visual description of the pattern of increase in autism cases (Figure 6–3, bottom). No inferences (for example, statistical tests or confidence intervals) based

Table 6–15. Three-parameter Poisson quadratic regression model: autism by year of diagnosis

Variables	Terms	Estimates*	Std. errors
Constant	a	4.700	–
Year	b	0.462	–
Year^2	c	–0.031	0.004

LogLikelihood $= -10.283$
* $= Years$ coded 1, 2, ... , 8 for computation accuracy

Table 6–16. Cases of autistic children for the years 1987–1994 predicted by a quadratic Poisson model

	1987	1988	1989	1990	1991	1992	1993	1994
Observed (n_i)	192	248	293	382	559	623	633	599
Predicted ($\log[\hat{n}_i]$)	5.132	5.502	5.811	6.059	6.246	6.372	6.437	6.441
Predicted ($\hat{n}_i$)	169.3	245.2	334.0	428.0	516.0	585.2	624.5	626.8

on estimated variances are made. Chance variability in the counts is not a primary issue, and it is the assessment of this variation that is sensitive to assumptions about the sampled populations.

One additional point: A quadratic term in a regression model is a specific kind of interaction. The model is no longer additive. Rewriting the Poisson quadratic regression model as

$$log\text{-}frequency = a + b\,year + c\,year^2$$
$$= a + (b + c\,year) \times year$$

shows that the influence of the variable *year* depends on the level of the variable itself. No longer does a single coefficient reflect the increase in autism. The increase in influence of variable *year* on the count of autism cases decreases as the *year* increase because the coefficient $(b + \hat{c}\,year)$ decreases $(c < 0)$. For example, for the *year* = 1987, the coefficient is $\hat{b} + \hat{c}\,year = 0.462 - 0.031(1) = 0.431$ and for the *year* = 1994, the coefficient is $\hat{b} + \hat{c}\,year = 0.462 - 0.031(8) = 0.214$, half the 1987 influence. The quadratic term in the model causes variable *year* to "interact" with itself. That is, the variable *year* and $(year)^2$ have a joint (nonadditive) influence.

POISSON REGRESSION EXAMPLE: ADJUSTED PERINATAL MORTALITY RATES

A Poisson regression model provides a statistically rigorous answer to the question: Do African-America newborn infants experience lower perinatal mortality than white infants after accounting for their generally lower birth weights?

A perinatal mortality "rate" is defined as the number of infant deaths occurring between birth and 28 days of life, plus the number of fetal deaths divided by the number of live births, plus the number of fetal deaths. A perinatal "rate" is not a rate but rather an estimate of the probability of a perinatal death, traditionally called a rate. All African-American and white live births plus fetal deaths reported during the year 1988 on California birth and death certificates allow the comparison of race-specific perinatal mortality risk. During 1988, a total of 448,379 births and fetal deaths occurred (44,356 African-America and 404,023 white infants). Birth certificates contain the mother's race/ethnicity (reported by the mother) and her infant's weight at birth (recorded in grams). The California perinatal data are given in Table 6–17, where the number of births and deaths are tabulated by race and classified into 100-gram birth weight intervals (less than 800 grams, 801 to 900 grams, ..., 4201 to 4300 grams).

The 70 race- and weight-specific categories contain the number of perinatal deaths, the number of live births plus fetal deaths (labeled "births"), and the perinatal mortality rates for white and black infants. The overall perinatal mortality rate among black infants is $(520/44,356) \times 1000 = 11.723$ deaths per 1000 births and among white infants it is $(2,897/404,023) \times 1000 = 7.170$ deaths per 1000 births. Thus, the overall black/white perinatal mortality rate-ratio is $11.723/7.170 = 1.635$.

Black newborn infants weigh less, on average, than white newborn infants (mean values: $\bar{x}_{black} = 3143.2$ grams and $\bar{x}_{white} = 3403.4$ grams) and for all infants, lower birth weight is associated with higher mortality. The two birth-weight distributions are displayed in Figure 6–4 (kernel smoothing, Chapter 10).

An important question, therefore, is: What racial differences in perinatal mortality would exist if the birth-weight distributions were the same for black and white infants? More technically, the question becomes: What is the weight-adjusted black/white perinatal mortality rate-ratio?

First Approach: Weight-Specific Comparisons

A direct and easily applied contrast of perinatal mortality risk essentially unaffected by differences in birth-weight distributions is accomplished by directly comparing black to white mortality rates within each birth-weight category

Table 6–17. Perinatal deaths, births, rates/1000 and rate-ratio (black/white) for 35 birth-weight categories (grams)

Weights	White infants			Black infants			Ratio
	Deaths	Births	Rate	Deaths	Births	Rate	
800–900	173	322	537.27	65	131	496.18	0.924
901–1000	148	337	439.17	40	122	327.87	0.747
1001–1100	134	398	336.68	30	131	229.01	0.680
1101–1200	106	381	278.22	29	137	211.68	0.761
1201–1300	103	444	231.98	21	143	146.85	0.633
1301–1400	86	427	201.41	19	143	132.87	0.660
1401–1500	108	597	180.90	19	165	115.15	0.637
1501–1600	85	560	151.79	20	167	119.76	0.789
1601–1700	84	682	123.17	24	219	109.59	0.890
1701–1800	86	722	119.11	12	194	61.86	0.519
1801–1900	100	935	106.95	26	298	87.25	0.816
1901–2000	81	978	82.82	15	299	50.17	0.606
2001–2100	74	1589	46.57	21	420	50.00	1.074
2101–2200	87	1714	50.76	10	453	22.08	0.435
2201–2300	82	2322	35.31	14	603	23.22	0.657
2301–2400	80	2885	27.73	12	763	15.73	0.567
2401–2500	80	4149	19.28	13	977	13.31	0.690
2501–2600	77	4916	15.66	14	1189	11.77	0.752
2601–2700	93	7455	12.47	10	1654	6.05	0.485
2701–2800	93	8855	10.50	17	1796	9.47	0.901
2801–2900	100	14,197	7.04	11	2545	4.32	0.614
2901–3000	86	17,903	4.80	9	2947	3.05	0.636
3001–3100	92	19,969	4.61	12	2851	4.21	0.914
3101–3200	90	27,068	3.32	9	3557	2.53	0.761
3201–3300	96	29,107	3.30	9	3324	2.71	0.821
3301–3400	79	35,627	2.22	11	3577	3.08	1.387
3401–3500	67	32,926	2.03	1	3119	0.32	0.158
3501–3600	69	36,360	1.90	9	2952	3.05	1.607
3601–3700	58	30,612	1.89	7	2250	3.11	1.642
3701–3800	59	32,119	1.84	2	2176	0.92	0.500
3801–3900	40	24,004	1.67	3	1573	1.91	1.145
3901–4000	35	23,217	1.51	1	1348	0.74	0.492
4001–4100	30	16,232	1.85	3	909	3.30	1.786
4101–4200	19	14,233	1.33	1	735	1.36	1.019
4201–4300	17	9,781	1.74	1	489	2.04	1.177
Total	2,897	404,023	7.17	520	44,356	11.72	1.635

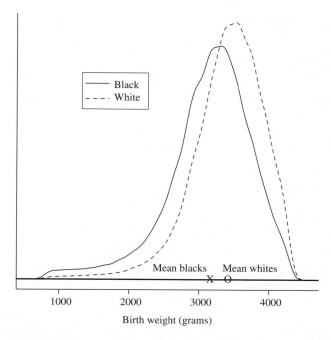

Figure 6–4. The distributions of birth weights of white and African-American infants.

(weight stratum). Differences between black and white birth weights within a 100-gram range are small and negligible. In terms of the weight-specific rate-ratios (*black rate/white rate*), 27 out of 35 perinatal mortality rate-ratios are less than 1 (*black rate < white rate*). These ratios are not influenced by differences in black–white birth weights because each of the 35 comparisons is between groups of infants with mean birth weights that are essentially the same (balanced). The fact that about 80% of weight-specific rates or rate-ratios show black infants with lower perinatal mortality is a persuasive indication that, after equalizing for birth-weight differences, black infants have consistently lower perinatal mortality. In other words, when infants of the same birth weights are compared, the black infants are more likely to survive, particularly black infants with low and extremely low birth weights. Figure 6–5 displays the black and white perinatal mortality rates by birth weight. Clearly, the black perinatal mortality rates (solid line) are generally below the white rates (dashed line) for most birth weights.

A more detailed view of these strata-specific differences is achieved by comparing the logarithms of the rates. Figure 6–6 is a plot of the logarithms of the perinatal mortality rates by birth weight over a reduced range, creating a clearer picture of the black–white mortality patterns, especially for the extreme birth weights. Contrasting log-rates, birth weight for birth weight, necessarily produces

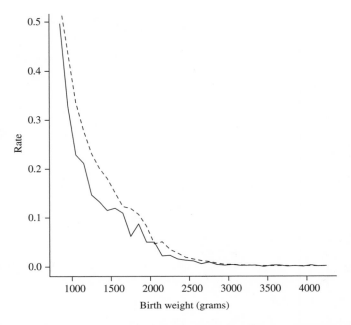

Figure 6–5. Perinatal mortality rates by birth weight for African-American versus white infants, 1988.

the same number of observed black–white mortality differences (27 lower black log-rates out of 35) but on a more visually sensitive scale. For example, on the log-scale, black perinatal mortality rates clearly fluctuate above the white rates among infants only in the neighborhood of birth weights of 4,000 grams, where these rates are highly unstable due to extremely small numbers of black perinatal deaths (a total of five black and 2133 white deaths). This feature of the relationship between white and black mortality rates among the high-birth-weight infants is essentially invisible when the rates are directly plotted (Figure 6–5).

The last column in Table 6–17 contains the weight-specific white–black perinatal rate-ratios for the 35 birth-weight categories. To accurately summarize these values with a single rate-ratio, it is necessary that the underlying ratio be the same for all birth-weight categories. The issue of a constant rate-ratio is directly explored with a graphic and simple approach. A line describing these ratios is estimated by assuming the ratios are constant and is compared to a line constructed directly from the rates themselves. Comparing these two lines gives an indication of the extent of homogeneity among the observed rate-ratios. The line representing constant rate-ratio is estimated from the simplest possible regression

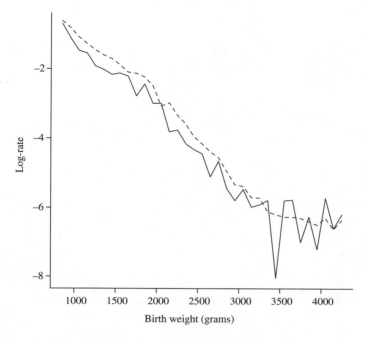

Figure 6–6. Perinatal mortality log-rates by birth weight for African-American versus white infants, 1988.

model, where the intercept is made equal to zero and

$$r_i^{(black)} = b r_i^{(white)} \quad \text{or} \quad \frac{r_i^{(black)}}{r_i^{(white)}} = b.$$

The notation $r_i^{(race)}$ represents the ith race- and weight-specific perinatal mortality rate. Ordinary least-squares estimation produces an estimate of the slope b (denoted $\hat{b}$) that accurately reflects the rate-ratio if in fact the rate-ratios are constant. Figure 6–7 displays the 35 pairs of white and black perinatal mortality rates $(r_i^{(white)}, r_i^{(black)})$ connected by a line (solid line), and the straight line is estimated as if the rate-ratios are constant (dashed line).

For the California perinatal mortality data, the estimate of the slope b is $\hat{b} = 0.782$ and is an accurate estimate of the constant perinatal mortality rate-ratio when the 35 differences between the observed ratios $r_i^{(black)}/r_i^{(white)}$ and the estimated value 0.782 are strictly random. In the following sections, two additional approaches describe estimates of this ratio and its statistical evaluation.

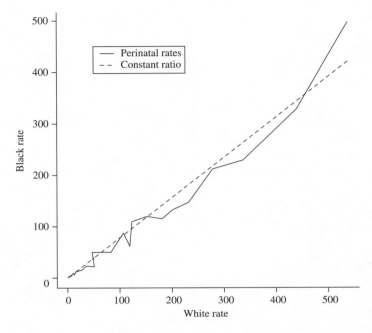

Figure 6–7. White and black perinatal mortality rates and the line estimated as if the rate-ratio is constant for all birth weights.

Second Approach: A Model-Free Summary

The 35 race- and weight-specific rate-ratios clearly reflect the black–white differences in perinatal risk but they are not a parsimonious summary description of the perinatal mortality pattern. In addition, no simple way exists to identify the influences of sampling variation on these 35 comparisons. A weighted average of the weight-specific rate-ratios, however, provides a single comprehensive summary ratio. Unlike 35 individual stratum comparisons, the influence of sampling variation is directly estimated, allowing a rigorous statistical evaluation.

Parallel to estimating a summary odds ratio (Chapter 2), it is statistically advantageous to consider the logarithms of the rate-ratios rather than the ratios themselves. Three specific reasons for this frequently used statistical strategy are:

1. A reduced range (less variability) makes a graphic display clearer by increasing the visibility of differences in the extreme ranges.
2. Log-rate-ratios convert multiplicative risk to an additive scale, making differences easier to describe and to statistically manipulate [ratios a/b become differences $log(a) - log(b)$].

3. Log-rates tend to have more symmetric and, therefore, more normal-like distributions producing more intuitive descriptions of their statistical properties.

Again, the symbol $r_i^{(race)}$ denotes the perinatal race-specific mortality rate from the ith birth weight category. Then, the estimated weight-specific rate-ratio contrasting black to white perinatal mortality rates is

$$\hat{R}_i = \frac{r_i^{(black)}}{r_i^{(white)}}$$

for the ith weight category. A weighted average of the logarithms of these estimated rate-ratios yields a single summary perinatal mortality log-rate-ratio of

$$\overline{log\text{-}R} = \frac{\sum w_i log(\hat{R}_i)}{\sum w_i}$$

where the weights w_i are the reciprocal values of the estimated variance of $log(\hat{R}_i)$.

In symbols, the weights are $w_i = 1/S^2_{log(\hat{R}_i)}$. Specifically, the estimated variances of the distributions of these weight-specific estimated log-rate-ratios are

$$S^2_{log(\hat{R}_i)} = \frac{1}{d_i^{(black)}} + \frac{1}{d_i^{(white)}}$$

where $d_i^{(race)}$ represents the number of race-specific perinatal deaths in the ith birth-weight category (Chapter 3).

For example, for the birth-weight category 2,501–2,600 grams ($i = 18$), the rate-ratio is

$$\hat{R}_{18} = \frac{\hat{r}_{18}^{(black)}}{\hat{r}_{18}^{(white)}} = \frac{14/1189}{77/4916} = \frac{11.775}{15.663} = 0.752,$$

and the log-rate-ratio becomes

$$log(\hat{R}_{18}) = log\left[\hat{r}_{18}^{(black)}\right] - log\left[\hat{r}_{18}^{(white)}\right]$$
$$= log(11.775) - log(15.663) = log(0.752) = -0.285.$$

An estimate of its associated variance is

$$S^2_{log(\hat{R}_{18})} = \frac{1}{d_{18}^{(black)}} + \frac{1}{d_{18}^{(white)}} = \frac{1}{14} + \frac{1}{77} = 0.084.$$

The weighted average of the logarithms of the 35 rate-ratios (Table 6–17, last column) is $log\text{-}\overline{R} = -0.261$, making $\overline{R} = e^{log\text{-}\overline{R}} = e^{-0.261} = 0.770$. That is, an estimate of the underlying ratio of black–white perinatal mortality rates is $\bar{R} = 0.770$. The black perinatal infant mortality rate is, on average, about three-quarters of the white rate after accounting for the influence of the remarkably lower birth weights among African-American infants.

This single weighted average is an unbiased summary of black–white perinatal mortality only when the rate-ratios from the 35 weight-specific categories are random fluctuations from the same underlying value. Said another way, the summary rate-ratio of 0.770 accurately indicates the black–white mortality differences only when race and birth weight have independent influences on perinatal mortality risk (homogeneous rate-ratios, no interaction). As always, for a single value to summarize usefully a series of values, it is necessary that the values combined are each an estimate of the same quantity.

The estimated variance of a weighed average in which the weights are the reciprocal of the estimated variances of the quantities being averaged is

$$variance(\overline{log\text{-}R}) = \frac{1}{\sum w_i} \qquad \text{(Chapter 2).}$$

For the black–white perinatal data, the estimated variance is

$$S^2_{\overline{log\text{-}R}} = \frac{1}{427.350} = 0.00234$$

making the standard error $S_{\overline{log\text{-}R}} = \sqrt{0.00234} = 0.048$.

The approximately symmetric (approximately normal) distribution associated with the logarithm of the summary rate-ratio allows the construction of an accurate but approximate confidence interval in the usual way. An approximate 95% confidence interval is

$$log\text{-}\bar{R} \pm 1.960 S_{\overline{log\text{-}R}} = -0.261 \pm 1.960(0.048) \quad \text{or} \quad (-0.355, \ -0.166),$$

based on the normal distribution and the estimate $\overline{log\text{-}R} = -0.261$. Because $\bar{R} = 0.770$ is $e^{\overline{log\text{-}R}}$, the approximate 95% confidence interval for the summary rate-ratio becomes

$$(e^{lower\ bound}, \ e^{upper\ bound}) = (e^{-0.355}, \ e^{-0.166}) = (0.701, \ 0.847).$$

Like all 95% confidence intervals, the probability that the interval $(0.701, 0.847)$ contains the value estimated by $\bar{R} = 0.770$ is approximately 0.95, providing a range of likely values for the underlying ratio of black to white perinatal mortality rates. The confidence interval provides definite assurance that the observed lower weight-adjusted mortality among the African-Americans is not an artifact of random variation.

Third Approach: Poisson Regression Model

Another approach to summarizing the black–white differences in perinatal mortality that accounts for the difference in birth-weight distributions is to employ a Poisson regression model. Such a model postulates a specific relationship between birth weight and race, thus making it possible to estimate, evaluate, and describe the separate influences on mortality from each of these two components. For the California birth/death certificate data, a potentially useful additive Poisson regression model is

$$log(r_{ij}) = a + bF_j + P(bwt_i) \quad j = 1, 2 \quad and \quad i = 1, 2, \cdots, 35$$

where $P(x) = c_1 x + c_2 x^2 + c_3 x^3 + c_4 x^4 + c_5 x^5$. The weight-specific perinatal mortality rate is denoted r_{ij} for the jth race in the ith birth-weight interval. The variable F is a binary indicator variable ($F_j = 1$ for African-American and $F_j = 0$ for white mother–infant pairs). A detailed description of the relationship between birth weight and perinatal mortality is not a primary interest and is pragmatically represented by a rather complex fifth-degree polynomial. Other functions could equally represent the independent (additive) influence of infant birth weight. The primary purpose of any expression chosen to characterize the pattern of mortality associated with birth weight is to provide a clear and focused description of the difference in black–white perinatal mortality. Geometrically, the complex polynomial function and the additive model allow the black and white log-rates to be accurately represented by the same relationship within both race categories; that is, two identical curves. The constant distance between these curves is a comparison of black–white perinatal mortality adjusted for birth weight. Thus, the model difference in log-rates (parameter denoted b) summarizes the black–white rate-ratio as if the perinatal mortality risk between infants were the same for all birth weights. In addition, the number of deaths in each of the 70 race- and weight-specific categories is postulated to have Poisson distributions. The additive regression model and the "Poisson assumption" make it possible to estimate the seven model coefficients and their standard errors (Table 6–18).

The Poisson model and its maximum likelihood estimated coefficients directly yield an estimate of the log-rate $[log(\hat{r}_{ij})]$ which, in turn, yields an estimate of the perinatal mortality rate ($\hat{r}_{ij}$), leading to model-estimated numbers of perinatal deaths in each race- and weight-specific category. For example, the white infant log-rate ($F = 0$) for the weight category 2001–2100 grams ($i = 18$) is estimated by

$$estimated\ log - rate = log(\hat{r}_{18}^{(white)}) = -3.994 - 0.290(0) + P(2050) = -4.152.$$

The model-estimated perinatal mortality rate is then $\hat{r}_{18}^{(white)} = e^{-4.152} \times 1000 = 15.732$ deaths per 1,000 births. The number of model-estimated perinatal

Table 6–18.   Estimated coefficients* from the Poisson regression model describing black–white perinatal mortality by birth weight

	Coefficient	Estimate	Std. error
Intercept	a	−3.994	–
Race	b	−0.290	0.048
Linear	c_1	−16.415	0.194
Quadratic	c_2	1.558	0.195
Cubic	c_3	2.035	0.186
Quartic	c_4	0.371	0.180
Quintic	c_5	−0.739	0.159

LogLikelihood $= -27.261$

* $=$ These coefficients result from a specialized numerical technique that allows for an extreme range of the values of the independent variables but does not change the analytic results.

deaths becomes this rate multiplied by the number of births or $\hat{d}_{18}^{(white)} = 0.0157(4916) = 77.3$. The corresponding observed quantities are $r_{18}^{(white)} = (77/4916) \times 1000 = 15.663$ deaths per 1000 births (perinatal mortality rate) and $d_{18}^{(white)} = 77$ perinatal deaths (Table 6–17).

Following the typical goodness-of-fit pattern, the 70 race- and weight-specific model-estimated numbers of perinatal deaths are compared to the 70 corresponding observed numbers of deaths. The comparison produces the chi-square test statistic of $X^2 = 56.216$ with 63 degrees of freedom. The degrees of freedom are the number of categories (rates) in the table minus the number of model parameters or $70 - 7 = 63$, yielding the p-value $P(X^2 \geq 56.216 \mid model\ is\ "correct") = 0.715$. As usual, the phrase "model is correct" means that all differences between observed and estimated numbers of deaths are due only to random variation. A p-value of 0.715 indicates a close correspondence between the model-estimated and the observed numbers of deaths, implying that the estimated coefficient ($\hat{b}$) from the additive model accurately summarizes the black–white perinatal mortality differences.

The generally excellent fit of the estimated Poisson regression model indicates that the relationships within the data are accurately separated into two components, one reflecting the influences of race and the other reflecting the influences of birth weight on the likelihood of a perinatal death. More specifically, the single coefficient $\hat{b}$ measures a constant black–white racial difference in risk. In terms of the model parameters, for the ith birth-weight category, the independent influence of race measured by the estimated log-rate difference is

$$log(\hat{R}_i) = log(\hat{r}_i^{(black)}) - log(\hat{r}_i^{(white)})$$
$$= [\hat{a} + \hat{b}(1) + \hat{P}(bwt_i)] - [\hat{a} + \hat{b}(0) + \hat{P}(bwt_i)] = \hat{b}.$$

Because the model is additive, the value of the complex polynomial $P(bwt_i)$ has no influence on the estimate of the coefficient $\hat{b}$. Therefore, the model-estimated and constant summary rate-ratio becomes $\hat{R} = e^{\hat{b}} = e^{-0.290} = 0.749$. As before, the estimated ratio indicates that the black perinatal mortality rate is about 75% of the white rate after accounting for the birth-weight differences. Thus, the estimated rate-ratio $\hat{R}$ is said to be adjusted for the influences from the differing white and Africa-American birth-weight distributions.

Because, like all estimates, the estimate $\hat{b}$ is subject to sampling variation, an assessment of this influence is always an important consideration. The test statistic

$$z = \frac{\hat{b} - 0}{S_{\hat{b}}} = \frac{-0.290 - 0}{0.048} = -6.009$$

has an approximate standard normal distribution when $b = 0$ (*rate-ratio* $= R = 1$). The estimated standard error $S_{\hat{b}} = 0.048$ is calculated as part of the maximum likelihood estimation process (Table 6–18). The p-value associated with the maximum likelihood estimate $\hat{b} = -0.290$ and, therefore, the approximately normally distributed z-value, yields a p-value of $P(|\hat{b}| \geq 0.290|b = 0) = P(|Z| \geq 6.009|b = 0) < 0.001$. The extremely small p-value again supplies clear evidence of a systematic racial difference in perinatal mortality between white and African-American infants, independent of infant birth weight, as suspected from the previous model-free analyses.

The influence of sampling variation on the estimated summary rate-ratio is additionally described by a confidence interval. An approximate 95% confidence interval is

$$\hat{b} \pm 1.960 S_{\hat{b}} = -0.290 \pm 1.960(0.048) \quad \text{and} \quad (-0.384, -0.195),$$

based on normal distribution and the model-estimated $\hat{b} = -0.290$. Because the summary rate-ratio $\hat{R} = 0.749$ is estimated by $e^{\hat{b}} = e^{-0.290}$, the confidence interval bounds for the underlying single rate-ratio R become

$$(e^{lower\ bound}, e^{upper\ bound}) = (e^{-0.384}, e^{-0.195}) = (0.681, 0.823).$$

This model-based confidence interval hardly differs from the previous model-free (weighted average) approximate 95% confidence interval $(0.701, 0.847)$.

Figure 6–8 displays the geometry of the log-rates calculated from the additive model. As dictated by an additive model, the distance (on a log-scale) between the polynomial curves describing the birth weight–mortality pattern for black and white infants is constant for all birth weights, $|\hat{b}| = 0.290$. Also, because $\hat{b}$ is less than zero, the model-estimated black perinatal mortality log-rates are less than the estimated white log-rates for all birth weights, again dictated by the model.

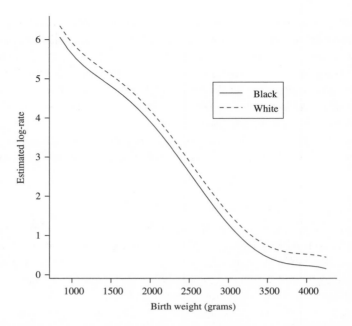

Figure 6–8. Estimated perinatal black–white mortality log-rates by birth weight.

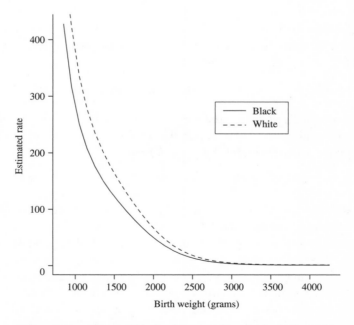

Figure 6–9. Estimated black–white mortality rates by birth weight.

Figure 6–9 displays the same estimated log-rates but exponentiated to produce estimated perinatal mortality rates for each birth weight and, necessarily, the black infants again have consistently lower estimated mortality (estimated rate-ratio = $\hat{R} = 0.749$) for all birth weights. A clear and simple summary of black–white perinatal mortality risk is produced by the additive Poisson model. Furthermore, the assessment of the model ("goodness-of-fit") indicates that this summary is likely an accurate reflection of the underlying difference in black–white risk.

7

ANALYSIS OF MATCHED CASE–CONTROL DATA

The analysis of matched pairs data is little more than a special case of the usual of case–control approach [22]. The fact that the data are made up of pairs produces some apparently different analytic methods. However, on close examination, these too are special cases of classical case–control analysis techniques. For example, the estimated odds ratio in the matched case–control context appears different from the more typical odds ratio used to summarize a series of 2×2 case–control tables (Chapter 2) but, as will be seen, it does not differ in principle. Nevertheless, the special case of matched pairs yields useful insights into the general issues of analyzing case–control data.

THE 2 × 2 CASE–CONTROL TABLE

Matched pairs case–control data collected to identify an association between a binary risk variable and a binary outcome are usually displayed in a 2×2 summary table. This 2×2 table differs in important ways from a 2×2 table generated by unmatched case–control data because it is itself a summary of a series of these traditional 2×2 tables.

Suppose F again represents the presence of a risk factor and $\overline{F}$ the absence of a risk factor, then matched pairs are usually classified into a summary 2×2 table such as Table 7–1.

Table 7–1. Notation for case–control matched pair case-control data classified by a binary risk factor

	Control F	Control $\overline{F}$	**Total**
Case F	a	b	$a+b$
Case $\overline{F}$	c	d	$c+d$
Total	$a+c$	$b+d$	N

The symbols a, b, c, and d represent counts of pairs where $N = a+b+c+d$ represents the total number of pairs consisting of a total $2N$ individuals.

The relationship between matched pairs and case–control data emerges from the more fundamental view of matched data as a series of 2×2 tables in which each table contains one matched pair. Each pair is a stratum consisting of two observations, making the number of strata equal to the number of matched pairs. These strata are constructed so that the members of each pair have essentially the same level of a confounding variable or variables. There are only four different kinds of matched pairs (Table 7–2), producing four kinds of typical case–control 2×2 tables (Chapter 1). The counts of these four kinds of tables make up the summary Table 7–1, where a represents the number of type 1 pairs, b represents the number of type 2 pairs, c represents the number of type 3 pairs, and d represents the number of type 4 pairs (Table 7–2).

Table 7–2. The four possible kinds of matched pairs tables (strata)

Type 1: Case and control both have the risk factor.

	F	$\overline{F}$	**Total**
Case	1	0	1
Control	1	0	1
Total	2	0	2

Type 2: Case has the risk factor and the control does not.

	F	$\overline{F}$	**Total**
Case	1	0	1
Control	0	1	1
Total	1	1	2

Type 3: Case does not have the risk factor and the control does.

	F	$\overline{F}$	**Total**
Case	0	1	1
Control	1	0	1
Total	1	1	2

Type 4: Case does not have the risk factor and control does not have the risk factor.

	F	$\overline{F}$	**Total**
Case	0	1	1
Control	0	1	1
Total	0	2	2

Data are frequently stratified to create homogeneous groups. For example, data stratified by race allow the study of smoking and birth weight (risk factor and outcome) within that stratum, free from the influence of race (Chapters 2 and 6). The variable race is the same for all individuals within a stratum. Therefore, summary statistics calculated from the data within each stratum are uninfluenced by race. These strata-specific measures are frequently combined creating a "race-free" overall summary (Chapter 2). Matched case–control pairs are created for the same reason. It is not important that each stratum contains the minimum possible number of observations, namely two. Simply, case–control matched pairs data are no more than a special case of N strata each containing two observations made homogeneous with respect to a single variable or several variables.

The probability that a case possesses the risk factor is estimated by $\hat{p}_1 = (a + b)/N$, where N represents the total number of pairs sampled. Similarly, the probability that a control possesses the risk factor is estimated by $\hat{p}_2 = (a + c)/N$. The essential question addressed by the analysis of all case–control data is: Does the distribution of the risk factor differ between cases and controls? Thus, from a 2×2 matched pairs table (Table 7–1), the quantity $\hat{p}_1 - \hat{p}_2 = (b - c)/N$ measures the difference in the distribution of the risk factor between cases and controls. The symbol b represents the number of pairs in which the case has the risk factor and the control does not (type 2, Table 7–2). The symbol c represents the number of pairs in which the case does not have the risk factor and the control does (type 3, Table 7–2). Thus, a measure of the influence of the risk factor is the difference between the proportions of these two kinds of case–control pairs, called *discordant pairs*.

For example, to study the influence of maternal smoking on the likelihood of low birth weight in newborns, an infant who weighs less than 2500 grams at birth (case) is matched to an infant who at birth weighs 2500 grams or greater (control), so that the mother of each infant has essentially the same prepregnancy weight ($\pm$ 0.1 kilograms). The risk factor is the mother's smoking exposure ($F =$ smoker and $\overline{F} =$ nonsmokers). The "matching-variable" is maternal prepregnancy weight. These two binary variables are part of the $N = 167$ matched-pairs data set represented in Table 7–3. The case–control array tabulated from the data displayed in Table 7–3 (columns 2 and 3) contains the counts of the four kinds of case–control prepregnancy weight-matched pairs (Table 7–4).

Because the value of the matching variable is essentially the same within each pair (stratum), differences within pairs are not influenced by the matching variable. The pairs are formed for just this reason. Furthermore, a summary created by combining the N strata-specific differences is also not influenced by the matching variable or variables. For the example data, a case–control difference between smoking and nonsmoking mothers within a matched pair is not influenced by the mother's prepregnancy weight. The case and control mothers are the same weight.

Table 7–3.   Representative data from a matched-pairs study of $N = 167$
low-birth-weight infants

Id	Status	Parity	Smk	Ppwt	Gest	Gain
1	1	1	1	40.9	1	6.1
1	0	0	1	40.9	0	21.0
2	1	1	0	43.0	1	9.2
2	0	1	1	43.0	1	10.0
3	1	0	0	44.5	1	3.4
3	0	0	0	44.5	0	15.4
4	1	0	1	44.5	1	4.4
4	0	0	1	44.5	0	18.1
5	1	0	1	44.5	1	6.1
5	0	0	0	44.5	0	19.3
6	1	0	0	45.5	0	1.0
6	0	1	0	45.5	0	1.5
7	1	0	0	45.5	0	8.4
7	0	0	1	45.5	0	8.9
8	1	1	0	45.5	1	6.5
8	0	0	0	45.5	1	8.8
.	.	.	.	.	.	.
.	.	.	.	.	.	.
.	.	.	.	.	.	.
165	1	1	0	97.7	1	10.6
165	0	1	0	97.7	0	18.7
166	1	0	0	105.0	0	3.6
166	0	1	1	105.0	0	10.7
167	1	1	0	118.0	1	0.0
167	0	1	0	118.0	0	5.5

id = matched pairs indicator
status: control = 0 or case = 1
parity: first child = 0 or one or more children = 1
smoking exposure (smk): nonsmoker = 0 or smoker = 1
prepregnancy weight (ppwt): prepregnancy weight, reported in kilograms
gestational age (gest): gestation <37 weeks = 0 or gestation ≥37 weeks = 1
maternal weight gained (gain): maternal weight gained during pregnancy, reported in
kilograms

Table 7–4.   Matched pairs data: case–control status (<2500 grams or ≥2500 grams) by
the risk factor (presence (F) or absence ($\bar{F}$) of maternal smoking) matched on maternal
prepregnancy weight

	Control F	Control $\bar{F}$	**Total**
Case F	$a = 15$	$b = 40$	$a+b = 55$
Case $\bar{F}$	$c = 22$	$d = 90$	$c+d = 112$
Total	$a+c = 37$	$b+d = 130$	$N = 167$

Therefore, a summary created from combining these 167 pairs is not influenced by maternal prepregnancy weight. A cost of removing the confounding influence of the matching variable is the inability to study its influence on the outcome variable.

The difference in the proportion of discordant pairs $\hat{p}_1 - \hat{p}_2 = b/N - c/N$ contrasts the distributions of the risk factor between cases and controls. More technically, it reflects the degree of symmetry or marginal homogeneity of the 2×2 case–control array (Table 7–4). If the risk factor is associated with case–control status, then p_1 differs from p_2 and the estimates of these two quantities likely reflect this difference. Conversely, if the risk factor is unrelated to case–control status, then estimates $\hat{p}_1$ and $\hat{p}_2$ differ only because of the influence of sampling variation.

The distribution of the observed differences $\hat{p}_1 - \hat{p}_2$ has estimated variance given by the expression

$$\hat{v} = variance(\hat{p}_1 - \hat{p}_2) = \frac{(b+c)N - (b-c)^2}{N^3}.$$

To repeat, the symbol b represents the observed number of discordant pairs in which the case has the risk factor and the control does not, and the symbol c represents the observed number of discordant pairs in which the control has the risk factor and the case does not ($N = a+b+c+d =$ total number of pairs). This estimated variance allows the usual construction of an approximate 95% level confidence interval based on the normal distribution. Specifically, the confidence interval bounds are

$lower\ bound = (\hat{p}_1 - \hat{p}_2) - 1.960\sqrt{\hat{v}}$ and $upper\ bound = (\hat{p}_1 - \hat{p}_2) + 1.960\sqrt{\hat{v}}.$

For the case–control birth-weight data (Table 7–4),

$$\hat{p}_1 = \frac{55}{167} = 0.329 \quad \text{and} \quad \hat{p}_2 = \frac{37}{167} = 0.222$$

and the difference $\hat{p}_1 - \hat{p}_2 = (40 - 22)/167 = 0.108$ has an estimated variance of $\hat{v} = 0.002$. An approximate 95% confidence interval is then

$$lower\ bound = 0.108 - 1.960\sqrt{0.002} = 0.017$$

and

$$upper\ bound = 0.108 + 1.960\sqrt{0.002} = 0.199.$$

The value zero is not contained in the confidence interval, indicating a plausibly systematic difference between p_1 and p_2. Thus, evidence exists that the underlying summary 2×2 table is not symmetric or, equivalently, the distributions of the row marginal frequencies (cases) and the column marginal frequencies (controls) systematically differ. From either point of view, it appears that maternal smoking is associated with the likelihood of a low-birth-weight infant. In addition, this association is not due to possibly differing influences in prepregnancy weights between the smoking and nonsmoking mothers. That is, the distributions of maternal prepregnancy weight are identical for cases and controls (exactly balanced).

ODDS RATIO FOR MATCHED DATA

The *Mantel-Haenszel summary odds ratio* calculated from a series of 2×2 tables is a specially constructed weighted average of the table-specific odds ratios. The estimated odds ratio are, as usual, $\hat{o}r_i = (a_i d_i)/(b_i c_i)$, one for each table. A weighted average summary odds ratio is

$$odds\ ratio = \hat{o}r_{MH} = \frac{\sum w_i \hat{o}r_i}{\sum w_i} = \frac{\sum \frac{b_i c_i}{n_i} \times \hat{o}r_i}{\sum \frac{b_i c_i}{n_i}} = \frac{\sum \frac{a_i d_i}{n_i}}{\sum \frac{b_i c_i}{n_i}} \qquad weights = w_i = \frac{b_i c_i}{n_i}$$

where $n_i = a_i + b_i + c_i + d_i$ is the total number of observations in each table, where $i = 1, 2, \cdots, k =$ number of tables (strata).

A special feature of the Mantel-Haenszel summary odds ratio is that it produces a summary value for a series of 2×2 tables regardless of the number of observations in each table ($n_i \geq 2$). Matched-pairs data, as noted, are a series of 2×2 tables (strata) each with two observations (Table 7–2). The Mantel-Haenszel estimate, therefore, provides a summary odds ratio, even for this minimum possible number of observations per table (stratum), namely $n_i = 2$. The summary of N matched pairs

Kind of pair	$a_i d_i / n_i$	$b_i c_i / n_i$	Number of pairs
1	0	0	a
2	1/2	0	b
3	0	1/2	c
4	0	0	d

shows the values and numbers of $a_i d_i / n_i$ and $b_i c_i / n_i$ terms among the four kinds of matched pairs (Table 7–2). Forming a weighted average from these N values produces the Mantel-Haenszel estimated summary odds ratio (denoted $\hat{o}r_m$), where

$$odds\ ratio = \hat{o}r_m = \frac{\sum \frac{a_i d_i}{n_i}}{\sum \frac{b_i c_i}{n_i}} = \frac{0a + (1/2)b + 0c + 0d}{0a + 0b + (1/2)c + 0d} = \frac{b}{c}$$

for $i = 1, 2, \cdots, N =$ pairs (tables). The estimated summary odds ratio $\hat{o}r_m = b/c$ measures the association between a risk factor and case–control status and is interpreted in the usual way. For the example data (Table 7–4), the estimated summary odds ratio is $\hat{or}_m = 40/22 = 1.818$. This ratio also reflects the extent of symmetry ($b = c$?) and marginal homogeneity ($p_1 = p_2$?) of the 2×2 case–control summary array. For example, when $\hat{or}_m = 1$, the case–control array is symmetric and the marginal frequencies are exactly equal.

CONFIDENCE INTERVAL FOR THE MATCHED-PAIRS ODDS RATIO

When both members of a matched pair have the same risk factor, observed differences between cases and controls are due to other influences. The pairs are "matched" for the risk factor and, like any variable that is the same within pairs, does not influence the observed within-pair case–control difference. For example, when both mothers smoke, the within-pair difference in birth weight is not due to smoking exposure. The same argument applies when both members of a pair do not have the risk factor. Therefore, like the matching variable, the pairs concordant for the risk factor (a and d, Table 7–1) are not relevant to assessing case–control status and are excluded from an analysis. The discordant pairs become the data set that now consists of $n = b + c$ pairs. Thus, the n discordant pairs collected in a matched-pairs design are typically treated as a sample from a binomial probability distribution.

When p represents the probability that a case possesses the risk factor among the discordant pairs [in symbols, $p = P(case = F \mid discordant\ pair)$], the probability that a sample of $n = b + c$ pairs contains b such discordant pairs is

$$binomial\ probability = \binom{n}{b} p^b (1-p)^{n-b}$$

where $b = 0, 1, 2, \cdots, n$. The natural and maximum likelihood estimate of the probability p is $\hat{p} = b/(b+c) = b/n$ (Chapter 3).

There are a number of ways in which confidence intervals are constructed for the binomial distribution parameter p based on its estimate $\hat{p}$ (Chapters 3 and 15). These confidence intervals lead to a number of ways to construct a confidence interval for an odds ratio estimated from matched-pairs data. Because the estimated odds ratio is a function of the estimate of p, where

$$\hat{or}_m = \frac{b}{c} = \frac{b/(b+c)}{c/(b+c)} = \frac{\hat{p}}{1-\hat{p}} ,$$

the confidence interval bounds for the odds ratio (denoted $\hat{or}_{bound}$) are the same function of the bounds created from the estimate $\hat{p}$ (denoted $\hat{p}_{bound}$), namely $\hat{or}_{bound} = \hat{p}_{bound}/(1 - \hat{p}_{bound})$. Therefore, the confidence interval bounds for an odds ratio can be directly calculated from the confidence interval bounds for the binomial probability p. From the maternal smoking matched-pairs data, an approximate 95% confidence interval based on $\hat{p} = b/n = 40/62 = 0.645$ is (0.518, 0.772) and produces the 95% confidence interval based on the estimated odds ratio $\hat{or} = b/c = 40/60 = 0.645/0.354 = 1.818$ of $(0.518/0.482, 0.772/0.228) = (1.075, 3.392)$. Figure 7–1 contains three expressions for estimating confidence bounds for the odds ratio from matched-pairs data.

1. Exact method

$$df_1 = 2c + 2 \quad df_2 = 2b \quad f_1 = f_{0.975, df_1, df_2} \text{ from a } f\text{-distribution}$$

$$t_{lower} = \frac{b}{b + (c+1)f_1}$$

$$or_{lower} = \frac{t_{lower}}{1 - t_{lower}}$$

$$df_1 = 2b + 2 \quad df_2 = 2c \quad f_2 = f_{0.975, df_1, df_2} \text{ from a } f\text{-distribution}$$

$$t_{upper} = \frac{(b+1)f_2}{c + (b+1)f_2}$$

$$or_{upper} = \frac{t_{upper}}{1 - t_{upper}}$$

2. Approximate method I

$$p_{lower} = \hat{p} - 1.960\sqrt{\frac{\hat{p}(1-\hat{p})}{n}} - \frac{1}{2n} \quad \text{where} \quad \hat{p} = \frac{b}{n}$$

$$or_{lower} = \frac{p_{lower}}{1 - p_{lower}}$$

$$p_{upper} = \hat{p} + 1.960\sqrt{\frac{\hat{p}(1-\hat{p})}{n}} + \frac{1}{2n}$$

$$or_{upper} = \frac{p_{upper}}{1 - p_{upper}}$$

3. Approximate method II

$$\hat{or}_m = \frac{b}{c}$$

$$\hat{v} = variance(log[\hat{or}_m]) = \frac{1}{b} + \frac{1}{c}$$

$$or_{lower} = \hat{or}_m e^{-1.960\sqrt{\hat{v}}} \quad \text{and} \quad or_{upper} = \hat{or}_m e^{+1.960\sqrt{\hat{v}}}$$

Figure 7–1. Three approaches to estimating a 95% confidence interval for an odds ratio from matched-pairs data (b and c are defined in Table 7–1 and $n = b + c$)

The case–control data (Table 7–4) describing the likelihood of a low-birth-weight infant and the risk from maternal smoking, give the following 95% confidence intervals for three methods of constructing a confidence interval. Based on the odds ratio $\hat{or}_m = b/c = 1.818$ estimated from the $n = 62$ discordant pairs (Table 7–4), they are:

1. Exact: lower bound $= 1.055$ and upper bound $= 3.212$,
2. Method I: lower bound $= 1.075$ and upper bound $= 3.392$ and
3. Method II: lower bound $= 1.081$ and upper bound $= 3.059$.

The exact method (Chapter 15) and method I are based directly on the binomial distribution, and method II results from the application of maximum likelihood estimation of the odds ratio (Chapter 3).

EVALUATING AN ESTIMATED ODDS RATIO

Continuing to rely on the binomial distribution as a statistical description of the distribution of matched-pairs data, tests can be created to assess the influence of sampling variation on the observed difference between the numbers of discordant pairs. When only random differences exist in the frequency of the risk factor between cases and controls, the underlying probability that a case possesses the risk factor among discordant pairs is 0.5 ($p = 0.5$). That is, it is equally likely that the risk factor is associated with either a case or a control observation. In symbols, when case status is unrelated to the occurrence of the risk factor,

$$p = P(case = F | discordant\ pair) = P(control = F | discordant\ pair) = 0.5.$$

In terms of the observed numbers of discordant pairs, when the risk factor has no influence, the numbers of discordant pairs b and c differ by chance alone.

A statistical test generated under this "no association" hypothesis using a normal distribution approximation instead of the exact binomial probabilities produces the most common evaluation of an observed association between risk factor and case–control status ($p = 0.5$? or $b = c$? or symmetric? or $p_1 = p_2$? or $or_m = 1$?). When $p = 0.5$, the expected number of discordant pairs is $np = n/2$, and its associated variance is $np(1 - p) = n/4$ from the binomial distribution, where again n represents the number of discordant pairs. Therefore, the test statistic Z

$$Z = \frac{|b - n/2| - 1/2}{\sqrt{n/4}}$$

has an approximate standard normal distribution when the risk factor is unrelated to case status ($p = 0.5$). Equivalently, the test statistic

$$X_m^2 = Z^2 = \frac{(|b - c| - 1)^2}{b + c}$$

has an approximate chi-square distribution with one degree of freedom. For a matched pairs analysis, the test statistic X_m^2 is called *McNemar's test*. In other situations, it is called the *binomial test*.

Using the smoking exposure and low-birth-weight matched-pairs data,

$$z = \frac{|40 - 62/2| - 1/2}{\sqrt{62/4}} = 2.159,$$

or

$$X_m^2 = \frac{(|40 - 22| - 1)^2}{40 + 22} = 4.661 = (2.159)^2,$$

and both test statistics necessarily yield the identical p-value of $P(|Z| \geq 2.159|no\ association) = P(X_m^2 \geq 4.661|no\ association) = 0.031$.

The correction factors used in these expressions (1/2 or 1) improve the correspondence between the continuous normal distribution (the approximate distribution) and the discrete binomial distribution (the exact distribution), particularly for small samples of data. As the sample size increases, the difference between the corrected and uncorrected test statistics becomes unimportant. For large sample sizes (no correction factor), the McNemar test statistic becomes

$$X_m^2 = \frac{(b - c)^2}{b + c}.$$

The uncorrected chi-square statistic for the smoking risk data is $X_m^2 = 5.226$ and yields a p-value of 0.022.

Although the concordant pairs are not relevant for assessing the influence of a risk factor, they remain a consideration in the collection of matched-pairs data. The term *over-matching* refers to matched data in which a loss of efficiency occurs because the risk factor distribution is similar for both cases and controls. For example, in a study of the influence of air pollution (binary risk factor) on respiratory illness (binary outcome) in which cases are matched to controls who live next door, the study will suffer from over-matching. For almost all pairs, both the case and the control will have the same level of air quality (concordant risk factors). That is, both members of a pair will be exposed to high levels of air pollution or both to low levels. This example of over-matching is extreme because the risk factor and the matching variable are almost perfectly associated,

Table 7–5. Case–control prepregnancy weight-matched data for mothers with one or more children (parity ≥ 1)

		Control smoker	Control nonsmoker	**Total**
Case	smoker	15	7	22
Case	nonsmoker	2	3	5
	Total	17	10	27

but it demonstrates one reason for the reduction of discordant pairs (counts b and c), because small numbers of discordant pairs make it less likely that influences associated with the risk factor will be detected (lower statistical power).

As noted, a typically effective strategy to reduce the influence of a confounding variable is to stratify the collected data and compare the distributions of the risk factor within these homogeneous subgroups (Chapter 2). This usually successful approach generally fails for matched-pairs data, unless large numbers of matched pairs are available. From the 167 matched pairs of mothers (Table 7–3), it might be of interest to investigate the influence of maternal smoking on the likelihood of a low-birth-weight infant, controlling for a potential confounding influence of a third variable, such as parity. From the example data (Table 7–3), a table is constructed so that both members of every matched pair have a previous child (parity ≥ 1); see Table 7–5.

The estimated odds ratio calculated from this table is $\hat{or} = 7/2 = 3.5$, where all 27 pairs of mothers both had a previous child (parity ≥ 1) and, of course, have the same prepregnancy weight. An odds ratio estimated from this table is not influenced by case–control differences in parity. However, it is estimated from only nine discordant pairs from the original 167 observations. Such a large loss of data is typical. When eliminating the influences from variables not included in the matching of the paired observations is an issue, employing a statistical model is frequently the only effective analytic strategy. As will be seen, a statistical model approach allows an analysis that accounts for the influence of one or more possibly confounding variables not included in the matching process, without an extreme loss of data.

DISREGARDING THE MATCHED DESIGN

Data collected in a matched design are sometimes analyzed as if the data were not matched. Ignoring the original design produces Table 7–6, when the risk factor and outcome are binary variables (Table 7–2).

The symbols a, b, c, and d again represent the counts of the four kinds of matched pairs (Table 7–2). For the maternal smoking data, the case–control counts

Table 7–6. The 2 × 2 case–control table resulting from ignoring the matched-pairs design

	Case	Control	**Total**
F	$a+b$	$a+c$	$2a+b+c$
$\overline{F}$	$c+d$	$b+d$	$2d+b+c$
Total	N	N	$2N$

Table 7–7. The 2 × 2 case–control table of smoking–birth weight data resulting from ignoring the matched-pairs design

	Case	Control	**Total**
F	55	37	92
$\overline{F}$	112	130	242
Total	167	167	334

of infants classified by their mother's smoking exposure (F and $\overline{F}$), ignoring the matching on maternal prepregnancy weight, are given in Table 7–7.

The resulting estimated odds ratio is $\hat{o}r = (55/112)/(37/130) = 1.725$, with an approximate 95% confidence interval of (1.060, 2.809). This odds ratio is somewhat lower than the matched pairs odds ratio of $\hat{o}r_m = 1.818$. However, the width of the confidence interval is reduced [(1.060, 2.809) vs. (1.081, 3.058)]. Although there is a gain in power (narrower confidence interval), ignoring the matched-pairs structure produces a biased estimate of the odds ratio. The bias occurs because of the failure to account for the confounding influence of prepregnancy weight on the birth weight–smoking association. Specifically, the bias associated with the matched and unmatched odds ratios is 1.818 versus 1.725. Such trade-offs between bias and precision are occasionally an issue in choosing an appropriate estimate.

The difference between the two odds ratios, $\hat{o}r$ and $\hat{o}r_m$, is proportional to $n(ad - bc)$. Thus, when $ad - bc = 0$ or $ad/bc = 1$, these two estimates are identical, ($\hat{o}r = \hat{o}r_m$). That is, the matching variable does not influence the estimated odds ratio. The effectiveness of a matching strategy to account for the influence of a confounding variable or variables is equally assessed by directly comparing the estimated odds ratios $\hat{o}r_m$ and $\hat{o}r$.

INTERACTION WITH THE MATCHING VARIABLE

To repeat, the influence of the variable or variables used to match the case–control pairs cannot be studied. However, measures of association between case–control status and a risk factor can be compared at different levels of the matching variable (interaction). From the example, the maternal smoking data matched for prepregnancy weight produces a simple question: Is the underlying odds

Table 7–8. Data on smoking exposure (F = smoker and $\overline{F}$ = nonsmoker) and case–control status stratified into two case–control arrays based on prepregnancy weight ($N = 167$ pairs)

Prepregnancy weight $\geq$ median of 56 kilograms ("high")

	Control F	Control $\overline{F}$	Total
Case F	10	23	33
Case $\overline{F}$	11	36	47
Total	21	59	80

Prepregnancy weight < median of 56 kilograms ("low")

	Control F	Control $\overline{F}$	Total
Case F	5	17	22
Case $\overline{F}$	11	54	65
Total	16	71	87

ratio measuring the association between low birth weight and smoking the same, regardless of the mother's prepregnancy weight? To start to address this question, the data can be divided into those pairs where the paired mother's prepregnancy weights are equal to or above the median weight (labeled "high") and those pairs below the median weight (labeled "low"). Unlike stratifying on a variable not used in the matching process (Table 7–5), no pairs are lost from the analysis ($n = 167$). Table 7–8 shows the 167 matched pairs stratified into two 2×2 case–control arrays created from the two maternal prepregnancy weight categories.

The estimated odds ratio $\hat{or}_{high} = 23/11 = 2.091$ measures the association between low birth weight and smoking exposure for the 80 pairs of mothers whose prepregnancy weight is equal to or greater than the median of 56 kilograms. The estimated odds ratio is $\hat{or}_{low} = 17/11 = 1.545$ for the 87 pairs of mothers whose prepregnancy weight is less than the median. Exact 95% confidence intervals (Figure 7–1) are $(0.979, 4.751)$ and $(0.683, 3.650)$, respectively. The overlapping confidence intervals suggest that no systematic difference likely exists between the two odds ratios estimated from two prepregnancy weight strata. Thus, little evidence exists of an interaction.

A formal test of the equality of these two estimated odds ratios ($or_{high} = or_{low} = or$?) is achieved with the usual chi-square test of independence applied to a 2×2 table created from the discordant pairs (counts b and c) from each subtable (Table 7–9).

A chi-square test of independence (Chapters 1 and 2) indicates the likelihood of equality between the two underlying matched-pairs odds ratios, as reflected by their estimates. The hypothesis of independence is identical to postulating

Table 7–9. Numbers of pairs* discordant for the smoking exposure data classified into high–low strata based on prepregnancy weight ($n = 62$ pairs)

	"High"	"Low"	Total
$F/\overline{F}$	23 (21.94)	17 (18.06)	40
$\overline{F}/F$	11 (12.06)	11 (9.94)	22
Total	34	28	62

* = Values in parentheses are the numbers of pairs expected when $or_{low} = or_{high} = or$ (no interaction).

that the underlying matched-pairs ratios within each stratum are equal (columns, Table 7–9). That is, the estimated matched-pairs odds ratios differ only by chance alone. This hypothesis ($or_1 = or_2 = or$) produces the theoretical expected values, where $21.94/12.06 = 18.06/9.94 = 40/22 = 1.818$ (Table 7–9). The resulting chi-square test statistic $X^2 = 0.322$ with one degree of freedom yields a p-value of $P(X^2 \geq 0.322 | or_{high} = or_{low}) = 0.570$. A p-value of 0.570 gives no reason to believe that the two odds ratios measuring the association between smoking exposure and case–control status differ between the high or low categories of maternal prepregnancy weight. In other words, the estimated odds ratios $\hat{or}_{high} = 2.901$ and $\hat{or}_{low} = 1.545$ likely differ by chance alone.

MATCHED PAIRS ANALYSIS: MORE THAN ONE CONTROL

The analysis of matched data with more than one control is technically a bit more extensive than a one-to-one matched design but differs little in principle. The case of two matched controls is presented. A similar pattern applies to any number of matched controls. Furthermore, a logistic model-based approach allows the analysis of matched data regardless of the number of controls for each case (following section).

When two controls are matched to each case, six possible kinds of matched sets exist. The case can have the risk factor or not. The two controls can both have the risk factor, one control can have the risk factor, or neither control can have the risk factor. Two possibilities for the cases and three possibilities for the controls produce a total of six different kinds of 1:2 matched sets, each made up of three observations ($n_i = 3$). These matched sets are displayed in Table 7–10 as six kinds of case–control 2×2 tables, each containing three observations.

The subscript indicate the number of cases and controls with the risk factor. For example, the symbol n_{02} represents the number of matched sets in which the case does not possess the risk factor and both controls do possess the risk

Table 7–10. The six possible kinds of 1:2 matched sets of data

Type 1: Case has the risk factor, and both controls have the risk factor.

	F	$\overline{F}$	**Total**
Case	1	0	1
Control	2	0	2
Total	3	0	3

Type 2: Case has the risk factor, and one control has the risk factor.

	F	$\overline{F}$	**Total**
Case	1	0	1
Control	1	1	2
Total	2	1	3

Type 3: Case has the risk factor, and both controls do not have the risk factor.

	F	$\overline{F}$	**Total**
Case	1	0	1
Control	0	2	2
Total	1	2	3

Type 4: Case does not have the risk factor, and both controls have the risk factor.

	F	$\overline{F}$	**Total**
Case	0	1	1
Control	2	0	2
Total	2	1	3

Type 5: Case does not have the risk factor, and one control has the risk factor.

	F	$\overline{F}$	**Total**
Case	0	1	1
Control	1	1	2
Total	1	2	3

Type 6: Case does not have the risk factor, and both controls do not have the risk factor.

	F	$\overline{F}$	**Total**
Case	0	1	1
Control	0	2	2
Total	0	3	3

Table 7–11. The notation for a 1:2 matched data set (n_{ij} = number of matched sets)

	Control F and F	Control $\overline{F}$ or F	Control $\overline{F}$ and $\overline{F}$
Case F	n_{12}	n_{11}	n_{10}
Case $\overline{F}$	n_{02}	n_{01}	n_{00}

factor. A 2×3 case–control array summarizes the data from a 1:2 matched sample (Table 7–11). The total number of sets (strata) is again denoted N. Much like the 2 × 2 matched pairs case–control summary array (Table 7–1), this 2 × 3 array is the tabulation of the six kinds of 2 × 2 tables (matched sets), a total of $3N$ individuals.

Again, as in matched-pairs analysis, each matched set (stratum) is a 2 × 2 table with the same level of a confounding variable or variables. The Mantel-Haenszel estimate again produces a summary odds ratio. The summary of N observed 2 × 2 tables

Kind of set	$a_i d_i / n_i$	$b_i c_i / n_i$	Number of sets
1	0	0	n_{12}
2	1/3	0	n_{11}
3	2/3	0	n_{10}
4	0	2/3	n_{02}
5	0	1/3	n_{01}
6	0	0	n_{00}

shows the values and numbers of $a_i d_i / n_i$ and $b_i c_i / n_i$ terms among the six kinds of matched sets. Applying the Mantel-Haenszel summary odds ratio to the N matched sets gives the summary odds ratio $\hat{o}r_m$ of

$$odds\ ratio = \hat{o}r_m = \frac{\sum \frac{a_i d_i}{n_i}}{\sum \frac{b_i c_i}{n_i}} = \frac{(0)n_{12} + (1/3)n_{11} + (2/3)n_{10}}{(2/3)n_{02} + (1/3)n_{01} + (0)n_{00}} = \frac{n_{11} + 2n_{10}}{2n_{02} + n_{01}}$$

for $i = 1, 2, \cdots, N = $ number of matched sets.

For an example, consider a small part of a study of birth defects and exposure to electromagnetic field (EMF) radiation conducted in rural France [23]. The cases (malformed infants) are matched to two controls for sex, date of birth, and location of maternal residence. Also recorded is a binary risk factor indicating whether the mother's residence was at a distance of less than 500 meters from a high-power electric line (exposed = F) or a distance equal to or more than 500 meters (not exposed = $\overline{F}$). These data are displayed by strata ($N = 12$ matched 1:2 sets from the original data) in Table 7–12. Each of the 12 strata constitutes a 2 × 2 table made up of three matched observations (one case and two controls). Table 7–13 summarizes these data in terms of the numbers of kinds of 1:2 matched sets among the six possibilities (the n_{ij}-values).

The 95% confidence interval based on the estimate $\hat{o}r_m = 2.0$ is $(0.464, 8.619)$, generated a from logistic model approach (to be discussed).

From the 1:2 matched sample of French birth defects data, the estimated odds ratio is

$$\hat{o}r_m = \frac{4 + 2(2)}{2(1) + 2} = \frac{8}{4} = 2.0.$$

Table 7–12. Binary case–control data ($N = 12$ matched sets) from a French study of birth defects and exposure to electromagnetic field radiation (F = exposed and $\overline{F}$ = not exposed)

Strata	Status	F	Strata	Status	F
1	1	0	7	1	0
1	0	1	7	0	1
1	0	0	7	0	1
2	1	1	8	1	0
2	0	1	8	0	1
2	0	0	8	0	0
3	1	0	9	1	1
3	0	0	9	0	0
3	0	0	9	0	1
4	1	1	10	1	1
4	0	0	10	0	0
4	0	1	10	0	1
5	1	1	11	1	1
5	0	0	11	0	0
5	0	0	11	0	0
6	1	0	12	1	1
6	0	0	12	0	1
6	0	0	12	0	1

For example, the stratum 4 matched set is (type 2) or

	F	$\overline{F}$	**Total**
Case	1	0	1
Control	1	1	2
Total	2	1	3

Table 7–13. Summary of the matched sets of birth defects data (Table 7–12) where EMF exposure is defined as a binary variable, distance <500 meters (F) and distance $\geq$500 meters ($\overline{F}$)

	Control F and F	Control $\overline{F}$ or F	Control $\overline{F}$ and $\overline{F}$
Case (F)	$n_{12} = 1$	$n_{11} = 4$	$n_{10} = 2$
Case ($\overline{F}$)	$n_{02} = 1$	$n_{01} = 2$	$n_{00} = 2$

As with the matched-pairs analysis, a chi-square test statistic is typically used to evaluate the hypothesis that the risk variable is unrelated to case–control status. The test statistic (denoted X_m^2) is a specific application of the test of independence of variables contained in a series of 2×2 tables, sometimes called the *Cochran-Mantel-Haenszel chi-square test for independence* [24]. An expression for this chi-square test statistic applied to the special case of 1:2 matched sets data is

$$X_m^2 = \frac{[(n_{11} + 2n_{10}) - (n_{01} + 2n_{02})]^2}{2(n_{11} + n_{10} + n_{02} + n_{01})}.$$

The value X_m^2 has an approximate chi-square distribution with one degree of freedom when the risk factor is unrelated to case–control status. For the birth defects example data (Tables 7–12 and 7–13), the chi-square statistic $X_m^2 = (8-4)^2/18 = 0.889$ yields a p-value of 0.346 (further discussed in the next section).

As with matched-pairs data, matched sets in which all members have or do not have the risk factor (n_{12} and n_{00}) are not included in the estimation or evaluation of the estimated odds ratio. Again, these sets are "matched" for the risk factor and do not provide information about its influence on case–control status.

A small issue: Statistical power increases as the number of controls per matched set increases. A mathematical argument demonstrates that the gain in efficiency relative to the matched pairs using McNemar's chi-square test is approximately $2R/(R+1)$ where R is the number of controls from a 1:R matched set [25]. For example, when five controls ($R = 5$) are used for each case (1:5), the analysis has $2(5)/(5+1) = 1.67$ times more statistical power than the 1:1 matched-pairs analysis ($R = 1$). An additional three controls per case (1:8), however, only increases the efficiency slightly (1.89).

Another small issue: As the number of controls, R, increases, the likelihood decreases of observing a matched set in which the case and all controls are concordant. Thus, using multiple matched controls can slightly increase the statistical power by producing a few more discordant sets.

MATCHED ANALYSIS: MULTILEVEL CATEGORICAL RISK FACTOR

A matched-pairs analysis of a binary risk factor produces a 2×2 case–control summary array. In a parallel fashion, a k-level categorical risk factor produces a $k \times k$ case–control summary array again containing counts of matched pairs. For example, it is thought that exposure to EMF radiation might be associated with increased likelihood of childhood leukemia [26]. To explore this conjecture, a categorical variable reflecting the extent of EMF exposure was created that combines a measure of EMF radiation strength with the distance of the case or control residence from the source of the exposure. The categories are called the *Wertheimer–Leeper wire codes* [26]. One version of this categorical variable, reflecting EMF exposure, has three levels [high current configuration (HCC), ordinary current configuration (OCC), and low current configuration (LCC)].

Data from a study of childhood leukemia conducted in northern California [27] illustrate the analysis of a multilevel categorical risk factor. These data consist

Table 7–14. The case–control matched-pairs array ($N = 126$ matched pairs) displaying childhood leukemia data at three levels of EMF radiation exposure (HCC, OCC, and LCC)

		Control HCC	Control OCC	Control LCC	Total
Case	HCC	0	5	17	22
Case	OCC	5	5	11	21
Case	LCC	13	9	61	83
	Total	18	19	89	126

of 126 pairs of children under the age of 15 matched for sex, age, and race, classified by the Wertheimer–Leeper scheme (Table 7–14). The resulting 3×3 case–control array allows an investigation of a possible association between the likelihood of childhood leukemia and EMF radiation exposure measured by a three-level categorical variable ($k = 3$).

For a k-level categorical variable, there are $k(k-1)/2$ sets of discordant pairs, but the statistical issues remain similar to the analysis of a binary variable. As with the 2×2 analysis, the primary question becomes: Is there a difference in the distribution of the risk factor between cases and controls among the discordant pairs? Differences between case and control distributions of a multilevel categorical risk factor are directly measured by the degree of symmetry or marginal homogeneity of the case–control array. Statistically, the question becomes: Do the pairs of counts within the $k(k-1)/2$ sets of discordant pairs differer by chance alone? For the example EMF data, the question is: Do the counts within the three kinds of discordant pairs (HCC/OCC, HCC/LCC, and LCC/OCC) differ by chance alone? For example, when no case–control association exists, the number of discordant pairs in which the case experiences an LCC exposure and the control an OCC exposure does not differ from the number of discordant pairs in which the case experiences an OCC exposure and the control an LCC exposure, except for the influence of random variation. For example (Table 7–14), the difference between the number of discordant LCC–OCC pairs $n_{32} = 9$ and $n_{23} = 11$ would be due strictly to chance when no case–control association exists. The same comparison made to evaluate discordant pairs classified into 2×2 case–control array remains an effective measure of association. However, the question of equality among three sets of discordant pairs translates into the question of whether the case–control array is symmetric. A perfectly symmetric array occurs when case–control status is exactly unrelated to the categorical risk factor variable. That is, for all sets of discordant pairs, the ratios n_{ij}/n_{ji} are 1.0 or for all pairs $n_{ij} = n_{ji}$, where n_{ij} again represents an observed cell frequency of the discordant matched pairs from the $k \times k$ case–control array.

When no association exists between case–control status and a risk variable, the counts within each cell of the case–control array deviate randomly from the

Table 7–15. The matched-pairs array displaying the distribution of case–control pairs for three levels of EMF radiation exposure (HCC, OCC, and LCC) as if exactly no association exists between leukemia case–control status and exposure (exactly symmetric)

	Control HCC	Control OCC	Control LCC	**Total**
Case HCC	0	5	15	20
Case OCC	5	5	10	20
Case LCC	15	10	61	86
Total	20	20	86	126

expected number of discordant pairs estimated by $\bar{n}_{ij} = (n_{ij} + n_{ji})/2$. For the EMF radiation example, such a symmetric array of theoretical counts is presented in Table 7–15. The three ratios within corresponding sets of discordant pairs are exactly 1.0 (5/5 = 15/15 = 10/10 = 1). The observed ratios are 5/5 = 1.0, 17/13 = 1.308 and 11/9 = 1.222. A formal comparison of the observed counts (Table 7–14) to the counts generated under the conjecture of no association (Table 7–15) is achieved with the usual Pearson chi-square test statistic or

$$X_S^2 = \sum \frac{(n_{ij} - \bar{n}_{ij})^2}{\bar{n}_{ij}} \qquad \text{(S for symmetry)}.$$

Like the 2×2 analysis, the concordant pairs (diagonal frequencies of the case–control array) provide no information about the risk factor ($n_{ii} = \bar{n}_{ii}$). The test-statistic X_S^2 has an approximate chi-square distribution with $k(k-1)/2$ degrees of freedom when no relationship exists between risk factor and case–control status; that is, when the underlying case–control array is symmetric. For the EMF data, the chi-square test statistic $X_S^2 = 0.733$ (degrees of freedom = 3) yields a p-value of $P(X_S^2 \geq 0.733 | no\ association) = 0.865$ (Table 7–14 vs. Table 7–15).

A little algebraic rearrangement of the chi-square test statistic X_S^2 produces a sum of three separate uncorrected McNemar summary values or

$$X_S^2 = \frac{(n_{12} - n_{21})^2}{n_{12} + n_{21}} + \frac{(n_{13} - n_{31})^2}{n_{13} + n_{31}} + \frac{(n_{23} - n_{32})^2}{n_{23} + n_{32}}$$

$$= \frac{(5-5)^2}{10} + \frac{(17-13)^2}{30} + \frac{(11-9)^2}{20} = 0.733.$$

This version of the chi-square statistic directly shows once again that the concordant pairs do not play a role in the analysis, and shows why the degrees of freedom are three.

At the heart of matched-pairs data analysis is the comparison of the row to the column marginal counts of the case–control array because they directly reflect case–control differences in the distributions of the risk factor. Therefore, the most

Table 7–16. The risk factor distributions (marginal frequencies) and their expected distributions when exactly no association exists between EMF radiation exposure and childhood leukemia data (last row)

	HCC	OCC	LCC	Total
Cases $(n_{.i})$	22	21	83	126
Controls $(n_{i.})$	18	19	89	126
Differences (d_i)	4	2	–6	0
Expected values $(\hat{N}_i)$	20	20	86	126

fundamental measure of case–control association is an assessment of the marginal homogeneity. When no association exists, the distribution of the marginal counts differ only by chance. The components of such a comparison are illustrated by the leukemia–EMF data (Table 7–16).

The expression for the theoretical marginal counts, generated as if no case–control association exists, is

$$\hat{N}_i = \frac{n_{i.} + n_{.i}}{2},$$

where $n_{i.}$ represents the sum of the ith row and $n_{.i}$ represents the sum of the ith column. For example, $\hat{N}_2 = (n_{2.} + n_{.2})/2 = (21 + 19)/2 = 20$ (Table 7–16, second column).

A chi-square statistic created to compare case and control marginal distributions when $k = 3$ is

$$X_H^2 = \frac{\bar{n}_{23}d_1^2 + \bar{n}_{13}d_2^2 + \bar{n}_{12}d_3^2}{2(\bar{n}_{12}\bar{n}_{13} + \bar{n}_{12}\bar{n}_{23} + \bar{n}_{13}\bar{n}_{23})} \qquad \text{(H for homogeneity)}$$

where again $\bar{n}_{ij} = (n_{ij} + n_{ji})/2$ and $d_i = n_{i.} - n_{.i}$. The expression X_H^2 is an explicit log-likelihood test statistic from a logistic model for the specific case of $k = 3$. This case and the analysis for $k > 3$ require a statistical model approach (to be discussed). The d_i-values are the differences between the corresponding row and column observed marginal totals (Table 7–16). If all d_i values are zero, the distributions of the marginal frequencies are identical. Incidentally, when the case–control array is symmetric, the marginal frequencies are necessarily identical (homogeneous). The converse property is not true. The test statistic X_H^2 has an approximate chi-square distribution with two degrees of freedom when the case–control array marginal distributions differ only because of sampling variation. For the EMF data, the test statistic $X_H^2 = 0.727$ yields a p-value of $P(X_H^2 \geq 0.727 | no\ association) = 0.695$. The marginal frequencies give no evidence of nonrandom differences in the case–control distributions of EMF radiation exposure using a three-level categorical Wertheimer–Leeper wire codes. The analysis of a $k \times k$ case–control matched pairs array is further discussed in the next section.

CONDITIONAL ANALYSIS OF LOGISTIC REGRESSION MODELS

A typical logistic regression analysis (Chapters 4 and 5) requires about one parameter for each level of a categorical variable included in the model. Precisely, k strata require $k - 1$ parameters and, in the case of matched-pairs data, is one less than the number of sampled pairs. For matched data or any data distributed into a large number of strata, estimates resulting from the application of standard logistic regression techniques are biased, often seriously biased [8]. An approach that produces estimates of the important parameters of the logistic regression model but does not incur the bias associated with estimating a large number of strata parameters is called a *conditional logistic regression analysis*. A conditional analysis produces unbiased estimates of the parameters that describe the relationships between risk factors and outcome, but does not produce estimates of the parameters necessary to identify the influences of the stratum variable. Typically, the influence of the "matching" variable (stratum-variable) is not an important issue in the analysis of matched data, making a conditional logistic model an effective statistical tool. The technical details describing the differences between standard (unconditional) logistic and conditional logistic estimation techniques are explored elsewhere [8]. In practical terms, two choices exist: If the number of strata is small, then an unconditional logistic analysis is appropriate and gives accurate estimates of the influences from all risk variables on the outcome variable, including the influences of any categorical (strata) variables. If the number of strata is large relative to the number of observations, conditional estimation is necessary to achieve accurate estimates of the influence of the risk variables. The cost of this second choice is that it is no longer possible to assess the variable or variables used to create the strata. Matched-pairs data always consists of a large number of strata (N pairs created from $2N$ observations) and, therefore, will always require conditional estimation of the logistic model parameters. Once again, the influence of the "matching" variable or variables on case–control status cannot be evaluated. Otherwise, the evaluation of the model parameters and the interpretation of the analytic results from the two approaches to describing the relationships between a binary outcome variable and the influence of one or more risk variables are not fundamentally different.

A roughly analogous strategy creates a matched-pairs t-test analysis from continuous data. For each pair (stratum), control values are subtracted from case values ($difference = x_{case} - x_{control}$). These within-pair differences become the focus of interest. Thus, the observed mean case–control difference is compared to zero. Similar to the conditional logistic model approach, the case–control differences are not influenced by the strata variable, and differences among strata do not play a direct role in the comparison.

CONDITIONAL LOGISTIC ANALYSIS: BINARY RISK FACTOR

Consider again matched-pairs data in which both the outcome and the risk variable are binary. A logistic regression model describing a series of 2×2 tables (one table for each matched set) is

$$log\text{-}odds = a_i + fF \quad i = 1, 2, \cdots, N = \text{number of pairs (strata)},$$

where F is a binary indicator variable (for the example data, $F = 1$ for smokers and $F = 0$ for nonsmokers). The symbol a_i denotes the level of the log-odds among nonsmokers within each matched pair ($N = 167$ strata), and the coefficient represented by f reflects the extent of a constant risk from smoking within each pair, relative to the log-odds a_i. Using the maternal smoking–birth-weight data, a conditional logistic analysis yields an estimate of the logistic model parameter $\hat{f} = 0.598$, with a standard error of $S_{\hat{f}} = 0.265$. The variance associated with the estimate $\hat{f}$, as before (Figure 7–1, method II), is estimated by $variance(log[\hat{or}_m]) = variance(\hat{f}) = 1/b + 1/c$. An approximate 95% confidence interval is (0.078, 1.118), based on the estimate $\hat{f}$, its estimated variance, and the normal distribution. The estimated matched-pairs odds ratio $\hat{or}_m = e^{\hat{f}} = e^{0.598} = 1.818$ generates the approximate 95% confidence interval $(e^{0.078}, e^{1.118}) = (1.081, 3.059)$ from the smoking exposure data.

The conditional logistic model yields an unbiased estimate of the model parameter, f, avoiding the issue that a standard logistic model would require about one parameter for each matched pair. As noted, the cost of an unbiased estimate of the regression coefficient f is that the influences of the matching variable cannot be studied. Technically, unbiased estimates of the 166 a_i-parameters are not possible.

Evaluating the estimated regression coefficient $\hat{f}$ for evidence of an association between smoking exposure and low birth weight presents nothing new. The hypothesis $f = 0$ generates the test statistic

$$z = \frac{\hat{f} - 0}{S_{\hat{f}}} = \frac{0.598}{0.265} = 2.252$$

where, as usual, z has an approximate standard normal distribution when maternal smoking exposure is unrelated to the risk of a low-birth-weight infant. The associated p-value is 0.024.

This same issue ($f = 0$?) is also addressed by comparing log-likelihood statistics from two nested conditional logistic models. For the model approach to the smoking data, when $f = 0$, the log-likelihood statistic is $log(L_f = 0) = -115.756$, and when $f \neq 0$, the log-likelihood statistic increases to $log(L_{f \neq 0}) = -113.105$.

The log-likelihood ratio difference produces the test statistic

$$X^2 = -2[log(L_{f=0}) - log(L_{f\neq0})] = -2[-115.756 - (-113.105)] = 5.302,$$

with an approximate chi-square distribution with one degree of freedom when $f = 0$. The associated p-value is 0.021. This result is essentially the same as a Wald statistic since, $z^2 = (2.252)^2 = 5.072$ (p-value of 0.024).

The logistic model analysis of the influence of smoking exposure on the likelihood of a low-birth-weight infant is identical to the estimates and analysis from the previous model-free approach (Table 7–4, $\hat{or}_m = b/c = 40/22 = 1.818$). The primary difference is that the conditional estimation of the parameters from logistic regression models can be extended to the analysis of a wide variety of matched-design situations.

MULTIPLE CONTROLS PER CASE

Conditional logistic regression tools directly apply to matched data even when the number of controls varies among the N sets. The minimum data that is needed consists of three values for each matched set; a value that identifies the members of each set, a value that indicates case–control status (case $= 1$ or control $= 0$), and a value that indicates the presence or absence of the risk variable ($F = 1$ or $F = 0$). The data are once again a series of 2×2 tables (strata), each containing any number of matched-control observations for each pair.

Consider again the 1:2 matched sets from the birth defects study carried out in rural France (Table 7–12). The analysis of these $N = 12$ matched sets using the conditional logistic model $log\text{-}odds = a_i + fF$ yields the parameter estimate $\hat{f} = 0.693$, with estimated standard error $S_{\hat{f}} = 0.745$ (from the computer estimation algorithm). The estimated odds ratio $\hat{or}_m = e^{0.693} = 2.0$ is the same as the previous Cochran-Mantel-Haenszel estimate. An evaluation of the hypothesis of no association between EMF radiation exposure and the likelihood of a newborn with a birth defect using the test statistic $z = 0.693/0.745 = 0.930$ yields a p-value of $P(|\hat{f}| \geq 2.0|f = 0) = P(|z| \geq 0.930|f = 0) = 0.352$. This result is expectedly similar to the previous Mantel-Haenszel chi-square test based on the chi-square statistic $X^2 = 0.889$, where the p-value is 0.346.

In addition, the conditional estimated parameter $\hat{f}$ and standard error yield the confidence interval

$$(\hat{A}, \hat{B}) = (\hat{f} - 1.960S_{\hat{f}}, \hat{f} + 1.960S_{\hat{f}})$$
$$= [0.693 - 1.960(0.745), 0.693 + 1.960(0.745)] = (-0.767, 2.123).$$

The associated 95% confidence interval based on the estimated odds ratio $\hat{or} = e^{0.693} = 2.0$ becomes $(e^{-0.767}, e^{2.123}) = (0.464, 8.619)$.

CONDITIONAL LOGISTIC ANALYSIS: A BIVARIATE REGRESSION MODEL

A bivariate logistic regression model allows an efficient and succinct assessment of an association between case–control status and two binary risk factors (denoted as F and G) from matched-pairs data. A conditional logistic model including the possibility of an interaction between a risk factor F and a second risk factor G is

$$log\text{-}odds = a_i + fF + gG + h(F \times G).$$

For this bivariate model, a specific illustration is generated when the binary variable $F = 0$ or 1 indicates again whether the mother is a nonsmoker or a smoker and the variable $G = 0$ or 1, also a binary variable, indicates whether her newborn infant is her first child or not. The outcome, matched for prepregnancy weight, is again the likelihood of a low-birth-weight infant (case) or a normal-weight infant (control). Using a conditional analysis based on this bivariate logistic regression model yields three parameter estimates (Tables 7–3 and 7–17). As before, no unbiased estimates of the a_i-values (166 strata variables) are possible.

The odds ratios for the four combinations of the two binary risk factors are estimated from the expression

$$\hat{or}_m = e^{\hat{f}F + \hat{g}G + \hat{h}(F \times G)} = e^{0.232F - 0.204G + 0.945(F \times G)}$$
$$= (1.261)^F (0.815)^G (2.572)^{F \times G}.$$

The model-estimated odds ratios (Table 7–18) are relative to nonsmoking mothers who are having their first child ($F = G = 0$ or $or_m = 1.0$).

When an interaction term is not included ($h = 0$), the bivariate model becomes

$$log\text{-}odds = a_i + fF + gG$$

Table 7–17. Coefficients estimated from a conditional analysis of a nonadditive logistic regression model relating the influence of smoking exposure and parity to the likelihood of a low-birth-weight infant

Variables	Parameters	Estimates	Std. errors	p-Values	Odds ratios
Smoking exposure	f	0.232	0.333	0.486	1.261
Parity	g	−0.204	0.260	0.432	0.815
Interaction	h	0.945	0.536	0.078	2.572

LogLikelihood = −111.486

Table 7–18. Odds ratio estimates from the nonadditive conditional logistic model regression analysis of the binary risk factors maternal smoking exposure and parity

	Smoker, $F = 1$	Nonsmoker, $F = 0$
Parity ≥ 1, $G = 1$	2.646	0.815
Parity $= 0$, $G = 0$	1.261	1.0

Table 7–19. Coefficients estimated from the additive logistic regression model relating the influence of smoking exposure and parity to the likelihood of a low-birth-weight infant

Variables	Parameters	Estimates	Std. errors	p-Values	Odds ratios
Smoking exposure	f	0.595	0.267	0.026	1.813
Parity	g	0.024	0.224	0.914	1.025

LogLikelihood $= -113.099$

and produces estimates of the separate influences of smoking exposure and parity based on conditional estimated coefficients from this additive logistic regression model (Table 7–19).

To evaluate the interaction term ($h = 0$?), a Wald test statistic or a comparison of log-likelihood statistics, as usual, are essentially equivalent when the comparison involves a single coefficient. The test statistic $z^2 = [\hat{h}/S_{\hat{h}}]^2 = (1.763)^2 = 3.108$ produces a p-value of 0.078 (Table 7–17). The log-likelihood approach, where $log(L_{h=0}) = -113.099$ when $h = 0$ (Table 7–19) and $log(L_{h \neq 0}) = -111.486$ when $h \neq 0$ (Table 7–17) yields the log-likelihood ratio chi-square test statistic

$$X^2 = -2[log(L_{h=0}) - log(L_{h \neq 0})] = -2[-113.099 - (-111.486)] = 3.227,$$

with an associated p-value of 0.073.

The additive model estimated influence of smoking on the likelihood of a low-birth-weight infant is reflected by the odds ratio $\hat{or}_m = e^{0.595} = 1.813$, adjusted for the influence of parity. An approximate 95% confidence interval is $(1.075, 3.058)$. These two summary statistics are suspect, to some extent, because no persuasive evidence exists of an absence of an interaction between smoking exposure and parity (p-value $= 0.073$).

CONDITIONAL LOGISTIC ANALYSIS: INTERACTIONS WITH THE MATCHING VARIABLE

To repeat once again, a conditional logistic analysis of the smoking exposure data (Table 7–3) does not produce information on the influence of maternal

Table 7–20. Coefficients estimated from a conditional analysis of a logistic regression model applied to the smoking exposure and low-birth-weight data, including an interaction with maternal prepregnancy weight

Variables	Parameters	Estimates	Std. errors	p-Values	Odds ratios
Smoking exposure	f	0.435	0.387	0.261	1.545
Smoking $\times$ weight	h	0.302	0.533	0.571	1.353

LogLikelihood $= -112.944$

prepregnancy weight on infant birth weight. However, questions concerning interactions with a matching variable remain relevant. For example: Does the odds ratio measuring the association between smoking exposure and low birth weight depend on maternal prepregnancy weight?

This question of an interaction was previously addressed by creating separate 2×2 tables stratifying the matched pairs into two groups based on the prepregnancy weights of the paired mothers (Table 7–8). A conditional logistic analysis produces the same results (Table 7–20). The logistic regression model is

$$log\text{-}odds = a_i + fF + h(F \times H)$$

where F is again a binary variable indicating nonsmoking or smoking mothers and H indicates whether the prepregnancy weights of the paired mothers are below or above the median prepregnancy weight. In addition, as before, the variable $H = 0$ indicates a maternal pair whose weights are less than 56 kilograms ("low") and $H = 1$ indicates a pair whose weights are 56 kilograms or greater ("high"). The distribution of prepregnancy weights among the cases is identical to the distribution among the controls (exactly balanced). Therefore, prepregnancy weight is guaranteed to have no confounding influence, and a term measuring its influence is not included in the logistic model.

The postulated logistic model applied to the smoking exposure and low-birth-weight data produces estimates of the model parameters f and h (Table 7–20). The odds ratios estimated from the logistic model are the same odds ratios that arise from analyzing two separate 2×2 tables (model-free). Again, for mothers whose prepregnancy weight is less than 56 kilograms, the estimated odds ratio is $\hat{o}r_{low} = e^{\hat{f}} = e^{0.435} = 1.545$ and for mothers whose prepregnancy weight is 56 kilograms or more, the estimated odds ratio is $\hat{o}r_{high} = e^{\hat{f}+\hat{h}} = e^{0.737} = (1.545)(1.353) = 2.091$.

Comparing log-likelihood statistics from the two nested models essentially duplicates the previous chi-square test of equality of the odds ratios (Table 7–9). For the interaction model, the log-likelihood value is $log(L_{h\neq0}) = -112.944$

(Table 7–20) and for the additive model, $log(L_{h=0}) = -113.105$. The difference

$$X^2 = -2[log(L_{h=0}) - log(L_{h\neq0})] = -2[-113.105 - (-112.944)] = 0.322$$

has an approximate chi-square distribution with one degree of freedom when the two log-likelihood statistics differ by chance alone. The associated p-value is $P(X^2 \geq 0.322|no\ interaction) = 0.571$. The previous model-free chi-square test of independence applied to the specially constructed 2×2 table (Table 7–9) produces almost the identical result ($X^2 = 0.322$).

CONDITIONAL LOGISTIC ANALYSIS: K-LEVEL CATEGORY RISK VARIABLE

Exploring the association between exposure to EMF radiation and the likelihood of leukemia provides an illustration of a conditional analysis using a logistic regression model applied to a three-level categorical variable. An additive logistic model is

$$log\text{-}odds = a_i + b_1 x_1 + b_2 x_2$$

where x_1 and x_2 are binary components of a design variable incorporating a three-level categorical variable (HCC, OCC, and LCC, Table 7–14) into the model. Estimates of the model coefficients b_1 and b_2 provide an assessment of the role of EMF radiation exposure as a risk factor for childhood leukemia. The two estimated model parameters and estimates of their standard errors (Table 7–21) are based on the 60 discordant pairs from the childhood leukemia data (Table 7–14).

When the case–control array is perfectly symmetric, then $b_1 = 0$ and $b_2 = 0$ (no case–control association) and the counts within the three kinds of discordant pairs (HCC–OCC, HCC–LCC, and OCC–LCC) have ratios of exactly 1.0. In addition, the marginal case–control distributions are identical. Specifically, the logistic model becomes $log\text{-}odds = a_i$. For this no association model and the EMF data, the log-likelihood value is $log(L_0) = -87.608$. When the values

Table 7–21. Coefficients estimated from the analysis of the childhood leukemia data used to assess the influence of EMF radiation exposure (three-level categorical variable) using a conditional logistic regression model

Variables	Coefficients	Estimates	Std. errors	p-Values	Odds ratios
X_1	b_1	0.037	0.428	0.932	1.037
X_2	b_2	0.256	0.333	0.442	1.292

LogLikelihood $= -86.972$

underlying one or both of the ratios of the discordant pairs are not 1.0 (b_1 and b_2 are not both equal to zero), the log-likelihood value is $log(L_1) = -86.972$ (Table 7–21). The difference between these two log-likelihood statistics measures the extent of association between the three-level categorical risk factor (EMF radiation exposure) and case–control status. As usual, this difference (multiplied by -2) has an approximate chi-square distribution when no association exists. For the EMF data, the likelihood ratio test statistic

$$X^2 = -2[log(L_0) - log(L_1)] = -2[-87.608 - (-86.972)] = 0.729$$

(two degree of freedom) produces a p-value of $P(X^2 \geq 0.729 | b_1 = b_2 = 0) = 0.695$. The chi-square distributed test statistic provides little evidence that the likelihood of leukemia is related to EMF radiation exposure. This likelihood ratio test and the previous chi-square test of marginal homogeneity (Table 7–16, $X_H^2 = 0.727$) are slightly different approaches to the same question and will always give approximately the same result.

In the case of a 3×3 case–control array, the goodness-of-fit assessment is identical to the assessment of an interaction. When an interaction term is included, the additive model becomes saturated, and the conditional logistic analysis applied to the case–control array ($k = 3$) produces estimated values identical to the observed data. Thus, the difference between the estimated values from additive model and the observed values (saturated interaction model) is a measure of the adequacy of the model to summarize the data. For the EMF data, the additive model hardly differs from the saturated model. The log-likelihood value for the saturated model is $log(L_{sat}) = -87.975$, and the log-likelihood value for the additive model is, as before, $log(L_{add}) = -86.972$. The small difference produces the likelihood ratio test statistic

$$X^2 = -2[log(L_{add}) - log(L_{sat})] = -2[-86.972 - (-86.975)] = 0.006.$$

The corresponding p-value is 0.938 (degrees of freedom $= 1$). Inferences from an additive model always require assurance that interactions are small and likely random (more details in Chapter 13), and this is certainly the case for the analysis of the EMF data.

CONDITIONAL LOGISTIC ANALYSIS: CONTINUOUS VARIABLES

An important feature of a statistical model is that continuous risk variables can be directly analyzed, as reported. To illustrate, consider a model postulated to explore an interaction between prepregnancy weight (denoted x and reported in kilograms)

Table 7–22. Coefficients estimated from a conditional logistic regression model reflecting a possible interaction between prepregnancy weight and smoking exposure

Variables	Parameters	Estimates	Std. errors	p-Values	Odds ratios
Smoking exposure	f	1.045	1.290	0.418	–*
Smoking × weight	h	−0.0075	0.021	0.723	0.993

LogLikelihood $= -113.042$
* = Depends on the prepregnancy weight

and smoking (F = binary indicator variable) using again the low-birth-weight data (Table 7–3) where

$$log\text{-}odds = a_i + fF + h(F \times x).$$

As before, the direct effect of prepregnancy weight is not part of the logistic model because it is the variable used to form the matched pairs (exactly balanced). In contrast to the previous analysis (Table 7–20), directly using reported prepregnancy weight allows the model parameters f and h to be estimated (Table 7–22) with a maximum efficiency and avoids the potential bias incurred from forming arbitrary categories based on maternal prepregnancy weight.

The estimated pattern of influence of prepregnancy weight (x) on the relationship between the likelihood of a low-birth-weight infant and maternal smoking exposure is summarized by a series of estimated odds ratios. For example, the model-estimated odds ratios among smokers ($F = 1$) for different prepregnancy weights (x) are given by the expression

$$\hat{o}r_m = e^{\hat{f}+\hat{h}x} = e^{1.045-0.0075x} = (2.843)(0.993)^x.$$

A nonadditive model dictates that the odds ratio measuring the association between smoking exposure and the likelihood of a low-birth-weight infant depends on maternal prepregnancy weight. Selected estimates of the model-generated odds ratios are:

Maternal weight (kg)	40	50	60	70	80
Odds ratio ($\hat{o}r_m$)	2.11	1.96	1.81	1.68	1.56

Evaluation of the importance of this interaction effect follows the usual pattern. The likelihood ratio chi-square test statistic with one degree of freedom is

$$X^2 = -2[log(L_{h=0}) - log(L_{h\neq0})] = -2[-113.105 - (-113.042)] = 0.125$$

making the associated p-value $P(X^2 \geq 0.125|h = 0) = 0.724$. Using an approach that is more powerful than the previous comparison of two odds ratios (Table 7–9),

Table 7–23. Coefficients estimated from a conditional logistic regression model reflecting the separate (additive) influences of smoking exposure and weight gained (as reported) on likelihood of a low-birth-weight infant

Variables	Parameters	Estimates	Std. errors	p-Values	Odds ratios
Smoking exposure	f	0.649	0.321	0.043	1.914
Weight gained	g	−0.257	0.050	<0.001	0.774

LogLikelihood = −80.271

again no apparent evidence emerges of an interaction between prepregnancy weight and smoking exposure.

The matched data displayed in Table 7–3 ($N = 167$ pairs) contain the reported maternal weight gained during pregnancy. In fact, the purpose of obtaining the data is to describe the influence of maternal weight gained on the likelihood of a low-birth-weight infant. An additive logistic regression model including both the influences of smoking (binary variable) and weight gained (in kilograms, as reported) is

$$log\text{-}odds = a_i + fF + gw$$

where w represents the reported maternal weight gained, abstracted from medical records, and again $F = 0$ indicates nonsmokers and $F = 1$ smokers. The evaluation of weight gained as an influence on the likelihood of a low-birth-weight infant using an additive conditional logistic model requires the estimation of two model coefficients (Table 7–23).

The relevance of weight gained to the likelihood of a low-birth-weight infant is once again assessed by comparing log-likelihood statistics. The chi-square likelihood ratio test statistic with one degree of freedom is

$$X^2 = -2[log(L_{g=0}) - log(L_{g \neq 0})] = -2[-113.105 - (-80.271)] = 65.566,$$

producing an associated p-value $= P(X^2 \geq 65.566 | g = 0) < 0.001$.

The extremely small significance level indicates an extremely plausible systematic decrease in likelihood of a low-birth-weight infant associated with maternal weight gained. Specifically, the estimated odds ratio $e^{-0.257} = 0.774$ indicates that the odds are reduced by a factor of $1/0.774 = 1.3$ for each kilogram increase in maternal weight, adjusted for smoking exposure and maternal prepregnancy weight. The 95% confidence interval is $(0.701, 0.854)$.

ADDITIVE LOGISTIC REGRESSION MODEL

In general, an additive logistic model for a sample of matched pairs is

$$log\text{-}odds = a_i + b_1x_1 + b_2x_2 + b_3x_3 + \cdots + b_kx_k$$

where each x_i-value represents one of k risk variables (continuous or discrete or categorical). Although conditional estimation techniques are required for a matched-pairs multivariable regression model, to repeat, the properties and the interpretation of analytic results are not fundamentally different from an unconditional logistic model (Chapter 5).

For both conditional and unconditional logistic models, the independent variables are unrestricted, which is the case for regression models in general. For example, a conditional logistic regression model employing four risk variables (three binary and one continuous) to study the likelihood of a low-birth-weight infant is represented by

$$log\text{-}odds = a_i + b_1x_1 + b_2x_2 + b_3x_3 + b_4x_4$$

where x_1 is binary (nonsmokers = 0 or smokers = 1), x_2 is binary (first child = 0 or one or more children = 1), x_3 is continuous (weight gained, as reported), x_4 is binary (less than term = gestation <37 weeks = 0 or full term = gestation $\geq$ 37 weeks = 1). The estimates of the additive model regression coefficients are given in Table 7–24 using the four variables contained in the 167 matched-pairs data set (Table 7–3).

The estimated regression coefficient $\hat{b}_3 = -0.244$ from the four-variable additive logistic model again indicates that weight gained during pregnancy has a strong influence on the likelihood of a low-birth-weight infant (p-value <0.001 and odds ratio = $e^{-0.244} = 0.783$).

The estimated regression coefficients are adjusted to be "free" from the confounding influences from maternal prepregnancy weight due to the matching structure of the data. The influences from the four risk variables (x_i) are "balanced" between case–control comparisons by including these variables in the additive

Table 7–24. Coefficients estimated from a four-variable additive conditional logistic model: smoking exposure, parity, weight gained, and gestation (Table 7–3)

Variables	Parameters	Estimates	Std. errors	p-Values	Odds ratios
Smoking exposure	b_1	0.629	0.325	0.053	1.877
Parity	b_2	−0.093	0.278	0.738	0.911
Weight gained	b_3	−0.244	0.052	<0.001	0.783
Gestation	b_4	0.796	0.776	0.305	2.216

LogLikelihood = −79.659

Table 7–25.   Results from the five-variable standard (unconditional) logistic regression analysis: smoking, parity, weight gained, gestation, and prepregnancy weight (Table 7–3)

Variables	Parameters	Estimates	Std. errors	p-Values	Odds ratios
Constant	a	0.309	0.696	–	-
Smoking exposure	b_1	0.549	0.269	0.041	1.731
Parity	b_2	−0.051	0.242	0.834	0.951
Weight gained	b_3	−0.105	0.021	<0.001	0.900
Gestation	b_4	0.588	0.257	0.022	1.800
Prepregnancy weight	b_5	0.004	0.010	0.712	1.004

LogLikelihood = −206.043

model. However, adding the parity and gestational age variables to the model has only a small influence on the association between weight gained and the likelihood of a low-birth-weight infant ($\hat{b}_3 = -0.244$, Table 7–24 and $\hat{b}_2 = -0.257$, Table 7–23).

When the matching variable or variables do not have a strong confounding influence, a matched and unmatched analysis produce similar results. A sense of the effectiveness of a matching strategy comes from comparing the conditional and unconditional logistic regression analyses. For the weight-gained data, a typical additive model (unconditional) is

$$log\text{-}odds = a + b_1x_1 + b_2x_2 + b_3x_3 + b_4x_4 + b_5x_5$$

and employs the same data and variables as the matched-pairs conditional analysis, but directly includes the measured prepregnancy weight as reported (x_5) and a single constant term (a). The matched structure of the data is ignored, yielding $2N = 2(167) = 334$ observations. The analysis using unconditional estimation produces the coefficients given in Table 7–25.

The estimated odds ratios from the unconditional analysis (Table 7–25) differ from the conditional analysis (Table 7–24). For the weight-gained variable, the matched-pairs estimated regression coefficient is $\hat{b}_3 = -0.244$ ($S_{\hat{b}_3} = 0.052$) and, ignoring the matched design, the estimated regression coefficient is $\hat{b}_3 = -0.105$ ($S_{\hat{b}_3} = 0.021$). In terms of odds ratios, the estimated odds ratios are $\hat{or}_m = 1/0.783 = 1.277$ and $\hat{or} = 1/0.900 = 1.111$, respectively. As expected, the standard errors associated with the "unmatched" coefficient are smaller, primarily due to the larger sample size ($n = 334$) that includes the concordant pairs. As previously noted, this trade-off (biased estimates with increased precision) is sometimes an issue in choosing between matched and unmatched approaches. It should also be noted that the influence of the matching variable (prepregnancy weight) in the unconditional model is decreased because the controls are not a random sample. Their distribution is necessarily similar to the cases because of the original matching process. Thus, the coefficient $\hat{b}_5$ is artificially reduced.

8

SPATIAL DATA: ESTIMATION AND ANALYSIS

The distribution of disease in a population is fundamental to epidemiology, as noted by Abraham Lilienfeld [28] who began his classic text:

> Epidemiology may be defined as the study of the distribution of disease or a pathological condition in human populations and the factors that influence this distribution.

Although Lilienfeld had in mind "distribution" in a broad sense, one of the earliest successes in epidemiology can be traced to the study of the spatial distribution of disease. Dr. John Snow (*b.* 1813) identified the source of cholera in the 19th century based in part on evidence from the spatial pattern of cases in a specific area of London.

> Note: British physician John Snow utilized what became a classic epidemiologic approach to study the origins of cholera in 1854. He postulated that cholera was caused by a contaminant in the water supply when bacterial disease was an unknown phenomenon. This remarkable insight was based on data collected from customers of two water companies, where one of these companies provided water relatively less contaminated with sewage. He also plotted the locations of cholera deaths in central London on a map. By comparing the mortality rates between the groups served by the two water companies and examining the spatial distribution of cases, Dr. Snow concluded that an "impurity" in the water was associated with the occurrence of cholera deaths. The complete account of this historical analysis of epidemiologic data is given in Snow's book *On the Mode of Communication of Cholera.*

197

Spatial distributions play a central role in the descriptions of a number of diseases and frequently are an essential element in the analysis of human data involving exposures to suspected environmental sources of disease risk. This chapter describes three approaches for identifying spatial patterns and, at the same time, introduces and illustrates the application of four valuable statistical techniques (test of variance, nearest-neighbor analysis, randomization tests, and bootstrap estimation) that additionally apply to a wide range of kinds of data.

POISSON PROBABILITY DISTRIBUTION: AN INTRODUCTION

The Poisson probability distribution provides a statistical description of objects distributed spatially at random. The spatial distributions of such diverse things as stars, weeds, bacteria, cases of rare diseases, and even World War II flying-bomb strikes are described, sometimes quite accurately, by Poisson probabilities.

The study of spatial patterns based on a Poisson probability distribution begins by dividing an area of interest into a series of equal-area and nonoverlapping subdivisions, so that the probability that a single random observation falls within a specific subdivision is small. In most cases this probability can be made small by creating a large number of subdivisions. When the probability that an observation is found in a specific subdivision is constant (denoted by p), the count of the subdivisions containing 0, 1, 2, 3, ... or more random observations has a Poisson probability distribution. Random means that the probability an observations falls into any one subdivision is proportional only to the size of the subdivision. The size of the subdivision and not its location completely determines this probability. More formally, the distribution of equal-area subdivisions containing k observations (denoted X) is given by the expression

$$\textit{number of subdivisions with k observations} = m \times P(X = k) = m \, \frac{\lambda^k e^{-\lambda}}{k!}$$

where m represents the total number of subdivisions and $P(X = k)$ represents a *Poisson probability*. A single parameter, denoted λ, completely determines the Poisson distribution. As noted (Chapter 3), for the Poisson distribution, the mean value and the variance are both equal to λ.

When spatial clustering exists, some subdivisions have large numbers of observations (cluster), whereas others to have relatively few observations. That is, the probability that an observation falls within a specific subarea varies. A Poisson distribution requires these probabilities to be constant. Failure of the Poisson distribution as a description of a spatial pattern provides evidence that the locations of at least some observations are not randomly distributed across the region under investigation.

Three kinds of spatial patterns are: uniform, random, and nonuniform (clustering). Specifically:

1. A uniform distribution has a pattern consisting of equal distances between all points.
2. A random distribution has no pattern of points.
3. A nonuniform distribution has a pattern of concentration and sparseness of points.

These three kinds of patterns (plus random variation) are displayed in Figure 8–1.

Spatial data distributed into a series of equal-area subdivisions produces a distribution of counts (such as Table 8–1). Comparison of the mean value to the variance of these spatial data characterizes the kind of pattern. For uniformly distributed points, the mean value is greater than the variance; for randomly distributed points, the mean value equals the variance; and for points that cluster, the mean value is less than the variance.

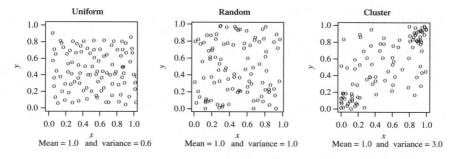

Figure 8–1. Three kinds of spatial patterns.

Table 8–1. Poisson probabilities ($\lambda = 2$) and counts of subdivisions with k points

k	0	1	2	3	4	5	6	7	**Total**
Theory:									
expected counts	13.5	27.1	27.1	18.0	9.0	3.6	1.2	0.5	100
probabilities	0.135	0.271	0.271	0.180	0.090	0.036	0.012	0.005	1.00
Data:									
observed counts	16	27	23	17	12	2	3	0	100
proportions	0.160	0.270	0.230	0.170	0.120	0.020	0.030	0.0	1.00

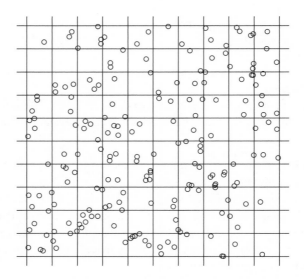

Figure 8–2. Two-hundred random points distributed over a unit square divided into 100 equal sub-squares.

Figure 8–2 displays $n = 200$ computer-generated random points distributed over a unit square. There are $m = 100$ sub-squares each with area $= 0.01$, so that each random point has the same probability of falling into a specific sub-square, namely $p = 1/m = 1/100 = 0.01$. The mean number of points per sub-square is then $\lambda = np = 200(0.01) = 2$. Or, more simply, since there are 200 points and 100 sub-squares, the mean number of random points per square is $n/m = 200/100 = 2$. Poisson probabilities from a distribution with a mean value of λ and the numbers of subdivisions with k points are the primary elements to assessing the randomness of a spatial pattern (Table 8–1 and Figure 8–2).

A classic study [29] of a spatial distribution was conducted during World War II to identify the pattern, if any, of flying-bomb strikes in south London. It was critical to know if the German flying bombs were falling at random ($p =$ constant) or whether these bombs possessed some sort of guidance system ($p \neq$ constant, clustering). South London was divided into $m = 576$ small subdivisions, each with an area of 0.25 square kilometers. The World War II flying-bomb data are reproduced in Table 8–2, where the number of subdivisions with k hits are recorded. For example, among the 576 areas, the number of subdivisions with three hits is 35.

Application of the Poisson distribution requires a value for the parameter λ or, more usually, an estimate of this defining parameter. The observed mean number of hits per subdivision ($\hat{\lambda} = \bar{x}$) is the maximum likelihood estimate of the unknown

Table 8–2. Flying-bomb hits in south London: data

k	0	1	2	3	4	5	Total
Count	229	211	93	35	7	1	576

Table 8–3. Flying-bomb hits data from south London: distributions of the observed and theoretical number of hits

k	0	1	2	3	4	5	Total
Observed counts	229	211	93	35	7	1	576
Probabilities	0.395	0.367	0.170	0.053	0.012	0.003	1.0
Theoretical counts	227.53	211.34	98.15	30.39	7.06	1.54	576

underlying mean number of hits, the parameter λ. Almost always, the sample mean $\bar{x}$ is used in place of the unknown population parameter λ to generate estimated Poisson probabilities from collected data. Specifically, for the World War II data,

$$
\hat{\lambda} = \frac{total\ number\ of\ hits}{number\ of\ subdivisions}
$$
$$
= \frac{0(229) + 1(211) + 2(93) + 3(35) + 4(7) + 5(1)}{576}
$$
$$
= \frac{535}{576} = 0.929
$$

is the estimated mean number of hits per subdivision (a bit less than one per subdivision). Or, the number $n = 535$ flying-bomb strikes among the $m = 576$ subdivisions produces the mean number of hits $\hat{\lambda} = \bar{x} = n/m = 535/576 = 0.929$. An estimate of the parameter λ makes it possible to estimate the Poisson probabilities and calculate the theoretical number of hits as if they were randomly distributed among 576 areas (Table 8–3). For the example, for $k = 3$ hits, the estimated Poisson probability is

$$
probability\ X\ equals\ three = \hat{P}(X = 3) = \hat{p}_3 = \frac{e^{-\hat{\lambda}}(\hat{\lambda})^3}{3!}
$$
$$
= \frac{e^{-0.929}(0.929)^3}{3!} = 0.053
$$

and the theoretical number of areas with three hits becomes $m\hat{p}_3 = 576(0.053) = 30.387$. The observed value is 35.

A chi-square statistic or any other goodness-of-fit measure used to evaluate the accuracy of the Poisson distribution as a description of the London data is hardly necessary. These World War II data appear in a number of textbooks because of the extraordinarily close correspondence between the observed and theoretically generated values. The conclusion more than 60 years ago would have been that the data from south London show no evidence that these weapons were guided with any accuracy.

Data certainly arise where it is not obvious whether a Poisson distribution accurately describes the variation among the sampled observations. In this situation, a summary value and its significance test are useful statistical tools. A summary test statistic to assess the Poisson distribution as a description of a spatial pattern is developed from the fact that the mean value and the variance are identical for randomly distributed spatial data. It follows that the sample mean value $\bar{x}$ and the sample variance S_X^2 should then be approximately equal when the data are randomly distributed (no spatial pattern) or, in symbols,

$$\frac{S_X^2}{\bar{x}} \approx 1$$

where $\bar{x}$ and S_X^2 are calculated in the usual way. The ratio $S_X^2/\bar{x}$ multiplied by $(m-1)$ has an approximate chi-square distribution when the sampled counts have a Poisson distribution (m represents again the total number of subdivisions). The degrees of freedom are the number of subdivision minus one or $m-1$.

The test statistic $X^2 = (m-1)S_X^2/\bar{x}$, called the *test of variance* for obvious reasons, is a specific version of the usual expression for the Pearson chi-square statistic. For the Poisson test of variance, the mean value represented by λ, is estimated by the sample mean value, $\hat{\lambda} = \bar{x} = \sum x_i/n$.

Substituting this estimate into the usual Pearson chi-square expression as the expected value ($expected_i = \bar{x}$) gives the test statistic

$$X^2 = \sum \frac{(observed_i - expected_i)^2}{expected_i} = \sum \frac{(x_i - \bar{x})^2}{\bar{x}} = (m-1)\frac{S_X^2}{\bar{x}}$$

where x_i represents one of n observations and $i = 1, 2, \cdots, n$. Again, the chi-square distribution is applied to assess the likelihood that the observed variation is random (Chapter 2).

To illustrate, the sample mean value of the data displayed in Figure 8–2 (also given in Table 8–1) is $\bar{x} = 2.0$, and the estimated variance is $S_X^2 = 2.242$, based on $n = 200$ observations. The ratio $S_X^2/\bar{x} = 2.242/2.0 = 1.121$ yields the test statistic $X^2 = 99(1.121) = 111.0$ that has an approximate chi-square distribution with $m - 1 = 99$ degrees of freedom when the 200 observations are distributed at random over the $m = 100$ subdivisions of the unit square (Figure 8–2). The associated p-value of $P(X^2 \geq 111.0 | p = constant) = 0.193$ indicates that an observed difference between $\bar{x}$ and S^2 (2.0 vs. 2.242) is not unusual when no spatial pattern exists. In other words, the observed variation is plausibly random.

A test of variance is effective for small samples of data and can be applied to assess randomness in a number of situations other than a spatial analysis. In addition, the test of variance can be modified to compare sampled data to other postulated probability distributions [30].

NEAREST-NEIGHBOR ANALYSIS

Employing counts from a series of subdivisions to identify spatial patterns has a weakness. Distance is a continuous measure. Analyzing tables constructed from grouping continuous values into a series of categories is rarely as effective as directly using the values themselves, particularly for samples containing small numbers of observations. One approach to the question of spatial randomness that directly utilizes the observed distances between points is a *nearest-neighbor analysis*.

A nearest-neighbor distance is basically what the name suggests. For a specific point, among a sample of n points, the distances to all other points are calculated. The nearest-neighbor value is the smallest distance among the $n - 1$ possibilities. For the ith point, the nearest-neighbor distance is denoted r_i. The collection of these n minimum distances, one for each of the n observations, constitutes a nearest-neighbor data set, denoted $\{r_1, r_2, \cdots, r_n\}$.

In a surprisingly simple way, the theoretical probability distribution of the nearest-neighbor distances can be justified under the condition that the spatial distribution of the observed points is random. A test of spatial randomness follows from comparing the mean value estimated from a sample of nearest-neighbor distances to the mean value derived from the theoretical probability distribution of a sample of nearest-neighbor distances among points with no spatial pattern.

Recall that Euler's constant, e, is defined by the expression

$$\left[1 + \frac{1}{n}\right]^n$$

and equals a value symbolized by e when n becomes infinitely large. A simple proof exists (in most calculus books) that Euler's expression is less than 3 for any value of n and is computed to be 2.71828 .... More generally, Euler's expression gives

$$\left[1 + \frac{x}{n}\right]^n = e^x$$

when n becomes infinite.

The importance of Euler's constant e in the nearest-neighbor context is that the product of n constant probabilities (denoted $p = 1 - q$) is simply expressed as

e^{-nq} or, specifically,

$$p^n = [1-q]^n = \left[1 - \frac{nq}{n}\right]^n \approx e^{-nq}$$

for moderate values of n, and is exact when n becomes infinite. For example, if $p = 0.99$ and $n = 200$, then

$$(0.99)^{200} = (1 - 0.01)^{200} = \left[1 - \frac{200(0.01)}{200}\right]^{200}$$

$$= 0.134 \text{ and } e^{-200(0.01)} = 0.135.$$

Consider a single point (x_0, y_0) and a circle of radius, r, with this point at the center. In addition, envision that this circle is contained in another circle with the same center but with larger radius, R $(r < R)$. The probability that a random point falls within the larger circle and also falls within the smaller circle is $\pi r^2/A$, where A represents the area of the larger circle $(A = \pi R^2)$. The complementary probability that a random point does not fall in the smaller circle is $1 - \pi r^2/A$. The probably that n independent random points fall within the circle A and do not fall into the smaller concentric circle is approximately

$$P(no\ points\ occur\ within\ radius\ r\ of\ the\ point\ [x_0,\ y_0]) =$$

$$\left[1 - \frac{\pi r^2}{A}\right]^n = \left[1 - \frac{n\pi r^2}{nA}\right]^n \approx e^{-n\pi r^2/A}.$$

Then, the complementary probability that at least one of n random points falls in the smaller circle is

$$F(r) = P(one\ or\ more\ points\ occur\ within\ radius\ r\ of\ the\ point\ [x_0,\ y_0])$$

$$\approx 1 - e^{-n\pi r^2/A}$$

where n/A represents the density of points (points per unit of area).

The probability that one or more of the n random points fall into the small circle is the same as the probability that a nearest-neighbor point falls within a radius of r units of the specific point (x_0, y_0). That is, if no points fall within the smaller circle, then the nearest-neighbor distance is greater than a distance r and, conversely, if one or more points fall in the smaller circle, then the nearest-neighbor distance is less than a distance r. The expression $F(r)$ is special case of a *cumulative probability distribution function*. For a selected nearest-neighbor value, r_0, the probability that a random nearest-neighbor distance is less than r_0 is $F(r_0)$. In symbols, this specific cumulative probability distribution function is

$$cumulative\ distribution\ function = F(r_0) = P(R \leq r_0) = 1 - e^{-n\pi r_0^2/A}$$

for a sample of n nearest-neighbor distances when the observed points are distributed spatially at random over an area A.

The cumulative distribution $F(r)$ defines the properties of the probability distribution of the random nearest-neighbor distances. For example, the theoretical median distance associated with a sample of n random nearest-neighbor distances is

$$F(r_m) = 1 - e^{-n\pi r_m/A} = 0.5, \quad \text{then} \quad median = r_m$$

$$= 0.470\sqrt{\frac{A}{n}} \quad (0.470 = \sqrt{log(2)/\pi}).$$

Along the same lines, using a calculus argument, the theoretical nearest-neighbor mean value and variance of the distribution of the nearest-neighbor sample mean value are

$$mean(\bar{r}) = 0.5\sqrt{\frac{A}{n}} \quad \text{with} \quad variance(\bar{r}) = 0.068\frac{A}{n^2} \quad \left(0.068 = \frac{1}{\pi} - \frac{1}{4}\right)$$

when the n points are randomly distributed over a region with total area A. The estimated sample mean value $\bar{r}$ is, as usual, $\bar{r} = \sum r_i/n$.

The similarity of the theoretical median and mean values of the distribution of the nearest-neighbor distances (mean/median $= 0.50/0.47 = 1.06$ for all sample sizes) indicates that the distribution of the nearest-neighbor distances is close to symmetric. A nearly symmetric distribution of nearest-neighbor distances essentially guarantees that the distribution of the sample mean value ($\bar{r}$) is accurately approximated by a normal distribution, even for relatively small samples of data ($n > 10$ or so).

To illustrate, the $n = 10$ hypothetical points plotted in Figure 8–3, contained in a total area $A = 15^2 = 225$ square units, generate 10 nearest-neighbor distances (Table 8–4).

The theoretical cumulative probability distribution function becomes $F(r) = 1 - e^{-0.140r^2}$ where $n\pi/A = 10(3.1416)/225 = 0.140$. For example, the probability that a random nearest-neighbor distance is within 2 units of a specific point is

$$P(R \leq 2) = 1 - e^{-0.104(2)^2} = 0.428$$

or the probability that nearest-neighbor distance is greater than 1 but less than 3 units is

$$P(1 \leq R \leq 3) = P(R \leq 1) - P(R \leq 3) = e^{-0.140(1)^2} - e^{-0.140(3)^2}$$
$$= 0.869 - 0.284 = 0.586,$$

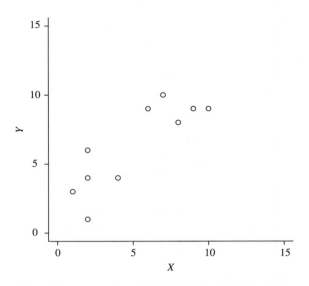

Figure 8–3. Ten hypothetical points distributed over a square 15 units on a side (A= 225) to illustrate nearest-neighbor calculations (Table 8–4).

Table 8–4. Nearest-neighbor distances from the example data displayed in Figure 8–3

	Point		Nearest		Distance
i	X	Y	X'	Y'	r_i
1	1	3	2	4	1.414
2	2	1	1	3	2.236
3	2	4	1	3	1.414
4	2	6	2	4	2.000
5	4	4	2	4	2.000
6	6	9	7	10	1.414
7	7	10	6	9	1.414
8	8	8	9	9	1.414
9	9	9	10	9	1.000
10	10	9	9	9	1.000

as long as the points are randomly distributed. The median value is $r_m = 0.470\sqrt{225/10} = 2.229$ or $P(nearest\text{-}neighbor\ distance \geq 2.229)=0.5$.

The mean value and the variance of the probability distribution of the mean nearest-neighbor distance, calculated under the conjecture that the 10 points occur randomly over the $A = 225$ square units of the xy-plane, are

$$mean(\bar{r}) = 0.5\sqrt{\frac{225}{10}} = 2.372 \text{ and}$$
$$variance(\bar{r}) = 0.068\frac{225}{10^2} = 0.153.$$

The observed mean value of the $n = 10$ nearest-neighbor distances $(\bar{r})$ is accurately approximated by a normal distribution, as mentioned, using these theoretical values $mean(\bar{r})$ and $variance(\bar{r})$, even for this rather small sample size. Specifically, the sample mean value is

$$\bar{r} = \frac{1}{n}\sum r_i = \frac{15.307}{10} = 1.531,$$

and applying the test statistic

$$Z = \frac{\bar{r} - mean(\bar{r})}{\sqrt{variance(\bar{r})}} = \frac{\bar{r} - 0.5\sqrt{A/n}}{\sqrt{0.068A/n^2}}$$

yields a typical summary statistic to assess the difference between sample and theoretical mean values $(\bar{r} = 1.531$ vs. $mean(\bar{r}) = 2.372)$. The test statistic Z is an observation from an approximate standard normal distribution when no spatial pattern exists.

Specifically, from the example data $(\bar{r} = 1.531)$, the value of the test statistic is

$$z = \frac{1.531 - 2.372}{\sqrt{0.153}} = -2.150.$$

The one-sided p-value associated with $z = -2.150$ is $P(Z \le -2.150 \,|\, no\ spatial\ pattern) = 0.016$ and indicates that it is not likely that the 10 points in Table 8–4 (Figure 8–3) are randomly distributed over the 225 square units of area. A one-sided statistical test is appropriate because small values of z are associated with small values of $\bar{r}$, and small values of $\bar{r}$ occur only when at least some of the observations cluster.

A nearest-neighbor analysis applied to the 200 points (Table 8–1 and Figure 8–2) confirms the previous Poisson analysis. The theoretical mean nearest-neighbor distance is $mean(\bar{r}) = 0.5\sqrt{1/200} = 0.035$, and the standard error of the distribution of the mean value is $\sqrt{variance(\bar{r})} = \sqrt{0.068(1/200^2)} = 0.00130$. The observed mean value calculated from the 200 observed nearest-neighbor distances is $\bar{r} = 0.0356$. Treating these data as if the observed points were distributed randomly over a unit square ($A = 1$), the test statistic becomes

$$z = \frac{0.0356 - 0.0354}{0.00130} = 0.206,$$

and the associated one-sided p-value is $P(Z \leq 0.206 | no\ spatial\ pattern) = 0.581$.

COMPARISON OF CUMULATIVE PROBABILITY DISTRIBUTION FUNCTIONS

An alternative to using a statistical test to compare a data estimated mean value ($\bar{r}$) to a theoretical derived mean value [$mean(\bar{r})$] is the comparison of two cumulative probability distribution functions. An empirical cumulative distribution function (estimated nonparameterically and denoted $\hat{F}$) is defined by the expression

$$\hat{F}(x) = P(X \leq x) = \frac{number\ of\ values\ less\ than\ or\ equal\ to\ x}{n}$$

for a sample of n observations. More simply, the values of the estimated cumulative distribution function denoted $\hat{F}(x)$ are the proportions of observations less than or equal to each value x for each of the n observations. This estimate is entirely assumption-free. Thus, the estimated cumulative probabilities are entirely determined by the data.

From the $n = 10$ nearest-neighbor values in Table 8–4, the estimated cumulative distribution function, denoted $\hat{F}(r_i)$, is

$$\hat{F}(r_i) = P(R \leq r_i) = \frac{i}{n} = \frac{i}{10} \qquad i = 1, 2, \cdots, 10$$

where the ten nearest neighbor distances r_i are ordered from low to high (Table 8–5).

For the same data, the theoretical cumulative probability function based on the assumption that the spatial distribution is random is again

$$F(r_i) = P(R \leq r_i) = 1 - e^{-n\pi r_i^2/A} = 1 - e^{-0.140r_i^2}.$$

Table 8–5. The nonparametric estimated cumulative distribution function ($\hat{F}_i$) for $n = 10$ example nearest-neighbor values (Table 8–4)

i	1	2	3	4	5	6	7	8	9	10
r_i	1.000	1.000	1.414	1.414	1.414	1.414	1.414	2.000	2.000	2.236
$\hat{F}(r_i)$	0.1	0.2	0.3	0.4	0.5	0.6	0.7	0.8	0.9	1.0

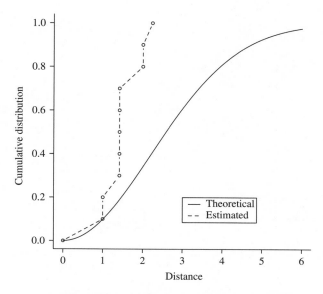

Figure 8–4. Comparison of two cumulative distribution functions: theoretical (F, data random) and nonparametric ($\hat{F}$, assumption-free) estimated from the $n = 10$ nearest-neighbor values (Table 8–4).

Methods exist to formally compare cumulative distribution $\hat{F}$ to F but in many cases a plot suffices to identify differences between the two distributions (particularly for this example). As with the comparison of mean values, the differences observed are either due to sampling variation or due to the fact that the spatial distribution of the observations is not random. The plot (Figure 8–4) leaves little doubt that the example data are not distributed spatially at random; in symbols, $F \neq \hat{F}$.

The spatially random points ($n = 200$) displayed in Figure 8–2 also illustrate the comparison of cumulative distribution functions ($\hat{F}$ to F). The nonparametric estimated distribution function $\hat{F}(r_i) = P(R \leq r_i)$ consisting of 200 probabilities is displayed in Figure 8–5 (dashed line). The parallel theoretical cumulative distribution function, again based on the assumption that no pattern exists within the spatial data (random),

$$F(r_i) = P(R \leq r_i) = 1 - e^{-n\pi r_i^2/A} = 1 - e^{-200\pi r_i^2/1.0},$$

is plotted on the same set of axes (solid line). The comparison shows essentially no difference, indicating that the conjecture that the data are spatially distributed at random is, as expected, supported by the random data.

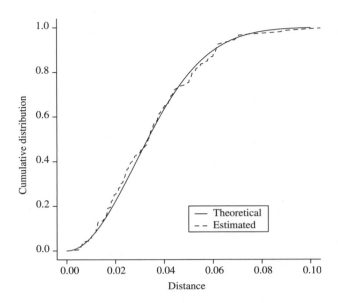

Figure 8–5. Comparison of the theoretical (*F*, data random) and data estimated (*F̂*, assumption-free) cumulative probability distributions for the *n* = 200 random points displayed in Table 8–1 and Figure 8–2.

Clearly, results less obvious than these two examples occur from the comparison of cumulative normal distribution functions ($\hat{F}$ vs. F). In the case where a plot is helpful but not conclusive, statistical tests exist, and the associated *p*-values indicate the likelihood that the observed difference arose by chance alone (for example, the previous test of mean values or the Kolmogrov test [31]).

The comparison of cumulative distribution functions is a general statistical technique and is useful in a large variety of situations ([32] and [33]). For example, the question of the normality of a set of observations is directly addressed by comparing theoretical and estimated cumulative distribution functions both graphically and with a Kolmogrov test.

A general issue encountered in spatial analysis of disease data must be considered in the application of the nearest-neighbor approach. The choice of the relevant geographic region is critical to the outcome of a spatial analysis and rarely do clear, unequivocal boundaries define the region of risk. Boundary determination is complicated because extending boundaries likely includes influential and noninformative observations that decrease the probability of detecting a spatial pattern when one exists (decreased statistical power). When an apparent "cluster" occurs within a specific town, it is likely that, when these data are combined with observations from the county, the significance of the "cluster" is reduced. The opposite is true. When the area under study is made sufficiently small, only a few observations appear to be a cluster. Clearly, the choice of boundaries for the area considered can, to a large extent, determine the results from a spatial analysis. Sometimes "natural" boundaries are appropriate, but the determination of the relevant area is usually a nonstatistical and difficult subjective issue.

A less important issue that applies specifically to nearest-neighbor analysis also concerns boundary influences. The justification of the expression for the cumulative probabilities explicitly requires that a circle of radius R is the study area. This theoretical requirement is violated to some extent in applied situations. However, adjustments to the expression for the mean value and its variance are available to correct this usually slight bias [34].

Perhaps the most important issue in an analysis of spatial data relates to why the studied area is chosen. When the area under investigation is chosen because a suspicious clustering of cases exists, the analysis is moot. An assessment of the likelihood that the distances among these cases occurred by chance alone is no longer possible. It is already the case that some clustering has occurred, making the probabilities associated with a nearest-neighbor analysis no longer correct nor useful. This kind of after-the-fact reasoning is referred to as "Texas sharp-shooting," where one shoots first and then draws the target based on the observed pattern.

A last note: As with the test of variance, the nearest-neighbor strategy used to identify nonrandom patterns is not only a spatial analysis technique. Nearest-neighbor distances widely apply to identifying clustering within other kinds of data. For example, when interest is focused on genetic characteristics, nearest-neighbor distances can be used to explore genetic similarities/dissimilarities among groups of individuals (Chapter 9). Nearest-neighbor distance also plays a role in the analysis of a wide variety of other situations, such as identifying genomic sequences, replacing missing observations, interpolating between numeric values, and even in spell checking.

RANDOMIZATION TEST

A randomization test is an assumption-free statistical technique that does not require sophisticated statistical distributions or theory. However, it does require the use of a computer for all but extremely small samples of data. A randomization test applies to numerous situations in addition to the analysis of spatial data. Before describing an application to spatial data, the randomization test analogous to the two-sample t-test and the chi-square test of independence illustrate this "computer-intensive" approach in familiar situations.

Table 8–6. Cholesterol levels of $n = 40$ men with weights greater than 225 pounds classified by A/B-behavior type (WCGS data, Chapters 4 and 11)

	Chol	A/B		Chol	A/B		Chol	A/B		Chol	A/B		Chol	A/B
1	344	B	9	246	B	17	224	A	25	242	B	33	252	A
2	233	A	10	224	B	18	239	A	26	252	B	34	202	A
3	291	A	11	212	B	19	239	A	27	153	B	35	218	A
4	312	A	12	188	B	20	254	A	28	183	B	36	202	B
5	185	B	13	250	B	21	169	B	29	234	A	37	212	A
6	250	A	14	197	A	22	226	B	30	137	B	38	325	A
7	263	B	15	148	B	23	175	B	31	181	A	39	194	B
8	246	A	16	268	A	24	276	A	32	248	A	40	213	B

Comparisons between individuals classified into two groups, sometimes referred to as *two-sample data*, using a randomization test parallels the classic two-sample t-test but, unlike the t-test, produces a completely assumption-free significance probability (p-value). That is, the statistical analysis depends entirely on the sampled data. In addition, a randomization test applies to any choice of a test statistic.

Data on cholesterol level and behavior type for the 40 heaviest Western Collaborative Group Study (WCGS) participants illustrate (Table 8–6) an application of the randomization approach. The observed mean cholesterol level is $\bar{y}_A = 245.050$ for the 20 type-A individuals and $\bar{y}_B = 210.300$ for the 20 type-B individuals. The classic two-sample Student's t-test applied to assess the influence of random variation on the observed difference of $\bar{y}_A - \bar{y}_B = 245.050 - 210.300 = 34.750$ yields a t-test statistic of $T = 2.562$ and a p-value of 0.0072 from a t-distribution with $n - 2 = 38$ degrees of freedom.

The natural null hypothesis that behavior type and cholesterol levels are unrelated is equivalent to considering the WCGS data as if 20 individuals were chosen at random and labeled "type-A" and the remaining 20 individuals were labeled "type-B." Of most importance, when 20 individuals are selected at random from the group of 40 subjects, the mean cholesterol level of these individuals and the mean level of the remaining 20 individuals differ by chance alone. The observed difference results strictly from the random differences among the individuals selected and not selected. Similar to randomly assigning individuals to treatment and control groups, before the treatment, the two randomized groups differ only because of sampling variation. Randomization guarantees that no systematic differences exist between any values compared between the two groups.

In principle, all possible samples of 20 could be selected from the 40 WCGS subjects and used to calculate all possible mean differences between 20 randomly sampled and 20 nonsampled cholesterol measurements. The mean value of this exactly symmetric distribution of sample mean differences, called the *null distribution*, would be exactly zero because all individuals would be equally distributed among the selected and nonselected groups when all possible samples are considered. In other words, for every positive difference in mean values, an identical negative difference exists. In most situations, the number of all possible differences is too large even for a modern computer to make such an extensive calculation (1.4×10^{11} samples for the cholesterol data). However, it is possible to repeat the process of randomly sampling the collected data a large number of times and calculating mean values from the sampled and unsampled individuals. The difference between a series of such mean values accurately characterizes the distribution of the mean differences as if the variable under study was unrelated to group membership. The resulting distribution is an estimate of the null distribution.

In terms of the WCGS data, comparing mean values calculated from repeatedly randomizing the 40 study participants, forming two groups of 20, produces an estimate of the null distribution of the differences in mean cholesterol levels. A total of 5000 random samples of 20 individuals produces 5000 random differences in mean levels of cholesterol (Table 8–7 and Figure 8–6). This estimated distribution is determined entirely by the process of repeatedly sampling 20 random values from the 40 observations. The data are randomly divided 5000 times into two groups of 20 individuals and 5000 times the difference in mean cholesterol values is calculated. Behavior type status is not considered and no assumptions are made about the sampled population. A histogram of these 5000 computer-generated random differences is displayed in Figure 8–6. The estimated null distribution is essentially symmetric with mean value near zero (–0.013) and accurately reflects a normal distribution. For example, the normal distribution predicts a 95th-percentile of 24.458 and the 95th-percentile of the randomization generated null distribution is 23.450.

Table 8–7. Summary values from the distribution of 5000 mean differences in cholesterol levels (null distribution) between two randomized groups

Number of samples	5000
Mean value	–0.013
Variance	211.300
Standard deviation	14.536
Minimum value	–45.150
Maximum value	58.250

Percentiles	1%	5%	10%	90%	95%	99%
Observed value	–33.650	–23.450	–18.550	18.950	23.450	32.750

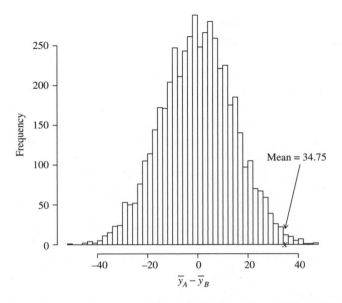

Figure 8–6. Histogram displaying the estimated null distribution of mean differences between randomized groups of WCGS data ($n = 40$ men with weights greater than 225 pounds).

The originally observed mean difference in cholesterol levels between type-A and type-B individuals is $\bar{y}_A - \bar{y}_B = 245.050 - 210.300 = 34.75$. It is a simple matter to count the number of more extreme values among the sample of 5000 randomized mean differences. Only 35 mean differences exceeded 34.75, directly indicating that an observed difference larger than 34.75 is not likely when behavior type and cholesterol level are unrelated. The empirical (no theory) p-value from the estimated null distribution is then $\hat{P}(\bar{Y}_A - \bar{Y}_B \geq 35.75 | no\ association) = 35/5000 = 0.007$ and almost exactly agrees with the previous parametric p-value of 0.0072 ($T = 2.562$) found using a t-distribution.

When the assumptions underlying a t-test hold, it is easily and directly applied. But when the assumptions do not hold, t-test results can become suspect while a randomization test continues to give an accurate statistical assessment. The t-test is designed to evaluate the difference between two mean values sampled from normal distributions with equal variances. The randomization procedure, on the other hand, allows the use of many kinds of summary values without assumptions about the population sampled. When, for example, the ratio of two mean values is a useful measure of the differences between two groups, an accurate t-test is not always possible because a ratio may not have even an approximate normal distribution. A randomization test, however, follows the previous pattern. Instead of mean differences, a large number of ratios are calculated from data randomized into two groups a large number of times. The originally observed ratio is then

Table 8–8. Pancreatic cancer and coffee consumption among male cases and controls (repeated from Chapter 2)

	Coffee consumption				
	$X = 0$	$X = 1$	$X = 2$	$X = 3$	**Total**
$Y = 1$ (case)	9	94	53	60	216
$Y = 0$ (control)	32	119	74	82	307
Total	41	213	127	142	523

evaluated against this estimated null distribution. The number of ratios created by the randomization process, for example, that exceed the originally observed sample value again is an assumption-free estimate of a one-sided p-value. The simplicity and the general applicability of the randomization test make it an extremely valuable statistical tool.

Another application of a randomization test is illustrated by the previous pancreatic cancer case–control data (Table 8–8, repeated from Chapter 2) consisting of $n = 523$ pairs of observations (X, Y). Each observation is a pair with a value X of 0, 1, 2, or 3 (cups of coffee) and a value Y of 0 or 1 (control–case). The values in the table are the counts of the eight different kinds of pairs (X, Y). A randomization test corresponding to the previous chi-square analysis (Chapter 2) illustrates this assumption-free approach applied to assess the relationships within a table, such as the evaluation of the association between coffee consumption and case–control status.

Both the classic chi-square and randomization approaches begin with the same null hypothesis that postulates that coffee consumption X and case–control status Y are unrelated (statistically independent). Using a computer program, the 523 values of $X = 0$, 1, 2, or 3 can be randomly associated with the 523 values of $Y = 0$ or 1. That is, a sample of X/Y-pairs is constructed consisting of 41 values of $X = 0$, 213 values of $X = 1$, 127 values of $X = 2$, and 142 values of $X = 3$ randomly paired with 216 values of $Y = 1$ and 307 values of $Y = 0$. Such a task is easily accomplished with a computer program by randomly ordering the 523 values of X and randomly ordering the 523 values of Y. The resulting set of 523 randomly paired values conforms perfectly to the null hypothesis. No X/Y-association exists. Thus, a 2×4 table constructed from these computer-generated 523 pairs is free of any association between variables X and Y. The distribution of any summary statistics calculated from these "no association" tables, therefore, reflects only random variation. A large number of these summary values, as before, creates an estimated null distribution.

For the pancreatic cancer data, 5000 randomized sets of X ("coffee consumption") and Y ("case–control status") values generate 5000 random

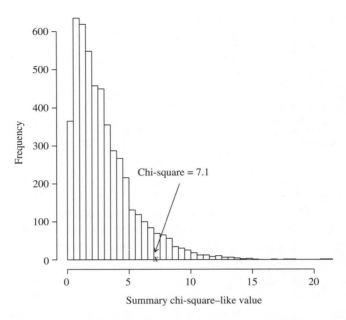

Figure 8–7. Histogram displaying the computer-generated null distribution of the chi-square–like summary statistic for the pancreatic cancer data as if X and Y were unrelated (Table 8–8).

2×4 tables containing values X and Y that are unrelated. Necessarily, the marginal frequencies are equal to those of the original table. To compare the randomization results to the originally observed Pearson chi-square statistic of $X^2 = 7.100$ (Chapter 2), the same chi-square test statistic is calculated for each table. The differences among these 5000 chi-square–like summary values reflect only random variation. They constitute an empiric estimate of the distribution of the chi-square summary statistic because the randomization process guarantees that no association exists between X and Y (displayed in Figure 8–7). Using this null distribution, the likelihood that a randomization test–generated value exceeds the originally observed value of 7.100 (Chapter 2) by chance alone is again simply a matter of counting the more extreme values. A total of 344 chi-square–like statistics generated from the 5000 randomized 2×4 tables (no association) exceeds the observed value 7.100. Thus, an empiric p-value from the pancreatic case–control data is estimated by $344/5000 = 0.069$.

As expected for a large sample of data ($n = 523$), the empirically estimated p-value hardly differs from the theoretical chi-square value calculated from the classic chi-square approach to evaluating an association in a table (p-value = 0.069, Chapter 2).

Unlike the Pearson chi-square test, a randomization approach does not depend on the theoretical and approximate chi-square distribution. In fact, a randomization procedure does not depend on any theoretical considerations (assumption-free). When the data are sparsely distributed in parts of a table or the sample size is generally small, the theoretical chi-square statistic potentially produces inaccurate results, but a randomization procedure based on an estimated null distribution continues to be an accurate assessment. Also note that the randomization procedure does not involve the degrees of freedom, an occasionally difficult value to calculate in analysis of data contained in multidimensional tables.

Randomization tests, for example, have become recently important in genetic studies, where tables frequently contain categories with few or no observations (haplotype analysis). Furthermore, summary measures of association between two categorical variables other than a chi-square statistic are readily calculated and evaluated with a randomization process. For example, Kendal's τ-correlation coefficient measuring association between ordinal variables (Chapter 13) is directly assessed with a randomization test without theoretical considerations. In fact, the influences of random variation on almost any summary statistic can be evaluated with a randomization test.

BOOTSTRAP ESTIMATION

The expression "pull yourself up by your bootstraps" originates from the book *The Surprising Adventures of Baron Munchausen*, by Rudolph Erich Raspe (1785). The Baron had fallen in a lake and, being a "surprising person," he saves himself by picking himself up by his bootstraps. In a statistical context, a *bootstrap estimate* refers to a statistical process that easily produces important results in an apparently effortless, simple, and self-contained way.

The concept of *sampling variation* is critical to bootstrap estimation. To start, consider a single sample from a normal distribution with mean $\mu = 10$ and variance $\sigma_X^2 = 4$. For a single sample of $n = 10$ independent observations, the estimated mean value is, as usual, $\bar{x} = \sum x_i / n$. The key to evaluating such an estimated sample mean is its associated variability reflected by its estimated variance. The variance of the probability distribution of a sample mean value can be directly calculated. It is the variance of the sampled population divided by the sample size. Thus, the sample variance of the mean estimated from 10 observations is $\sigma_{\bar{x}}^2 = \sigma_X^2 / n = 4/10 = 0.4$. This theoretical result allows the evaluation of the influence of sampling variation on the estimated mean value with, for example, a statistical test or a confidence interval using the estimated variance S_X^2 / n.

Another approach to measuring the influence of sampling variation on an estimated mean value is to repeatedly sample the population that produced the

Table 8–9. The first ten samples from 5000 random samples of $n = 10$ observations from a normal distribution with mean value $= \mu = 10$ and variance $= \sigma^2 = 4$

	Sampled values										Mean
i	1	2	3	4	5	6	7	8	9	10	$\bar{x}_i$
1	14.16	13.04	11.32	7.15	8.36	11.02	7.65	7.24	9.67	7.66	9.727
2	9.27	11.45	8.03	10.18	8.10	13.13	13.26	9.44	5.55	12.48	10.089
3	13.26	10.55	12.43	10.84	13.84	8.26	9.20	8.33	12.09	10.65	10.946
4	10.64	10.68	9.16	9.47	7.69	8.49	12.23	10.41	4.36	8.42	9.155
5	5.99	10.69	12.62	8.78	8.19	10.70	11.12	10.02	9.50	11.15	9.876
6	11.63	7.03	6.58	7.31	12.45	9.58	11.73	7.65	7.05	11.45	9.247
7	9.52	9.28	12.15	11.07	11.39	7.73	7.46	11.39	12.31	9.53	10.183
8	12.00	10.56	7.81	6.39	8.66	9.48	13.25	11.21	12.11	12.34	10.381
9	9.50	7.68	10.88	7.05	8.28	10.63	13.20	15.11	10.98	12.13	10.543
10	12.05	13.34	10.24	7.42	9.64	10.58	11.27	8.98	12.16	11.91	10.759

original estimate. Table 8–9 illustrates this artificial situation, where repeated samples of 10 observations are selected and mean values are calculated from each sample. The variability among these sampled mean values directly indicates the sampling variation associated with a single sampled mean value calculated from $n = 10$ observations. These values differ because the sampled values that make up each mean value differ. The first ten samples and their estimated mean values from a set of 5000 samples (denoted $\bar{x}_i$) are recorded in Table 8–9. A histogram displays the sampling variability of all 5000 estimated mean values (Figure 8–8).

The variance calculated from the $k = 5000$ sample mean values provides a direct (no theory) estimate of the sampling variation associated with the distribution of the mean value. It is

$$
\begin{aligned}
estimated\ variance &= \frac{1}{k-1}\sum(\bar{x}_i - \bar{x})^2 \\
&= \frac{1}{4999}(9.727 - 10.001)^2 + \cdots + (10.982 - 10.001)^2 \\
&= 0.409
\end{aligned}
$$

$i = 1, 2, \cdots, k = 5000$ where the overall estimated mean (the mean value of the 5000 sampled mean values) is $\bar{x} = 10.001$. The corresponding population values are again $\mu = 10$ and $\sigma_X^2/n = 4/10 = 0.4$.

This example is more conceptual than useful because resampling a population is rarely a practical way to assess variability. In applied situations, a single sample of n observations is collected and a single mean value is estimated. However, the example illustrates in concrete terms what is meant by sampling variation. It is the variation of a summary statistic that arises because the sampled observations

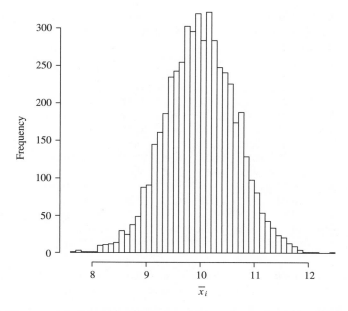

Figure 8–8. Distribution of 5000 computer-generated mean values ($n = 10$) sampled from a normal population with mean value $= \mu = 10$ and variance $= \sigma^2 = 4$.

randomly differ from sample to sample. Sampling variation occurs because each sample of observations consists of a different fraction, frequently a small fraction, of the possible population values.

Bootstrap estimates are possible because of a remarkable property of a sample of observations. The distribution of a sample mean value, illustrated in Figure 8–8, can be estimated from a single sample. Instead of resampling the original population, the sample itself is resampled. That is, the original sample of n observations is sampled to produce a *replicate sample*. After each observation is sampled, it is "returned" to the original set, so that the every sampled observation comes from exactly the same set of original observations. In statistical language, this process is called *sampling with replacement*. A replicate sample of n observations likely contains original observations that appear more than once and, therefore, other original observations do not appear at all. This sampling process is repeated a large number of times, producing a large number of replicate samples. The differences among the replicate samples are due only to sampling variation and, therefore, the differences among summary statistics calculated from these replicate samples are also due only to sampling variation. Thus, an assumption-free distribution of a summary statistic is estimated from a single sample of n observations.

Table 8–10. Ten samples from the 5000 computer-generated replicate samples from the original sample of $n = 10$ observations and their mean values

i	1	2	3	4	5	6	7	8	9	10	Mean $\overline{x}_{[i]}$
				Sampled values							
1	8.25	11.22	11.22	12.26	10.04	9.87	9.87	10.67	12.26	10.04	10.570
2	8.25	10.67	10.95	8.25	12.26	10.04	8.25	8.25	10.04	9.04	9.600
3	10.25	10.04	11.22	10.72	9.87	8.25	10.25	10.95	8.25	10.95	10.077
4	10.72	9.87	9.04	10.95	8.25	10.04	10.67	9.87	8.25	10.25	9.792
5	9.87	10.25	9.87	10.72	11.22	10.25	11.22	11.22	10.72	8.25	10.361
6	10.67	11.22	8.25	12.26	10.67	10.72	9.87	10.67	9.04	10.04	10.341
7	9.04	8.25	10.72	11.22	9.04	10.67	10.72	10.67	10.95	9.04	10.032
8	10.04	10.04	10.04	9.87	11.22	10.95	12.26	9.04	10.67	10.04	10.417
9	10.04	9.04	10.67	8.25	9.04	10.67	10.25	10.95	10.72	11.22	10.086
10	10.67	10.04	10.04	10.25	11.22	10.95	11.22	10.67	10.25	12.26	10.758

Consider again $n = 10$ observations sampled from a normal population with mean value $= \mu = 10$ and variance $= \sigma^2 = 4$. Specifically, the

$$observed\ sample = \{10.72, 10.25, 8.25, 11.22, 12.26, 9.04, 10.95, 10.67, 9.87$$
$$and\ 10.04\}$$

where the sample mean value is $\overline{x} = 10.327$ based on this single sample. Table 8–10 displays the first ten replicate samples from a total of $k = 5000$ (sampled with replacement).

When $\hat{g}$ represents an estimate of the parameter value denoted g (g for generic), and $\hat{g}_{[i]}$ represents the same estimate of the parameter g but calculated from a specific replicate sample, then the mean value of k such replicate estimates,

$$\hat{g}_{[.]} = \frac{1}{k} \sum \hat{g}_{[i]},$$

is the bootstrap estimate of the parameter g. From the example data ($n = 10$ and $k = 5000$), the bootstrap estimated mean value (denoted $\overline{x}_{[.]}$) is

$$\overline{x}_{[.]} = \frac{\sum \overline{x}_{[i]}}{k} = \frac{1}{5000}(\overline{x}_{[1]} + \overline{x}_{[2]} + \cdots + \overline{x}_{[5000]})$$
$$= \frac{1}{5000}(10.570 + 9.600 + \cdots + 10.621) = \frac{51,651}{5000} = 10.330.$$

The mean $\overline{x}_{[.]} = 10.330$ is the mean value of the 5000 replicate mean values.

In addition, the resampling process produces a general description of the behavior of the estimated value, namely an estimate of the distribution of the estimated value $\hat{g}$.

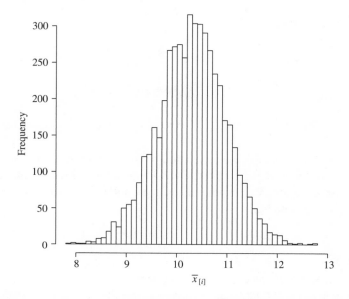

Figure 8–9. A bootstrap estimate of the distribution of the estimated mean value ($n = 10$) based on 5000 replicate samples.

The histogram (Figure 8–9) displaying the 5000 replicate mean values ($\bar{x}_{[i]}$-values) is an estimate of the distribution of the sample mean value based on resampling the original sample of ten observations. Both Figure 8–8, based on a population sampled 5000 times, and Figure 8–9, based on a single sample resampled 5000 times, display estimates of the same population distribution of the sampled mean value, namely a normal distribution with mean value $= \mu = 10$ and variance $= \sigma_{\bar{x}}^2 = 4/10 = 0.4$. However, the bootstrap estimated distribution is directly and easily estimated by replicate sampling of a single sample of n observations.

A key analytic tool, as always, is the estimated variance of the distribution of a summary statistic. It too is directly calculated from the replicate samples. In symbols, the estimated variance of the distribution of the estimate, $\hat{g}$, based on k replicate samples is

$$variance\ of\ \hat{g} = variance(\hat{g}_{[i]}) = \frac{1}{k-1}\sum(\hat{g}_{[i]} - \hat{g}_{[.]})^2.$$

An estimate of the variance of $\hat{g}$ is no more than the usual estimated variance calculated from the k replicate estimated values, $\hat{g}_{[i]}$. For the sample mean example, the estimated variance is

$$variance\ of\ \bar{x} = variance(\bar{x}_{[i]}) = \frac{1}{4999} \sum (\bar{x}_{[i]} - \bar{x}_{[.]})^2$$

$$= \frac{1}{4999} \sum (\bar{x}_{[i]} - 10.330)^2 = 0.447,$$

based on $k = 5000$ replicate samples from the original ten observations (Table 8–10 or Figure 8–9).

Two kinds of confidence intervals follow from a bootstrap estimated distribution of a summary statistic. First, the 2.5th and the 97.5th percentiles of the estimated bootstrap distribution directly estimate a 95% confidence interval.

Second, the bounds

$$\hat{g}_{[.]} \pm 1.960 \sqrt{variance(\hat{g}_{[i]})}$$

form an alternative estimate of a 95% confidence interval, based on the property that bootstrap estimates, like many estimates, typically have at least approximate normal distributions.

Based on the bootstrap estimated distribution of the mean value (Figure 8–9): 2.5th percentile (rank $= 125$) $= 8.950$ and 97.5th percentile (rank $= 4875$) $=$ 11.592 yields the 95% confidence interval of (8.950, 11.592).

The parallel normal distribution–based approach

$$\bar{x}_{[.]} \pm 1.960 \sqrt{variance(\bar{x}_{[i]})} = 10.330 \pm 1.960\sqrt{0.447}$$

yields the approximate 95% confidence interval of (9.020, 11.640). It is important to keep in mind that the sample size remains $n = 10$, and the 5000 replicates do not improve the precision of the original estimates ($\bar{x} = 10.327$ or $\bar{x}_{[.]} = 10.330$). Bootstrap estimation, however, does produce an estimate of their precision without assumptions or statistical theory.

Although the illustrated variance and confidence intervals apply to the mean value estimated from a specific sample, the process applies in general. That is, in a relatively effortless, simple, and self-contained way, the distribution of many kinds of summary statistics can be estimated and used to evaluate the influence of random variation on an estimated summary value.

Example: Bootstrap Estimation of a Percentage Decrease

Data from a small clinical trial of a drug ($n = 15$ participants) thought to reduce blood pressure illustrate a bootstrap approach [35]. Table 8–11 contains systolic blood pressure levels measured before taking the drug and 2 hours later. One

Table 8–11. Data from a small clinical trial ($n = 15$) of a potentially useful blood pressure lowering drug (captopril)

Observation	1	2	3	4	5	6	7	8
Before	130	122	124	104	112	101	121	124
after	105	112	112	106	110	105	90	95
$\hat{P}_j$	19.23	8.20	9.68	−1.92	1.79	−3.96	25.62	23.39

Observation	9	10	11	12	13	14	15
Before	115	102	98	119	106	107	100
after	103	98	118	108	110	108	102
$\hat{P}_j$	10.43	3.92	−20.41	9.24	−3.77	−0.93	−2.00

measure of effectiveness of the drug is each participant's percentage decrease in blood pressure over the 2-hour period or

$$percentage\ decrease = \hat{P}_j = 100 \times \frac{before_j - after_j}{before_j} \qquad \text{(for the } j^{th} \text{ person)}$$

and, summarizing all 15 patients, the mean percentage decrease is

$$mean\ percentage\ decrease = \overline{P} = \frac{1}{n}\sum \hat{P}_j = \frac{1}{15}(78.512) = 5.233\%.$$

The distribution of the mean percentage decrease, $\overline{P}$, is estimated from 5000 bootstrap samples of the $n = 15$ original observations (Table 8–11) and is displayed in Figure 8–10. The differences among these 5000 replicate estimates, $\overline{P}_{[i]}$, reflect the sampling variation associated with the observed mean percentage decrease in systolic blood pressure. The distribution of mean percentage decrease produces the bootstrap estimated percentage mean decrease, where

$$overall\ percentage\ decrease = \overline{P}_{[.]} = \frac{1}{5000}\sum \overline{P}_{[i]} = 5.269\%.$$

The bootstrap estimated variance of the distribution of the estimate $\overline{P}_{[i]}$ (Figure 8–10) is

$$variance\ of\ \overline{P} = variance(\overline{P}_{[i]}) = \frac{1}{k-1}\sum(\overline{P}_{[i]} - \overline{P}_{[.]})^2$$

$$= \frac{1}{4999}\sum(\overline{P}_{[i]} - 5.269)^2 = 8.801.$$

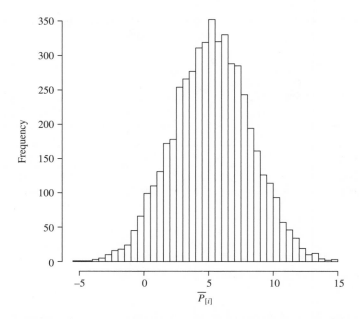

Figure 8–10. Bootstrap estimated distribution ($k = 5000$) of the mean percentage decrease ($\overline{P}$) based on $n = 15$ systolic blood pressure before/after measurements.

To assess the likelihood that the observed decrease in blood pressure occurred strictly by chance, a purely empiric estimate of the p-value is the count of the number of observations less than zero divided by the number of replicate samples or $191/5000 = 0.038$. The plot of the distribution of the estimated mean decrease appears normal-like (Figure 8–10).

Therefore, not surprisingly, the normal distribution based test statistic

$$z = \frac{0 - \overline{P}_{[.]}}{\sqrt{variance(\overline{P}_{[i]})}} = \frac{-5.269}{\sqrt{8.801}} = -1.776$$

yields the similar p-value of $P(Z \leq -1.776 | no\ change) = 0.042$. Both results produce essentially the same level of evidence that the observed decrease in blood pressure is not likely entirely due to sampling variation. Thus, random variation is not a plausible explanation of the observed decrease. It appears that the distribution of $\overline{P}$ is shifted away from zero (no effect) and toward a mean decrease estimated by $\overline{P}_{[.]} = 5.269\%$. From another point of view, changes in systolic blood pressure values less than zero (blood pressure increases) appear to be unlikely. Note that no assumptions are made about the sampled population, and summary measures other than the percentage change in blood pressure could be similarly evaluated.

Again two possible approaches to estimating a confidence interval are:

- Assumption free: the 2.5% and 97.5% percentiles from the bootstrap estimated distribution are (−0.755, 11.804), and

- Normal distribution based: $\overline{P}_{[.]} \pm 1.960\sqrt{variance(\overline{P}_{[i]})} = 5.269 \pm 1.960(2.967)$ yields the approximate 95% confidence interval (−0.546, 11.084).

A bootstrap estimated distribution can be viewed as repeated sampling of a "population." The "population" is the sampled observations. Furthermore, the size, the mean value and the variance of the sampled "population" are fixed and known values. The mean of the "population" of 15 blood pressure differences for the example data is $\overline{P} = 5.233\%$ and the bootstrap estimate of that value is $\overline{P}_{[.]} = 5.269\%$, based on 5000 replicate samples. As noted, bootstrap resampling of data is the same in principle as the impractical resampling of a population but is easily achieved with widely available computer tools when applied to a single sample of observations.

PROPERTIES OF THE ODDS RATIO AND THE LOGARITHM OF AN ODDS RATIO

Bootstrap strategies are fundamentally the same when applied to tabular or discrete data. Consider, the association between coronary heart disease (CHD) risk and behavior type (type-A versus type-B) described in a 2×2 table (Table 8–12).

Replicate sampling of the 3154 WCGS participants (sampling with replacement) creates a series of replicate 2×2 tables. Computing the odds ratios and the logarithms of the odds ratio from each of these tables provides a description of the distributions of these two measures of association. Again, an estimate of the distribution of the estimated odds ratio generated with bootstrap sampling requires no assumptions or sophisticated statistical theory. Five thousand replicate 2×2 tables provide the information needed to explore the properties of the odds ratio calculated from the A/B-behavior type data (Table 8–12). Table 8–13 contains

Table 8–12. Coronary heart disease and behavior type for $n = 3154$ WCGS participants (repeated from Chapters 4 and 6)

	CHD	No CHD	Total
Type-A	178	1411	1589
Type-B	79	1486	1565
Total	277	2897	3154

Table 8–13. Ten bootstrap replicate 2 × 2 tables from 5000 tables
generated by resampling the WCGS data to describe the properties of the odds ratio and
the log- odds ratio measures of association

	Tables									
Replicates (i)	1	2	3	4	5	6	7	8	9	10
$a_{[i]}$	154	195	201	176	173	195	181	176	194	199
$b_{[i]}$	1435	1394	1388	1413	1416	1394	1408	1413	1395	1390
$c_{[i]}$	79	81	89	72	62	78	79	85	79	84
$d_{[i]}$	1486	1484	1476	1493	1503	1487	1486	1480	1486	1481
$\hat{or}_{[i]}$	2.019	2.563	2.402	2.583	2.962	2.667	2.418	2.169	2.616	2.524
$log(\hat{or}_{[i]})$	0.702	0.941	0.876	0.949	1.086	0.981	0.883	0.774	0.962	0.926

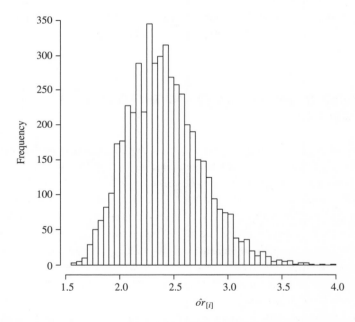

Figure 8–11. The bootstrap estimated distribution of the odds ratio ($k = 5000$) from the
WCGS data (Table 8–12).

the first 10 of 5000 bootstrap replicate 2 × 2 tables, the odds ratios, and log-odds
ratios. The total sample of 5000 bootstrap replicate tables produces the estimated
distributions shown in Figures 8–11 and 8–12.

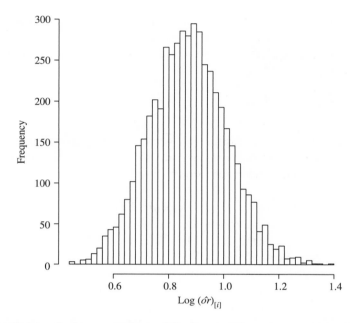

Figure 8–12. The bootstrap estimated distribution of the logarithm of the odds ratio ($k = 5000$) from the WCGS data (Table 8–12).

The bootstrap estimated distribution of the odds ratio is slightly asymmetric and has mean value

$$bootstrap\ estimated\ mean\ value = \hat{o}r_{[.]} = \frac{1}{k}\sum \hat{o}r_{[i]} = 2.405,$$

with estimated variance

$$variance\ (\hat{o}r_{[i]}) = \frac{1}{k-1}\sum (\hat{o}r_{[i]} - \hat{o}r_{[.]})^2 = 0.112$$

where again k represents the number of replicate samples ($k = 5000$).

The bootstrap estimated logarithm of the odds ratios produces a slightly more symmetric distribution (more normal-like distribution, Figure 8–12). The mean value and variance again are directly estimated from the bootstrap estimated distribution. Specifically, the mean value is

$$bootstrap\ estimated\ log\text{-}mean\ value = \overline{log(\hat{o}r_{[.]})} = \frac{1}{k}\sum log(\hat{o}r_{[i]}) = 0.867,$$

with estimated variance

$$variance[log(\hat{o}r_{[i]})] = \frac{1}{k-1}\sum [log(\hat{o}r_{[i]}) - \overline{log(\hat{o}r_{[.]})}]^2 = 0.021.$$

The bootstrap estimate of the variance is simply the variance calculated directly from the bootstrap estimated distribution (Figure 8–12). The previous estimate from a theoretical expression (Chapter 4) yields a similar estimate of the same variance where

$$variance(log[\hat{or}]) = \frac{1}{a} + \frac{1}{b} + \frac{1}{c} + \frac{1}{d} = \frac{1}{178} + \frac{1}{1411} + \frac{1}{79} + \frac{1}{1486} = 0.020.$$

However, the origins of this estimate are not as simple (Chapter 3) and requires a specific application of a rather sophisticated theory to derive the expression for the estimated variance. Bootstrap estimation only requires a series of replicate samples.

Taking advantage of the more symmetric distribution of the logarithm of the odds ratio, a normal distribution–based 95% confidence interval becomes $0.867 \pm 1.960\sqrt{0.0207}$ or $(0.586, 1.149)$. An estimated 95% confidence interval for the odds ratio is then

$$lower\ bound = e^{0.586} = 1.796 \quad and$$
$$upper\ bound = e^{1.149} = 3.155,$$

based on the bootstrap estimated odds ratio $e^{0.867} = 2.379$. The previously estimated 95% confidence interval (Chapter 4) is $(1.803, 3.123)$.

ESTIMATION OF ABO ALLELE FREQUENCIES

Commonly used statistical summaries have known distributions or approximate normal distributions or transformations producing approximate normal distributions. For methods based on these summaries, results from bootstrap estimation are similar to the parametric approaches. As illustrated, the bootstrap and the "theoretical" confidence intervals for the odds ratio are essentially the same. However, situations arise that are not as statistically tractable. In this case, a bootstrap estimate requires only that the original observations be repeatedly sampled to estimate the distribution of the summary value. Thus, the bootstrap pattern of estimation allows the evaluation of most summary statistics, not just those with known and easily applied theoretical properties.

A classic problem in genetics is the estimation of allele frequencies. Weinberg (circa 1910) derived a clever estimate of allele frequencies for the human ABO blood types using the observed numbers of phenotype (denoted: n_A = number of blood group A individuals, n_B = number of blood group B individuals, n_{AB} = number of blood group AB individuals, and n_O = number of blood group O individuals). An example of the counts of such phenotypes is given in Table 8–14.

Table 8–14. Counts of phenotype frequencies from the ABO blood group system
(n = 713 African-American individuals)

	Blood group phenotypes				
	A-type	B-type	AB-type	O-type	**Total**
Denoted	n_A	n_B	n_{AB}	n_O	n
Counts	187	137	30	359	713
Proportions ($\hat{P}$)	0.262	0.192	0.042	0.504	1.0

These data are part of a large study [36] of many kinds of red blood cell systems and consist of a sample of ABO-system determinations from 713 African-Americans.

When random mating occurs with respect to the ABO blood types, genetic theory predicts that the phenotype frequencies are simple functions of the ABO-allele frequencies. When the allele frequencies are represented as p (allele frequency of type A), q (allele frequency of type B), and $r = 1 - p - q$ (allele frequency of type O), then the expressions for the phenotype frequencies are:

frequency of phenotype A individuals is $P_A = p^2 + 2pr$,
frequency of phenotype B individuals is $P_B = q^2 + 2qr$,
frequency of phenotype AB individuals is $P_{AB} = 2pq$, and
frequency of phenotype O individuals is $P_O = r^2$.

Weinberg noted that when these relationships hold, estimates of the allele frequencies p and q are

$$\hat{p} = \sqrt{\hat{P}_A + \hat{P}_O} - \sqrt{\hat{P}_O} \quad \text{and} \quad \hat{q} = \sqrt{\hat{P}_B + \hat{P}_O} - \sqrt{\hat{P}_O},$$

and $\hat{r} = 1 - \hat{p} - \hat{q}$.

The phenotypic frequencies $\hat{P}_A = n_A/n = 0.262$, $\hat{P}_B = n_B/n = 0.192$ and $\hat{P}_O = n_O/n = 0.504$ are the observed proportions of the A, B, and O phenotypes among $n = 713$ observed individuals (Table 8–14). Therefore, the Weinberg estimates of the allele frequencies p and q become

$$\hat{p} = \sqrt{0.262 + 0.504} - \sqrt{0.504} = 0.166 \quad \text{(A–allele)}$$

and

$$\hat{q} = \sqrt{0.192 + 0.504} - \sqrt{0.504} = 0.124 \quad \text{(B–allele)},$$

making $\hat{r} = 1 - \hat{p} - \hat{q} = 1 - 0.166 - 0.124 = 0.710$ (O–allele).

The variances of these estimates are complicated and not easily derived, because the Weinberg classic estimates are not maximum likelihood estimates.

Table 8–15. The first ten bootstrap samples and estimates from $k = 2000$ replicate samples of the ABO-data (Table 8–14) to estimate the allele frequencies and their variances

	Replicate samples				Estimates		
i	A-type	B-type	AB-type	O-type	$\hat{p}_{[i]}$	$\hat{q}_{[i]}$	$\hat{r}_{[i]}$
1	178	142	41	352	0.160	0.130	0.711
2	197	128	41	347	0.176	0.119	0.706
3	192	151	28	342	0.173	0.139	0.688
4	202	135	27	349	0.179	0.124	0.696
5	181	131	28	373	0.158	0.117	0.724
6	188	133	25	366	0.165	0.120	0.715
7	187	130	29	366	0.164	0.117	0.719
8	193	137	31	352	0.172	0.126	0.703
9	163	124	40	386	0.142	0.110	0.748
10	186	134	26	366	0.163	0.121	0.716

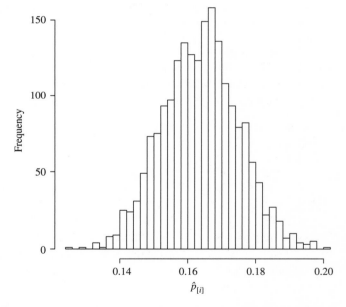

Figure 8–13. The bootstrap estimated distribution from 2000 replicate values of $\hat{P}$.

As noted, the variances of maximum likelihood estimates are directly obtained as part of the estimation process (Chapter 3). However, a bootstrap approach follows the usual pattern, producing the estimated distribution of each estimated allele frequency ($\hat{p}$, $\hat{q}$, and $\hat{r}$). Table 8–15 shows the first ten bootstrap replicate samples from the data (Table 8–14) among 2000 such replicate samples. Figure 8–13

Table 8–16. The estimated ABO allele frequencies among African-Americans ($n = 713$), their standard errors, and 95% confidence intervals calculated from bootstrap estimated distributions

Blood types	Allele frequencies	Estimates*	Standard errors	Upper bounds	Lower bounds
Type-A	p	0.166	0.011	0.142	0.185
Type-B	q	0.124	0.010	0.105	0.145
Type-O	r	0.710	0.015	0.680	0.740

* = Based on 2000 replicate bootstrap samples using the phenotype data in Table 8–14.

displays the distribution of the 2000 bootstrap estimates of the A-type allele frequency ($\hat{p}$). The similar distributions of $\hat{q}$ and $\hat{r}$ are not shown. Of more importance, the estimated standard errors and the percentile bootstrap estimated 95% confidence interval bounds are directly derived from these three bootstrap estimated distributions. As before, these calculations follow directly and simply without assumptions or statistical theory (Table 8–16).

AN IMPORTANT PROPERTY (BOOTSTRAP VERSUS RANDOMIZATION)

Randomization tests and bootstrap estimation are in fact not very different statistical tools. A summary statistic designed to contrast two populations, such as the mean difference $\hat{c} = \bar{x} - \bar{y}$ illustrates the similarity. The estimated summary value $\hat{c}$ measures the difference between the two sampled populations but, of course, the influence of sampling variation remains an issue. Furthermore, this sampling variation is often accurately described by a normal distribution.

For a bootstrap estimate, the difference between two sampled populations is measured by the likelihood that a summary value is less than zero when the bootstrap estimate $\bar{c}_{[.]}$ is treated as the mean value. Based on a normal distribution with a mean value $\bar{c}_{[.]}$, the bootstrap estimated p-value is

$$P(C \leq 0 | \textit{mean of the distribution of the } \hat{c}\textit{-values} = \bar{c}_{[.]}) = P\left[Z \leq \frac{0 - \bar{c}_{[.]}}{S_{\hat{c}}}\right]$$

where $S_{\hat{c}}^2$ represents the estimated variance of the estimate $\hat{c}$. The case in which the difference between the two sampled populations is measured by the likelihood that a summary value is greater than zero follows the same pattern.

For the randomization test, the difference between sampled populations is measured by the likelihood that a summary value is greater than the estimated

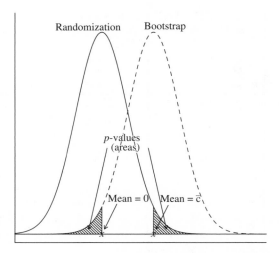

Figure 8–14. Illustration of the equivalence of a bootstrap analysis and the randomization test for a two-sample comparison.

value $\bar{c}_{[.]}$ when the mean value is zero. Based on a normal distribution with mean zero, the randomization estimated p-value is

$$P(C \geq \bar{c}_{[.]} \mid \textit{mean of the distribution of the } \hat{c}\textit{-values} = 0) = P\left[Z \geq \frac{\bar{c}_{[.]} - 0}{S_{\hat{c}}}\right]$$

again, where $S_{\hat{c}}^2$ represents the estimated variance of the estimate $\hat{c}$.

For the bootstrap distribution, the mean value is estimated by $\bar{c}_{[.]}$ and for the randomization distribution, the mean value is zero (Figure 8–14). In addition, the estimated variances of the distributions of the summary estimates $\hat{c}$ are approximately equal. Therefore, the symmetric normal distribution produces two approximately equal p-values. In symbols,

$$p - value = P(Z \leq -z) = P(Z \geq z) = P\left[Z \leq \frac{0 - \bar{c}_{[.]}}{S_{\hat{c}}}\right] \approx P\left[Z \geq \frac{\bar{c}_{[.]} - 0}{S_{\hat{c}}}\right].$$

The distribution generated by randomization describes the variation of a summary statistic under the classic null hypothesis that all variation is due to random sampling influences. It is the distribution parallel to the normal distribution, chi-square distribution, or t-distribution used extensively in parametric statistical testing procedures. Based on a null hypothesis, the estimated distribution provides the probability that a summary value differs from a theoretical value only because of the influence of random variation.

   The distribution generated by bootstrap resampling also describes the variation of a summary value derived entirely from the data. It is an empiric description of a summary statistic unconstrained by any hypothesis. For example, this hypothesis-free bootstrap distribution allows a direct calculation of a confidence interval. In the language of hypothesis testing, randomization produces an estimate of the null distribution and bootstrap replicate sampling produces an estimate of the alternative distribution.

   Bootstrap estimation can fail to be effective. An extreme example is an estimate of the distribution of the range *(maximum value − minimum value)*. The failure to produce an effective bootstrap estimate, even for a large number of replicate samples, occurs because replicate samples produce relatively few different summary values. Some examples of other familiar statistics whose distributions are not effectively described by bootstrap estimation are the median, the nearest-neighbor mean, the maximum value, and the minimum value. As with the range, a bootstrap sampling produces relatively small numbers of different values for these summary statistics, which does not allow an effective estimate of their distributions.

   More technically, the effectiveness of resampling is a question of "smoothness." A "smooth" statistic is one in which small changes in the composition of the replicate sample produce correspondingly small changes in the estimated summary value. The median value is an example of an "unsmooth" statistic. Based on a sample of $n = 10$ and $k = 5000$ replicate samples, Figure 8–15 displays the bootstrap estimated distribution of the median value contrasted to the distribution of the median estimated from 5000 independent samples of the original normal distribution ($\mu = 10$ and $\sigma^2 = 4$). The basic difference is that bootstrap resampling of the ten observations yields only about 40 different median values, whereas the repeated sampling of ten values from the original distribution yields 5000 different median values.

   The bootstrap estimate of the distribution of the sample mean compared to the distribution created by resampling the population (Figures 8–8 and 8–9) illustrates the case of a "smooth" estimate. The two estimated distributions are essentially the same.

A LAST EXAMPLE: ASSESSMENT OF SPATIAL DATA

The conceptually simple problem of determining whether 24 lymphatic cancer cases are associated with the location of a microwave tower (source of electromagnetic field [EMF] radiation exposure) is difficult using a traditional statistical approach. First, a summary measure sensitive to clustering around a point must be created. The distribution of this summary statistic then must be estimated under

Bootstrap distribution (median)

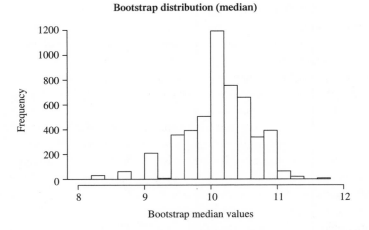

Bootstrap median values

Resampled normal distribution (median)

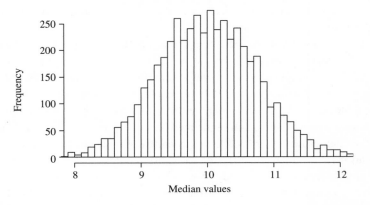

Median values

Figure 8–15. Bootstrap estimated distribution of the median comparing 5000 replicate samples ($n = 10$) to the directly estimated distribution of the median from 5000 samples of $n = 10$ from a normal distribution ($\mu = 10$ and $\sigma^2 = 4$).

the hypothesis that no spatial pattern exists. A summary value estimated from the observed data is then compared to a theoretical value derived from this null distribution of no association. Finally, the likelihood that the observed difference occurred by chance alone is estimated. This process is familiar and practical in many situations. However, a bootstrap-based analysis produces a parallel assessment without statistical theory using only a computer to resample the spatial data.

Table 8–17 and Figure 8–16 show the locations of 24 cases of lymphatic cancer observed during the period 1977 to 1986 in the city/county of San Francisco

Table 8–17. The locations* of cases of lymphatic cancer occurring during the period 1977–1987 among San Francisco residents age less than 20 years ($n = 24$)

X	Y	X	Y	X	Y	X	Y	X	Y
0.30	−4.33	−0.99	0.87	−1.96	−1.13	2.33	−0.63	0.35	2.39
−4.17	0.37	−1.96	1.30	−3.11	0.55	2.02	1.29	−2.60	−2.23
0.60	−2.49	0.12	−2.38	−0.41	0.70	−0.32	−2.60	1.48	0.30
−3.56	−0.03	−1.48	−4.39	1.48	−2.57	−1.91	−0.41	−1.67	−2.22
−1.73	−3.02	0.01	2.38	−0.80	1.75	−3.07	1.80		

*= X and Y are values transformed from the original longitude and latitude coordinates to yield distances in kilometers.

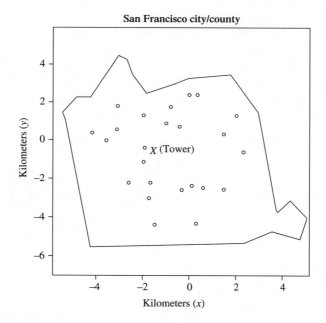

Figure 8–16. The locations of 24 cases of lymphatic cancer in San Francisco city/county, 1977–1987.

among individuals less than 20 years old. The "X" on the map indicates the location of a large communication tower that has been suggested as a source of possible cancer-causing electromagnetic radiation exposure.

To assess possibility that the spatial pattern of cases of lymphatic cancer are associated with the microwave tower, a natural summary measure is the observed mean distance to the tower. That is, from the case location (x_i, y_i) the distance is

$$distance = d_i = \sqrt{(x_i - x_0)^2 + (y_i - y_0)^2}$$

to the location of the tower $(x_0, y_0) = (-1.540, -0.540)$. The observed $n = 24$ observations (kilometers) are:

{4.214, 1.517, 0.727, 3.871, 3.484, 2.782, 1.889, 1.907, 4.005, 1.989, 2.891, 2.473, 1.679, 2.394, 3.133, 2.079, 3.852, 3.642, 0.394, 1.686, 2.489, 3.305, 2.408, 2.794}.

The estimated bootstrap mean distance to the tower is $\overline{d}_{[.]} = \sum d_i/n = 2.572$ kilometers. The statistical question becomes: Is the observed mean distance sufficiently small to be unlikely to have occurred by chance?

A bootstrap sampling of the 24 distances produces an estimate of the distribution of the estimated mean distance to the tower. The estimated distribution based on 2000 replicate samples from the 24 original distances is displayed in Figure 8–17. From theoretical considerations, the distance between a random point and the tower location is $d_0 = 2.731$ kilometers.

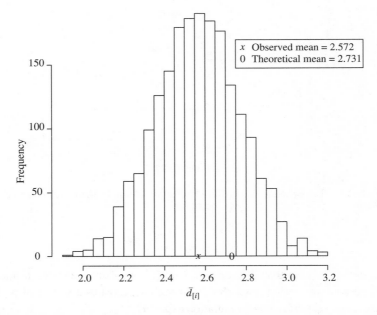

Figure 8–17. The bootstrap distribution of the mean distance of lymphatic cancer cases from the San Francisco microwave tower ($k = 2000$ replicates).

It now becomes straightforward to judge whether this observed distance $\overline{d}_{[.]} = 2.572$ is substantially smaller than $d_0 = 2.731$; that is, unlikely by chance.

As indicated by Figure 8–17, the replicate mean values $\overline{d}_{[i]}$ have an approximate normal distribution. Using the bootstrap estimated variance, $variance(d_{[i]}) = 0.041$, the test statistic

$$z = \frac{\overline{d}_{[.]} - d_0}{S_{\overline{d}_{[i]}}} = \frac{2.564 - 2.731}{\sqrt{0.041}} = -0.825$$

has an approximate standard normal distribution when the observed difference $(\overline{d}_{[.]} - d_0)$ occurs by chance alone. The one-sided p-value based on the normal distribution is $P(Z \leq -0.825 | no\ difference) = 0.205$. The parallel and purely empiric bootstrap one-sided p-value is $P(\overline{D} \leq 2.564 | no\ difference) = 420/2000 = 0.210$. Thus, the distribution of the mean distance to the tower $\overline{d}$ is shifted toward smaller values (shorter case distances) but a substantial likelihood remains that random variation is the explanation.

From another point of view, the estimated 95% confidence interval is the 2.5th percentile (observation rank 50) and the 97.5th percentile (observation rank 1950) from the bootstrap estimated distribution and is (2.163, 2.953). The theoretical mean distance $d_0 = 2.731$, based on the assumption that the spatial distribution of cases is strictly random, is contained in the confidence interval and, therefore, is a plausible value for the underlying mean distance between cases of lymphatic cancer and the microwave tower, estimated by $\overline{d}$ or $\overline{d}_{[.]}$.

9

CLASSIFICATION: THREE EXAMPLES

Three statistical tools, one based on *dendrograms*, another based on *principal components*, and a third based on a purely graphical approach, introduce a few of the issues encountered in classifying multivariate observations. Rather than discuss this complex and wide-ranging topic in general, classifying human populations based on the similarities/differences in the frequencies of genetic variants provides an instructive example. Frequencies of 13 genetic variants from three major red blood cell systems (ABO-system, Rh-system, and MN-system) collected from a variety of sources are used to identify similar and dissimilar multivariate observations. Data consisting of summary values (such as frequencies of genetic variants) rather than individual measurements are commonly referred to as *aggregate or ecologic data*.

The presence of genetic variation in human blood was first established by Lansteiner in 1901, with the identification of different blood group types, now called the ABO-system. The Rh- and MN-systems also contain well-known and reliably identified genetic variants. Based on these three red blood cell systems (a total of 13 genetic variants), the "genetic distances" between the members of the 26 populations can be estimated (325 "distances"). These "distances" allow an extensive 13-component variable to be simplified and then used to order the populations from similar to different based on an intuitive process.

The complete genetic data set is displayed in a 26 by 13 array (Table 9–1). The rows are 26 race/ethnicity groups and the columns contain the frequencies

Table 9–1. Gene frequencies* for 26 race/ethnicity groups

Group	ABO-system				Rh-system							MN-system	
	A	B	AB	O	CDE	CDe	Cde	cDE	cdE	cDe	cde	M	N
French	0.21	0.06	0.06	0.67	0.00	0.43	0.01	0.14	0.01	0.02	0.39	0.55	0.45
Czech	0.25	0.04	0.14	0.57	0.01	0.42	0.01	0.15	0.00	0.01	0.40	0.53	0.47
German	0.22	0.06	0.08	0.64	0.02	0.38	0.03	0.12	0.01	0.03	0.41	0.55	0.45
Basque	0.19	0.04	0.02	0.75	0.00	0.38	0.01	0.07	0.00	0.01	0.53	0.54	0.46
Chinese	0.18	0.00	0.15	0.67	0.00	0.74	0.00	0.19	0.00	0.03	0.04	0.62	0.38
Ainu	0.23	0.00	0.28	0.49	0.00	0.56	0.00	0.21	0.19	0.00	0.04	0.40	0.60
Aboriginal	0.22	0.00	0.00	0.78	0.03	0.63	0.04	0.14	0.00	0.16	0.00	0.22	0.78
Guinean	0.22	0.00	0.14	0.64	0.00	0.95	0.00	0.04	0.00	0.01	0.00	0.21	0.79
Maori	0.34	0.00	0.00	0.66	0.00	0.48	0.01	0.48	0.00	0.03	0.00	0.51	0.49
Icelander	0.13	0.06	0.06	0.75	0.00	0.43	0.00	0.16	0.02	0.02	0.37	0.57	0.43
Eskimo	0.30	0.00	0.06	0.64	0.03	0.59	0.00	0.33	0.00	0.050	0.00	0.83	0.17
Indian (Brazil)	0.00	0.00	0.00	1.00	0.03	0.55	0.00	0.40	0.00	0.02	0.00	0.74	0.26
Bantu	0.10	0.08	0.11	0.71	0.00	0.08	0.05	0.06	0.00	0.61	0.20	0.56	0.44
North Africa	0.17	0.06	0.15	0.62	0.00	0.43	0.00	0.14	0.00	0.09	0.34	0.54	0.46
India	0.16	0.03	0.22	0.59	0.01	0.57	0.00	0.14	0.00	0.04	0.24	0.69	0.31
Spanish	0.27	0.04	0.06	0.63	0.02	0.44	0.01	0.11	0.00	0.04	0.38	0.53	0.47
Norwegian	0.26	0.06	0.06	0.62	0.00	0.43	0.01	0.13	0.01	0.02	0.40	0.55	0.45
Indian (Mex)	0.02	0.00	0.01	0.97	0.00	0.68	0.00	0.30	0.00	0.02	0.00	0.79	0.21
Egyptian	0.21	0.05	0.20	0.54	0.00	0.46	0.01	0.14	0.00	0.24	0.15	0.52	0.48
Chinese (U.S.)	0.21	0.00	0.18	0.61	0.00	0.71	0.00	0.20	0.00	0.02	0.07	0.58	0.42
Japanese (U.S.)	0.28	0.00	0.18	0.54	0.00	0.63	0.00	0.32	0.00	0.00	0.05	0.56	0.44
Navajo	0.03	0.00	0.00	0.97	0.04	0.38	0.09	0.31	0.01	0.17	0.00	0.91	0.09
white (U.S.)	0.20	0.07	0.07	0.66	0.01	0.38	0.01	0.14	0.01	0.04	0.41	0.56	0.44
Black (Calif)	0.13	0.04	0.13	0.71	0.01	0.16	0.03	0.11	0.00	0.40	0.30	0.41	0.59
Mexican (U.S.)	0.11	0.02	0.06	0.81	0.06	0.50	0.01	0.24	0.02	0.04	0.14	0.70	0.30
Asian (U.S.)	0.24	0.01	0.17	0.58	0.00	0.63	0.01	0.26	0.00	0.02	0.06	0.56	0.44

* = The term *gene frequency* is technically a combination of phenotype (ABO) and allele (Rh and MN) frequencies.

of 13 genetic variants from the three red cell blood systems. These 13 observed frequencies constitute a single multivariate observation and become the basis for classifying the 26 race/ethnicity groups in terms of their genetic make-up.

DENDOGRAM CLASSIFICATION

Two components of a classification process are a definition of distance between observations and, once distance is established, a method to classify similar and dissimilar distances.

The distance between two points (x_1, y_1) and (x_2, y_2) is given by the expression

$$d_{12} = \sqrt{(x_1 - x_2)^2 + (y_1 - y_2)^2} \quad (Pythagorean\ theorem).$$

This well-known geometric definition of distance is directly extended to multi-dimensional observations. The distance between one p-dimensional point represented as $\{x_{i1}, x_{i2}, x_{i3}, \cdots, x_{ip}\}$ and another represented as $\{x_{j1}, x_{j2}, x_{j3}, \cdots, x_{jp}\}$ is

$$d_{ij} = \sqrt{\sum (x_{ik} - x_{jk})^2} \quad k = 1, 2, 3, \cdots, p.$$

This distance between the ith and j^{th} points is referred to as *Euclidean distance*. For example, if "point i" is $\{x_{i1}, x_{i2}, x_{i3}, x_{i4}\} = \{1, 2, 3, 4\}$ and if "point j" is $\{x_{j1}, x_{j2}, x_{j3}, x_{j4}\} = \{4, 3, 2, 1\}$, then the Euclidean distance between these two four-dimensional ($p = 4$) observations is

$$d_{ij} = \sqrt{(1-4)^2 + (2-3)^2 + (3-2)^2 + (4-1)^2} = \sqrt{20} = 4.472.$$

Euclidean distance reflects, somewhat arbitrarily but effectively, the genetic difference between race/ethnicity groups. Summarizing differences in terms of Euclidean distance provides a numeric comparison between groups but is only one of a number of choices for defining multivariate "distance." However, it is, perhaps, the simplest.

To illustrate, the 13 genetic frequencies observed in Chinese born in the U.S. (Table 9–1, row 20) are

$\{0.21, 0.0, 0.18, 0.61, \cdots, 0.42\}$ (a 13-component multivariate observation),

and the frequencies of the same 13 genetic frequencies observed in Chinese born in China (Table 9–1, row 5) are

$\{0.18, 0.0, 0.15, 0.67, \cdots, 0.38\}$ (also a 13-component multivariate observation), making the genetic/Euclidean distance between these two groups ($p = 13$)

$$distance(Chinese[U.S.], Chinese[China])$$
$$= \sqrt{(0.21 - 0.18)^2 + \cdots + (0.42 - 0.38)^2} = 0.103.$$

For contrast, the frequencies of the same 13 genetic frequencies observed in white Americans (Table 9–1, row 23) are

$$\{0.20, 0.07, 0.07, 0.66, \cdots, 0.44\},$$

and the genetic/Euclidean distance between Chinese born in the U.S. and white Americans is

$$distance(Chinese[U.S.], white[U.S.])$$
$$= \sqrt{(0.21 - 0.20)^2 + \cdots + (0.42 - 0.44)^2} = 0.499.$$

In terms of genetic/Euclidean distance, the U.S.-born Chinese are "closer" to the Chinese born in China than to U.S. white Americans.

To classify multivariate observations it is necessary to define similarity. One approach consists of reducing the 325 distances between groups to 26 nearest-neighbor genetic/Euclidean distances characterizing proximity between race/ethnicity groups. For each of the 26 race/ethnicity groups, the Euclidean distances to the other 25 race/ethnicity groups are calculated. Then, similarity is defined in terms of nearest-neighbor genetic distance. For example, if the Spanish race/ethnicity group is selected, then, among the genetic distances to the other 25 race/ethnicity groups, the smallest distance is to the Norwegians (*nearest-neighbor distance* = 0.057). Table 9–2 lists the 26 nearest-neighbor genetic/Euclidean distances from smallest to largest.

U.S. white and German genetic frequencies produce the smallest nearest-neighbor distance (0.047, rank 1). The largest nearest-neighbor distance is between Guinean and Aboriginal genetic frequencies (0.420, rank 26).

The nearest-neighbor distance from group "A" to "B" is not necessarily the nearest-neighbor distance from group "B" to "A". The nearest-neighbor distance from the Czechs to the Norwegians is 0.105, but the nearest-neighbor distance associated with the Norwegians is 0.057 and is the nearest-neighbor distance to the Spanish.

Calculating the nearest-neighbor distances is the first step in sorting out the similarities and differences among the 26 race/ethnicity groups. The next step is to construct a specialized plot displaying a classification process, called a *dendrogram* (*dendro−*, from the Greek meaning "tree"). A dendrogram displays a hierarchical

Table 9–2. Nearest-neighbor distances for the 26 race/ethnicity groups ordered from smallest to largest

From	To	Distance
German	white (U.S.)	0.047
white (U.S.)	German	0.047
Spanish	Norwegian	0.057
Norwegian	Spanish	0.057
French	white (U.S.)	0.063
Japanese (U.S.)	Asians (U.S.)	0.087
Asians (U.S.)	Japanese (U.S.)	0.087
Chinese	Chinese (U.S.)	0.103
Chinese (U.S.)	Chinese	0.103
Czech	Norwegian	0.105
Icelander	French	0.121
North Africa	French	0.141
Basque	white (U.S.)	0.181
Indian (Brazil)	Indian (Mex)	0.185
Indian (Mex)	Indian (Brazil)	0.185
Egyptian	North Africa	0.266
India	Chinese (U.S.)	0.287
Mexican (U.S.)	India	0.324
Maori	Japanese (U.S.)	0.327
Bantu	Black (Calif)	0.334
Black (Calif)	Bantu	0.334
Ainu	Asians (U.S.)	0.341
Navajo	Indian (Brazil)	0.357
Eskimo	Mexican (U.S.)	0.369
Aboriginal	Guinean	0.420
Guinean	Aboriginal	0.420

classification process that orders the 26 nearest-neighbor genetic distances based on their similarity (Figure 9–1).

The following description gives a partial description of the mechanics of constructing the dendrogram.

The dendrogram plot based on all 13 genetic variants (Figure 9–1) is constructed by first identifying the "closest" nearest-neighbor pair of race/ethnicity groups (German, U.S.-whites). This pair forms the first cluster. The next race/ethnicity group to be classified is either the nearest-neighbor to the first cluster or is the nearest-neighbor to another race/ethnicity group. The latter is the case, creating a second cluster (Spanish-Norwegian). This same comparison is repeated. The French genetic frequencies are closer to the first cluster than any other pair of race/ethnicity groups are to each other, forming two classification clusters (German-U.S. white-French and Spanish-Norwegian). On the fourth step, these two clusters are closer nearest-neighbors than any two race/ethnicity groups and, therefore, becomes a single cluster. The fifth step

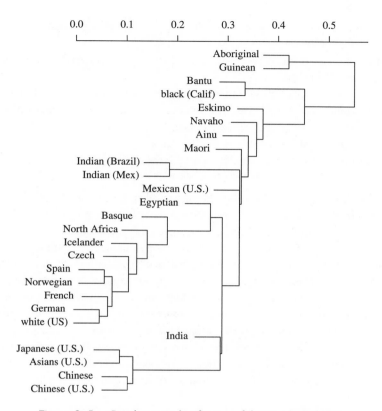

Figure 9–1. Dendrogram classification of the 26 race/ethnicity groups based on nearest-neighbor genetic distances.

produces a new cluster between the Japanese and Asians born in the U.S. The sixth step produces an additional member of the first cluster, the Czech population. Then, a third cluster is formed [Chinese (U.S) and Chinese (China)]. Next, the two Asian clusters are closer to each other than any remaining pairs of race/ethnicity groups. The process continues until the least similar race/ethnicity group or groups are included (Aboriginal-Guinean). The classification process begins with 26 groups and ends with one. The dendrogram is the graphic record of the process. It shows which race/ethnicity groups are "close" and which are not. Nearest-neighbor Euclidean distance is recorded on the horizontal axis (top).

Properties of the multivariate genetic data are easily recognized from the dendrogram (Figure 9–1). Some examples are:

- Closest race/ethnicity groups are the Germans and U.S. whites (smallest nearest-neighbor distance).

- Europeans are members of a tight cluster {Germans-French-Norwegian-Spanish-Czech}.
- Asians also form another tight cluster {Japanese(U.S.)-Asian(U.S.)-Chinese (U.S.)-Chinese(China)}.
- A clear pattern of clustering is centered in Europe, starting with France and Germany, and genetic distance smoothly increases as geographic distance from central Europe increases (Germany < France < Spain-Norway < Czechoslovakia < Iceland < North Africa).
- The most distant race/ethnicity groups are Guinean, Bantu, and Aboriginal.

The grouping process identifies the very similar, the similar, the different, and the very different multivariate observations. Such results are not possibly achieved by directly comparing the 26 groups, each characterized by a 13-component multivariate observation (rows, Table 9–1). However, choices other than Euclidean distance exist to describe multivariate "distance." A variety of definitions of "closeness" also exist, other than nearest-neighbor distance. For example, a correlation coefficient could be used to reflect similarity between pairs of groups. In addition, a number of methods exist to measure distance between groups of observations, such as the distance between their centroids (two-dimensional mean values), the largest distance between the two sets of observations, or the smallest distance between two sets of observations. Therefore, a variety of possibilities are available to classify multivariate data and to construct dendrogram plots [37].

PRINCIPAL COMPONENT SUMMARIES

A variable created by combining the components of a multivariate observation to construct a simpler summary is called a *canonical variable*. Mathematically, it is said that the dimensionality of the multivariate observation is reduced. Euclidean distances are one kind of canonical variable, and principal components are another.

To illustrate the properties and the geometry of principal component summaries, a small fictional data set consisting of six bivariate ($p = 2$) observations, denoted x and y, serve to describe principal component analysis in detail (Table 9–3), followed by a realistic application using the genetic data in Table 9–1.

For bivariate variables, one kind of description of their joint distribution is an elliptical region with center ($\bar{x}$, $\bar{y}$). Such an ellipse is generated from the estimated variance of x (S_x^2), the estimated variance of y (S_y^2), and the estimated covariance of x and y (S_{xy}). These data ellipses estimated from the six data points are displayed in Figure 9–2 [$\times$ = bivariate data value = (x_i, y_i)]. The construction and interpretation of such an ellipse is further discussed in Chapters 14 and 15.

Table 9–3. Six bivariate observations to illustrate a principal component analysis

i	1	2	3	4	5	6	Means	Variances
x_i	5	8	8	10	14	15	$\bar{x} = 10$	$S_x^2 = 14.8$
y_i	6	11	8	14	9	12	$\bar{y} = 10$	$S_y^2 = 8.4$

Estimated covariance $= S_{xy} = 5.6$.

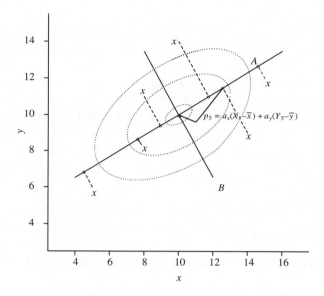

Figure 9–2. Three representative data ellipses with major axis A and minor axis B and the first principal component values (circles) based on the six example data points ($S_x^2 = 14.8$, $S_y^2 = 8.4$, and $S_{xy} = 5.6$, Table 9–3).

As with a simple linear regression analysis, a natural summary of a bivariate distribution is a straight line.

The first principal component is derived from the line that is the major axes of an ellipse (Figure 9–2, labeled A). This summary line represents "typical" observations in the sense that it is the line closest to all the points in the data set. More specifically, it is the line that minimizes the sum of the squared perpendicular distances from the six points to the line (dashed lines, Figure 9–2). The estimation of this line is fully discussed in Chapter 14. Technically, it is said that the points on the line (circles) corresponding to each observed pair (x_i, y_i) are each *projections* of a bivariate data point. For example, from Table 9–3, the first point ($x_1 = 5$, $y_1 = 6$) is projected onto the line yielding the point ($X_1 = 4.523, Y_1 = 6.822$). The other five projected points are similarly calculated (denoted X and Y, Table 9–4)

Table 9–4. The six data values and their corresponding projections on the major axes of the data ellipse

i	1	2	3	4	5	6	Means
x_i	5	8	8	10	14	15	10
Y_i	6	11	8	14	9	12	10
X_i	4.523	8.938	7.636	11.736	12.558	14.609	10
Y_i	6.822	9.384	8.628	11.008	11.485	12.674	10

and displayed in Figure 9–2 (circles). Two-dimensional data are then summarized by points on a one-dimensional line. The values on the line create a canonical summary.

The first principal component summary consists of the six distances of these x_i/y_i-points to the center of the ellipse, the point $(\bar{x}, \bar{y}) = (10, 10)$. For example, for the point $(14, 9)$ or $i = 5$, the value of the first principal component summary is

$$P_5 = \sqrt{(X_5 - \bar{x})^2 + (Y_5 - \bar{y})^2}$$
$$= \sqrt{(12.558 - 10)^2 + (11.485 - 10)^2} = 2.958$$

where the projected x/y-point $(14, 9)$ is $(12.558, 11.485)$. From a more direct expression, the same first principal component values are also given by

$$first\ principal\ component = P_i = a_x(x_i - \bar{x}) + a_y(y_i - \bar{y}),$$

based on the bivariate observation (x_i, y_i) and two coefficients a_x and a_y. For example, the first principal component summary of the observation $(14, 9)$ is again

$$P_5 = 0.865(14 - 10) + 0.502(9 - 10) = 2.958$$

where $a_x = 0.865$ and $a_y = 0.502$. The coefficients a_x and a_y are found by a complex estimation process, and for multivariate observations with more than two or three components, are calculated with a computer program [37]. Thus, the six values (denoted P_i) in Table 9–5 are the distances on the line A from the projected point to the point $(10, 10)$ and constitute the first principal component summary for the example x/y-data.

The variance of the six principal component values is $S_P^2 = 18.050$ and is the maximum possible variance of any linear combination (sum) of the variables x and y. This property results from the choice of the major axes of the ellipse as the summary line because it spans the longest possible distance within the ellipse, producing the greatest possible variability among the set of projected points. Any other line produces six points with less variability. The mathematical/technical name for this variance is the *largest eigenvalue*.

Table 9–5. The first principal component from the six example data points

i	1	2	3	4	5	6	Means	Variances
x_i	5	8	8	10	14	15	10	14.8
y_i	6	11	8	14	9	12	10	8.4
P_i	−6.332	−1.228	−2.734	2.008	2.958	5.328	0	18.050

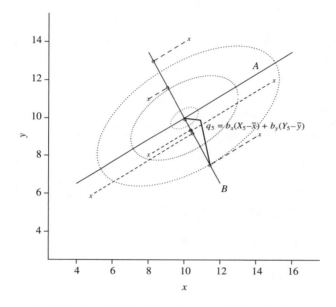

Figure 9–3. Three representative data ellipses with major axes A and minor axes B and the second principal component values (circles) based on six example data points $S_x^2 = 14.8$, $S_y^2 = 8.4$, and $S_{xy} = 5.6$, Table 9–3).

A second summary of the bivariate x/y-data is constructed from the minor axes of the data ellipse. In the two variable case, it is the only possibility. However, for the case with more than two variables, the second longest axes is chosen. The six values of this second principal component (denoted Q_i) and the complete geometry of its properties are shown in Figure 9–3. All six data points are projected (again denoted X, Y) on the minor axes (B) of the data ellipse (Table 9–6).

As before, the perpendicular distance from the data points to the line creates the projected points that are used to construct the second principal component summary (Figure 9–3, labeled B). Parallel to the first principal component, for the point (14, 9) or $i = 5$, the value of the second principle component is

$$Q_5 = \sqrt{(11.442 - 10)^2 + (7.515 - 10)^2} = 2.873$$

Table 9–6. The six data values and their corresponding projections on the minor axes of the data ellipse

i	1	2	3	4	5	6	Means
x_i	5	8	8	10	14	15	10
y_i	6	11	8	14	9	12	10
X_i	10.477	9.062	10.364	8.264	11.442	10.391	10
Y_i	9.178	11.616	9.372	12.992	7.515	9.326	10

Table 9–7. The second principal component from the six example data points

i	1	2	3	4	5	6	Means	Variances
x_i	5	8	8	10	14	15	10	14.8
y_i	6	11	8	14	9	12	10	8.4
Q_i	0.950	−1.869	0.726	−3.460	2.873	0.780	0	5.150

where the projected x/y-point $(14, 9)$ is $(11.442, 7.515)$. Again from a more general expression, the second principal component based on the two coefficients, $b_x = 0.502$ and $b_y = −0.865$, is also given by

$$second\ principal\ component = Q_i = b_x(x_i − \bar{x}) + b_y(y_i − \bar{y})$$

and, for the point $(14, 9)$,

$$Q_5 = 0.502(14 − 10) − 0.865(9 − 10) = 2.873.$$

The six distances (Q_i) to the point $(\bar{x}, \bar{y}) = (10, 10)$ constitute the second principal component summary (Table 9–7).

The bivariate variable $(p = 2)$ example illustrates two fundamental properties of principal component summaries in general. First, the correlation between the first and the second principal components is zero $[correlation(P, Q) = 0]$. The choice of the perpendicular axes of an ellipse as summary lines guarantees that these two sets of points (principal component values) are uncorrelated. Note that the covariance between P_i (Table 9–6) and Q_i (Table 9–7) is exactly zero. Second, the total variance given by $S_x^2 + S_y^2 = 14.80 + 8.40 = 23.2$ is redistributed among the principal component summary values. That is, the components of the total variation become $S_P^2 + S_Q^2 = 18.050 + 5.150 = 23.2$. As noted, the first principal component has maximum variability. The relative worth of each principal component as a summary of the data is often reported in terms of its percentage of this total variation. For the example, the percentage associated with the first principal component is $percent = (18.050/23.2) \times 100 = 77.8\%$.

GENETIC CLASSIFICATION

For the genetic data (Table 9–1), a 13-component multivariate observation is reduced to a summary made up of two principal components (a 13-dimensional observation is reduced to a two-dimensional canonical variable). This considerably simpler bivariate variable calculated from each of the 26 race/ethnicity groups provides an efficient as well as intuitive statistical tool to classify multivariate observations and, in the case of classifying the 26 race/ethnicity groups based on genetic frequency data, yields results similar to the dendrogram approach.

The most valuable summary variable (denoted P_i), as always, is the first principal component and is the linear combination of the 13 genetic components given by

$$P_i = a_1 A_i + a_2 B_i + a_3 AB_i + \cdots + a_{12} N_i + a_{13} M_i$$

where A_i, B_i, AB_i, $\cdots$, N_i and M_i represent the 13 genetic frequencies (a row of Table 9–1 for the ith race/ethnicity group). The 13 coefficients a_j are determined so this canonical variable has maximum variability among all possible linear combinations of the 13 genetic frequencies.

Variability is a desirable feature of a summary statistic used as a tool for classification, and the first principal component has maximum variability. A summary measure with little or no variability is not much use. When a summary takes on similar values under all circumstances, it poorly reflects a multivariate observation. If the Dow-Jones stock market index (another kind of canonical variable), for example, barely changes when the component stocks themselves change, it would not usefully reflect the general stock market activity. A highly variable summary potentially captures, even with a single value, much of the information contained in a less tractable and certainly more complex multivariate observation. Although the first principal component, P_i, is the most variable linear combination, it is not necessarily an effective summary.

The second principal component summary is similarly created. Again, a linear combination of the 13 multivariate components produces another canonical variable, denoted

$$Q_i = b_1 A_i + b_2 B_i + b_3 AB_i + \cdots + b_{12} N_i + b_{13} M_i.$$

The second principal component is again a linear combination summarizing the genetic frequencies. The 13 coefficients b_j are chosen so that this second principal component has two properties. First, as with the bivariate data ($p = 2$), the correlation between the first and second principal components is exactly zero ($correlation(P, Q) = 0$). Because these two linear combinations are uncorrelated, they potentially reflect different aspects of a multivariate observation. Thus, the second principal component is not only an additional summary but likely

Table 9–8. The 13 coefficients used to construct of the two principal components, P and Q, summarizing the genetic variation among the 26 race/ethnicity groups

j	Gene	a_j	b_j
1	A	0.16	–0.14
2	B	0.06	0.08
3	AB	0.11	–0.10
4	O	–0.33	0.15
5	cde	–0.03	0.01
6	CDe	–0.17	–0.69
7	Cde	–0.01	0.04
8	cDE	–0.32	–0.10
9	cdE	0.02	–0.03
10	cDe	0.12	0.30
11	cde	0.39	0.47
12	M	–0.53	0.27
13	N	0.53	–0.27

summarizes characteristics of the multivariate observation not reflected by the first principal component. Second, the principle component Q is the second most variable summary among all possible linear combinations ($variance(P) >$ $variance(Q) > variance(R)$, where R represents any other linear combination of the multivariate components. Table 9–8 contains the coefficients for the first two principal components calculated from the gene frequency data (the 13 a_j- and b_j-coefficients).

For the example, the 13 French genetic frequencies (row 1 in Table 9–1) produce the two canonical principal component summaries

$$P_1 = 0.16(0.21) + 0.06(0.06) + 0.11(0.06) + \cdots - 0.53(0.55) + 0.53(0.45)$$
$$= -0.191$$

and

$$Q_1 = -0.14(0.21) + 0.08(0.06) - 0.10(0.06) + \cdots + 0.27(0.55) - 0.27(0.45)$$
$$= -0.021.$$

The values $P_1 = -0.191$ and $Q_1 = -0.021$ succinctly summarize much of the information contained in the 13 French genetic frequencies using a far simpler bivariate measure. The other 25 bivariate summaries are similarly calculated (principal component pairs (P_i, Q_i), Table 9–9) and are plotted in Figure 9–4 (standardized so that $\bar{P} = \bar{Q} = 0$). The 13 genetic frequencies ($p = 13$) are "reduced" to 26 summary values each consisting of two components

Table 9-9. The 26 values of the first two principal components, denoted P and Q^*

I	Group	P_i	Q_i
1	French	-0.124	0.121
2	Czech	-0.192	0.087
3	German	-0.161	0.162
4	Basque	-0.184	0.236
5	Chinese	0.152	-0.229
6	Ainu	-0.185	-0.289
7	Aboriginal	-0.257	-0.317
8	Guinea	-0.290	-0.615
9	Maori	0.088	-0.166
10	Icelander	-0.050	0.143
11	Eskimo	0.387	-0.051
12	Indian (Brazil)	0.484	0.014
13	Bantu	-0.168	0.485
14	N. Africa	-0.143	0.102
15	India	0.070	0.013
16	Spain	-0.172	0.092
17	Norwegian	-0.155	0.112
18	Indian (Mex)	0.512	-0.047
19	Egyptian	-0.139	0.004
20	Chinese (U.S.)	0.070	-0.237
21	Japanese (U.S.)	0.050	-0.240
22	Navaho	0.574	0.272
23	white (U.S.)	-0.135	0.176
24	black (Calif)	-0.316	0.316
25	Mexican (U.S.)	0.239	0.066
26	Asians (U.S.)	0.044	-0.210

$* =$ Standardized so the mean values $\overline{P} = \overline{Q} = 0$.

($p = 2$). In mathematical language, a 13-dimensional variable is projected onto a two-dimensional plane. Thus, a 13-component observation is summarized by a bivariate value with a simple geometry. The two uncorrelated principal component summary values produce a bivariate summary that potentially identifies the similarities/differences among 26 multivariate observations in a simple and intuitive fashion.

The magnitudes of the principal component coefficients (Table 9–8) indicate the elements of the multivariate measurement that are important in creating the summary values P and Q. The first principal component is dominated by the alleles of the MN-system ($a_{12} = a_{13} = \pm0.53$). The largest coefficients in the second principal component are associated with the Rh-system (CDe-allele; $b_6 = 0.69$ and the cde-allele; $b_{11} = -0.47$).

These genetic variants are, therefore, the most influential elements of a multivariate classification of the genetic data based on the P_i, Q_i pairs. Similarly,

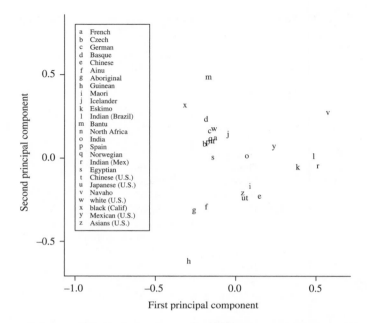

Figure 9–4. The bivariate canonical values of the first two principal components describing the genetic distance between 26 race/ethnicity groups.

gene frequencies with correspondingly small coefficients are the least important in classifying the race/ethnicity groups (CDE, Cde, and cdE, for example). In addition, the percentage of the total variation associated with the first two principal components is 68.2% ($P = 36.5\%$ and $Q = 31.7\%$, where $S_P^2 = 0.065$ and $S_Q^2 = 0.056$ from a total variance of 0.177). From this point of view, a measure of the "loss of information" incurred from using a two-variable principal component to summarize the genetic data, rather than a 13-variable multivariate observation, is 31.8%. The gain is a simple and easy to understand value.

The principal components for each of the 26 race/ethnicity groups (projected points on a plane) are displayed in Figure 9–4. Many of the same features of the blood group data seen in the dendrogram are also seen in this graphic canonical description. The cluster containing the Europeans and the U.S. whites once again is a dominant feature ({c, w, q, a, b, p and n} = {Germany, U.S. (white), Norway, France, Czechoslovakia, Spain, and North Africa}). The Asian cluster is also obviously present ({u, t, z, e and i} = {Japanese (U.S.), Chinese (U.S.), Asians (U.S.), Chinese (China) and Maori}). A cluster not apparent from the dendrogram (Figure 9–1) is suggested by the principal component approach. Three North American native populations ({k, l and r} = {Eskimo, Indian (Brazil) and Indian

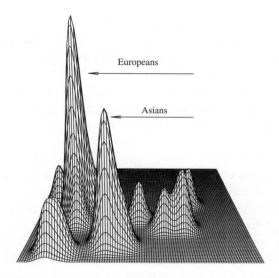

Figure 9–5. A three-dimensional plot of Figure 9–4 again displaying the principal component classification of the 26 genetic groups.

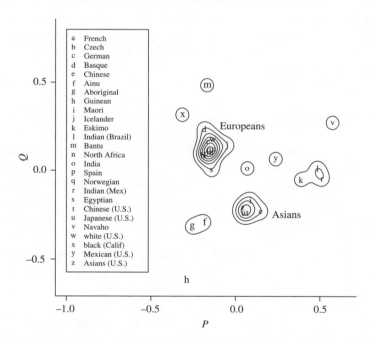

a	French
b	Czech
c	German
d	Basque
e	Chinese
f	Ainu
g	Aboriginal
h	Guinean
i	Maori
j	Icelander
k	Eskimo
l	Indian (Brazil)
m	Bantu
n	North Africa
o	India
p	Spain
q	Norwegian
r	Indian (Mex)
s	Egyptian
t	Chinese (U.S.)
u	Japanese (U.S.)
v	Navaho
w	white (U.S.)
x	black (Calif)
y	Mexican (U.S.)
z	Asians (U.S.)

Figure 9–6. A contour plot combining Figures 9–4 and 9–5, displaying the classification of the 26 race/ethnicity groups.

(Mexico)}) form a not extremely tight but, nevertheless, a notable cluster that has some historical basis. The genetically most different race/ethnicity groups are again clearly identified on the perimeter of the plot (for example, {m, v and h} = {Guinean, Bantu, and Navajo}).

The principal component summary is further enhanced by using a smoothing algorithm, producing a three-dimensional representation (Figure 9–5) of the principal component summaries P and Q (bivariate kernel estimation, Chapter 15). The "floor" of the three-dimensional smoothed distribution represents the race/ethnicity groups located by values of their first two principal component summaries. The "hills" indicate the areas of high concentration of similar race/ethnicity groups, and the "valleys" indicate the areas of low or no concentration. The extent of clustering is proportional to the heights of the "hills." The two tallest "hills" reflect the dominant European and Asian clusters that contain large proportions of genetically similar race/ethnicity groups.

To further describe the membership of the race/ethnicity clusters, a "contour map" of the three-dimensional representation is valuable (Figure 9–6). A contour plot contains no new information but provides an alternative perspective by combining both Figures 9–4 and 9–5, producing a visually appealing and easily interpreted representation. Similar to a geographic map, contours readily identify the groups that make up specific clusters (the "hills"). These plots, like most descriptive statistical techniques, are only one of a number of ways to display the classification of multivariate data.

A MULTIVARIATE PICTURE

An extremely simple graphic description of multivariate data produces an entirely visual comparison of a series of multivariate observations. A canonical "star" is constructed with p-points, where the distance from each point to the center of the star is proportional to one of the p-components of the multivariate measurement.

To illustrate, three multivariate measurements with $p = 13$ components produce the three "stars" displayed in Figure 9–7.

Measurement 1 is twice the size of measurement 3 and in reverse order, which is directly seen in the plot. Measurement 2 is entirely different from the other two 13-variate observations, and this too is obvious from the plot.

For the genetic data, 26 star-summaries constructed with 13 points proportional to the 13 gene frequencies represent each of the race/ethnicity multivariate observations. When these 26 star-summaries are plotted, each multidimensional measurement is viewed as the single entity. Differences and similarities naturally emerge.

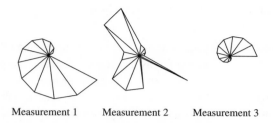

Measurement 1   Measurement 2   Measurement 3

Multivariate measurement 1 = {0, 1, 2, 3, 4, 5, 6, 7, 8, 9, 10, 11, 12}
Multivariate measurement 2 = {0, 1.5, 2, 2.5, 11.5, 10.5, 3.5, 4, 8, 8.5, 0.5, 12}
Multivariate measurement 3 = {6, 5.5, 5, 4.5, 4, 3.5, 3, 2.5, 2, 1.5, 1, 0.5, 0}

Figure 9–7. A simple illustration of a "star" plot.

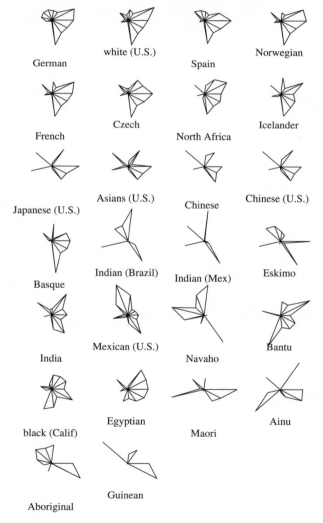

Figure 9–8. The genetic data displayed as star-summaries providing commensurate geometric representations of the 26 multivariate observations (ordered by nearest neighbor distance, Table 9–2).

The plot of 26 star-summaries from the genetic data (Figure 9–8) provides essentially the same description as the dendrogram and the principal component plots, but is created in an extremely intuitive fashion. This plot is an entirely visual comparison of the genetic frequencies that gives a simultaneous impression of all 13 components of the multivariate observation characterized by different but simple and commensurate geometric forms. Consistent with the dendrogram and principal component analyses, Germany, white (U.S.), Norway, Spain, and France are clearly similar (Figure 9–8, first two rows). The Asian groups (third row) are similar among themselves but different from the European groups. The groups such as Ainu, Aboriginal, and Guinean, are easily identified as different from each other and entirely different from the other race/ethnicity groups (last three "stars").

10

THREE SMOOTHING TECHNIQUES

A conceptual model representing the primary issues encountered in smoothing data is

$$y = f(t) + \varepsilon.$$

The symbol $f(t)$ represents a specific but unrestricted relationship over a range of values of t that can be as simple as a horizontal line or more complicated than a high-degree polynomial. For one reason or another, this unknown pattern is obscured by a degree of uncertainty, represented by ε. Together, these two components produce an imperfectly observed value, represented by y. The goal of smoothing techniques is to improve the description of these frequently obscured relationships within collected data.

The "error term" ε is sometimes assumed to have a specific structure (for example, a normal distribution with a mean value of zero), or it can just represent the inability to clearly observe the function $f(t)$. The term "smoothing" refers to reducing these obscuring influences, thus making the pattern and properties of the underlying relationship $f(t)$ more visible. When it is sensible to attribute a specific and known mathematical form to $f(t)$, parametric estimation is typically more effective. However, in many situations it is desirable to describe underlying relationships without assumptions or a mathematical structure. The estimate of the function $f(t)$ and its properties are then entirely determined by the characteristics of the data. Smoothing methods balance a decreasingly detailed description against an increasingly parsimonious picture, producing a focus on underlying relationships. A clear "picture" of the essential features of a relationship potentially becomes a key to understanding the issues that the data were collected to study. It is this assumption-free description that is the topic of this chapter and referred to as *smoothing*.

SMOOTHING: A SIMPLE APPROACH

Figure 10–1 (top) displays U.S. annual age-adjusted Hodgkin disease incidence and mortality rates of African-American males and females per 100,000 persons-years-at-risk during the period 1973–1990 (Table 10–1). These incidence and mortality rates vary considerably over the 18-year period. This variation occurs primarily because the small numbers of new cases and deaths recorded each year are highly sensitive to random variation, extreme deviations, and disproportionate influences of a variety of reporting biases. A three-step process applied to the originally observed rates of Hodgkin disease creates a smooth description of

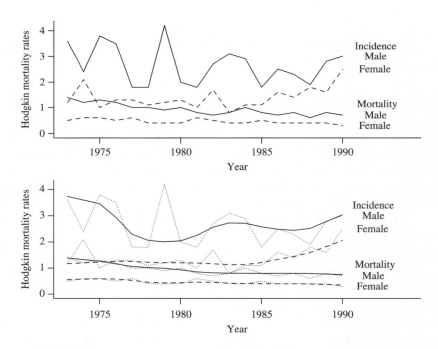

Figure 10–1. U.S. age-adjusted annual incidence and mortality rates of Hodgkin disease per 100,000 person-years during the period 1973–1990 for male and female African-Americans.

Table 10–1. U.S. age-adjusted annual incidence and mortality rates of Hodgkin disease per 100,000 person-years-at-risk during the period 1973–1990 for male and female African-Americans

Year	Incidence Male	Incidence Female	Mortality Male	Mortality Female
1973	3.6	1.2	1.4	0.5
1974	2.4	2.1	1.2	0.6
1975	3.8	1.0	1.3	0.6
1976	3.5	1.3	1.2	0.5
1977	1.8	1.3	1.0	0.6
1978	1.8	1.1	1.0	0.4
1979	4.2	1.2	0.9	0.4
1980	2.0	1.3	1.0	0.4
1981	1.8	1.0	0.8	0.6
1982	2.7	1.7	0.7	0.5
1983	3.1	0.8	0.8	0.4
1984	2.9	1.1	1.0	0.4
1985	1.8	1.1	0.8	0.5
1986	2.5	1.6	0.7	0.4
1987	2.3	1.4	0.8	0.4
1988	1.9	1.8	0.6	0.4
1989	2.8	1.6	0.8	0.4
1990	3.0	2.5	0.7	0.3

incidence–mortality relationship (Figure 10–1, bottom) with one of the simplest kinds of smoothing methods.

First, extreme rates are removed, then each annual rate is made more like its neighboring values, and finally new end-points are established by extrapolation. In symbols, for rates denoted $r_1, r_2, r_3, \cdots, r_n$, the three steps are:

1. Median moving-average smoothing

$$r_i^{(1)} = median(r_{i-1}, r_i, r_{i+1}) \quad \text{for } i = 2, 3, \cdots, n-1 \text{ followed by}$$

2. Mean moving-average smoothing where

$$r_i^{(2)} = w_1 r_{i-1}^{(1)} + w_2 r_i^{(1)} + w_3 r_{i+1}^{(1)} = 0.25 r_{i-1}^{(2)} + 0.50 r_i^{(1)} + 0.25 r_{i+1}^{(1)}$$

for $i = 2, 3, \cdots, n-1$, then

3. End points calculations

$$r_1^{(3)} = 2r_2^{(2)} - r_3^{(2)} \quad \text{and} \quad r_n^{(3)} = 2r_{n-1}^{(2)} - r_{n-2}^{(2)}.$$

Table 10–2. The intermediate values from the process of smoothing the male Hodgkin incidence rates (column 1, Table 10–1)

Rate	Iteration 1	Iteration 2	Iteration 3	Iteration 4
3.6	3.600	3.600	3.600	3.721
2.4	3.575	3.569	3.541	3.507
3.8	3.525	3.425	3.348	3.293
3.5	3.075	2.975	2.936	2.913
1.8	2.225	2.369	2.433	2.477
1.8	1.850	2.019	2.106	2.181
4.2	1.950	1.962	2.022	2.085
2.0	2.000	2.031	2.078	2.123
1.8	2.175	2.231	2.256	2.275
2.7	2.575	2.531	2.508	2.489
3.1	2.850	2.744	2.686	2.641
2.9	2.800	2.737	2.694	2.656
1.8	2.550	2.562	2.566	2.564
2.5	2.350	2.400	2.441	2.472
2.3	2.300	2.369	2.420	2.461
1.9	2.425	2.481	2.520	2.553
2.8	2.725	2.719	2.730	2.745
3.0	3.000	3.000	3.000	2.937

Table 10–2 illustrates the details of this three-step smoothing process applied to the African-American male Hodgkin incidence rates. The *median moving-average* (step 1) removes extreme and possible outlier observations. For the example, the largest incidence rate 4.2 is replaced by 2.0. Applied to all 18 rates, this produces new incidence "rates" with less variability ($r_i^{(1)}$, column 2). This first step, however, tends to leave level spots in the resulting curve and has no influence on sequences of three consecutively increasing or decreasing values. The second step removes the levels spots and further decreases the local variability by increasing the similarity among neighboring observations (said to be "made locally similar"). Step 2 is a special case of a general technique called a *moving-average*. A mean moving-average further smoothes the already once smoothed incidence "rates" ($r_i^{(2)}$, column 3). This two-step process applied again to the once smoothed values yields a yet smoother set of "rates." Repeating the process several times creates a stable curve describing the essential pattern of male Hodgkin incidence risk over the 18-year period (iteration 4, last column). Since a median smoothing followed by a mean smoothing does not effect the first and last observations, smoothed values are found by a simple linear extrapolation from the estimated curve, producing smoothed first and last "rates" ($r_1^{(3)}$ and $r_n^{(3)}$). These 18 smoothed male incidence rates and three similarly smoothed incidence and mortality rates are displayed as continuous curves in Figure 10–1 (bottom).

For the Hodgkin disease application, the median moving-average is based on observed rates grouped into sets of three. There is nothing special about this choice except that it yields a smooth, yet not too smooth, representation of the pattern of Hodgkin disease. Along the same lines, the choice of the weights used in the mean moving-average is also rather arbitrary. The three chosen weights ($w_1 = w_3 = 0.25$ and $w_2 = 0.5$) further smooth the incidence and mortality patterns but other choices yield equally useful and similarly smooth sequences. This kind of weighed averaging is sometimes called "hanning" after Julius von Hanning ($b.$ 1839), a famous 19th century Austrian scientist. Smoothing methods, in general, depend heavily on these kinds of subjective decisions. Statistical techniques exist to make rigorous comparisons among rates and to assess the influence of random variation (for example, statistical tests and confidence intervals, Chapter 6). The primary goal of smoothing methods, however, is to produce a clear and uncomplicated description of the pattern underlying the collected data, such as the age-specific Hodgkin rates (Figure 10–1), without imposing a statistical structure.

Hodgkin disease incidence data from the Surveillance Epidemiology End Results (SEER) national cancer registry further illustrate the median/mean moving-average smoothing technique. Sex- and age-specific rates smoothed over a life span of 85 years are shown in Figure 10–2 for African-America and white SEER populations. The properties and patterns of these incidence rates are not as obvious from the direct plot (top). Considerable variation exists, and three rates are zero. However, the second plot (bottom) consisting of median/mean moving-average smoothed curves is simple, easily interpreted, and provides a far more descriptive contrast of the black–white age-specific patterns of male and female Hodgkin disease incidence.

KERNEL DENSITY ESTIMATION

A strategy different from median/mean moving-average produces a smooth curve representation of the distribution of a sample of observed values based on the pattern typically used to create a histogram. To start, consider a small illustrative set of ten observations (ordered):

$$y = \{2.6, 3.2, 4.6, 4.8, 5.6, 6.2, 7.6, 8.4, 10.2, \text{ and } 13.6\}$$

and its histogram representation (Figure 10–3).

One kind of histogram consists of creating a sequence of numeric intervals and counting the number of observations that fall within each interval and then constructing a rectangle with area equal to the proportion of the total number of

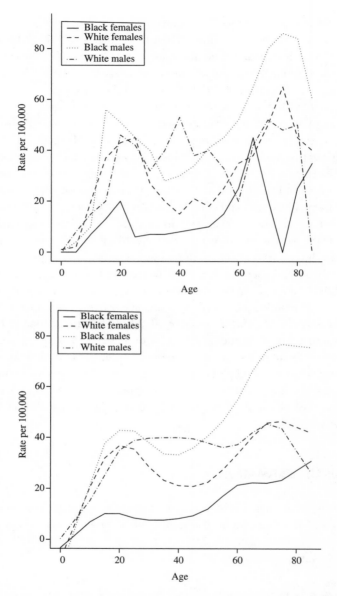

Figure 10–2. The sex- and age-specific incidence rates of Hodgkin disease among African-America and whites for males and females (SEER cancer registry data).

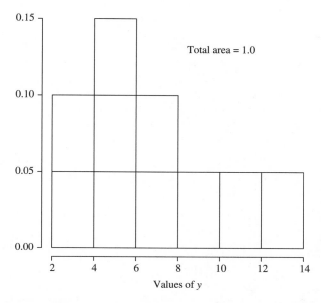

Figure 10–3.   Histogram of the $n = 10$ observations labeled y.

observations contained in each of these intervals. The rectangles are then displayed on a horizontal axis. For the "data" labeled y, six intervals between the smallest and largest values (2 and 14, Figure 10–3) result from selecting an interval length of two. Each interval becomes the location of one of six rectangles. In fact, each of these six rectangles are themselves made up of a series of smaller rectangles placed one on top of another (a sum). The size of these smaller rectangles, one for each observation, is chosen so that the total area of the histogram is 1.0.

Thus, for n observations, each sub-rectangle has an area equal to $1/n$ or *height* × *interval-width* $= 1/n$. For example, the observations $\{3.2, 4.6,$ and $4.8\}$ generate three sub-rectangles and combined (added) form the larger rectangle representing the proportion of observations between values 4 and 6 (*area* $= 3(1/n) = 3(1/10) = 0.30$, Figure 10–3). The display of these six rectangles produces a "picture" of the distribution of the sampled observations.

A cohort of 8280 women who served in the armed forces during the Vietnam war era (July 1956–March 1973) was studied to detect possible increases in gender-specific health problems. Women who served in Vietnam ($n_1 = 4140$, "cases") were compared to military women who served elsewhere ($n_0 = 4140$, controls). A small part of this study is a comparison of the age distributions of these two groups of military veterans (displayed by two histograms, Figure 10–4). As with

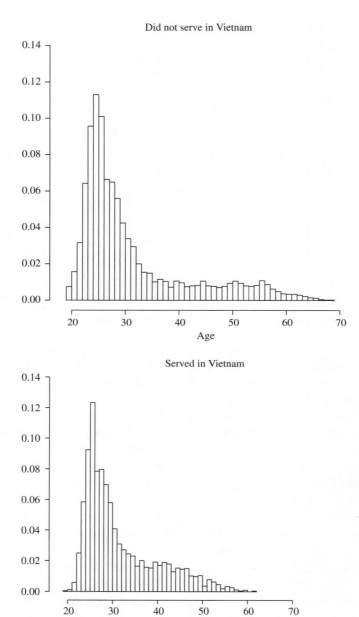

Figure 10–4. Histograms of the age distributions of armed forces women who did not serve and did serve in Vietnam (1956–1973).

all histograms, the rectangle heights identify where the data are concentrated and where they are not. For example, the histograms of these skewed age distributions show that the vast majority of military women are between ages 20 and 30, and only a few are over the age of 60 or under the age of 20. Comparing women ages 35–50, a higher proportion of these women appear to have served in Vietnam.

A parallel approach to displaying the distribution of collected data is called *kernel density estimation*. This smoothing technique is not very different from a histogram approach. In fact, the construction of a histogram can be viewed as a special case. The fundamental difference lies in the choice of the geometric representation of each observation. A histogram employs a rectangle to represent each of the n observations to create a graphical display by combining these rectangles. A kernel estimate similarly combines n continuous distributions to create a smoothed graphical display. There are a number of choices for these kernel distributions. For the following description, normal distributions are selected (mean values = observations = y_i with standard deviation = σ). These n normal distributions (one for each observation) are combined (a sum), creating a graphic description of the collected data with properties much like a histogram. Figure 10–5 indicates the process. The three curves at the bottom of Figure 10–5, each describing the distribution of the ten observations from the example data (labeled y), result from combining ten normal distributions each with mean value of y_i for three selected standard deviations, $\sigma = 0.2$, 1.0, and 2.0 (columns). In this smoothing context, the standard deviation σ is called *the bandwidth* and is sometimes given special notation, such as the letter h. The size of the bandwidth h controls the degree of smoothness. A continuous curve produced by a sum of the n heights of these normal distributions over the range of interest creates a "picture" of the distribution based on the observed data. The heights of these sums reflect the concentration of the data. Like a histogram, large values occur where the data are concentrated and small values where the data are sparse. Unlike a histogram, the height of the estimated distribution varies continuously over the range of the data (even beyond). These sums, therefore, produce a continually varying curve characterizing the distribution of the sampled observations.

The bandwidth determines the degree of smoothness and is controlled by the selection of the standard deviation of the normal distributions. A small standard deviation creates normal distributions that vary little from their mean values, and sums of these kernel distributions essentially indicate the location of each observation ($h = \sigma = 0.2$, Figure 10–5). As the bandwidth increases, these kernel distributions are spread further from their mean values and, when added, produce a summary curve created by blending neighboring observations into a smoother representation ($h = 1.0$, Figure 10–5). Further increases in the bandwidth, further smooths the curve ($h = 2$, Figure 10–5). For extremely large bandwidths, the smoothed curve becomes essentially a horizontal line. Therefore,

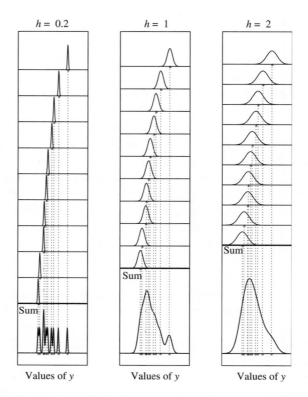

Figure 10–5. Estimated distributions based on $n = 10$ observations (y) using three choices of bandwidths ($h = 0.2$, $h = 1.0$, and $h = 2.0$).

the bandwidth parameter h determines the smoothness of the estimated curve somewhere between a series of "spikes" (one "spike" for each data point) to a horizontal line. Systematic methods exist to choose a bandwidth [38]. However, a trial-and-error approach allows control over the decision of the "best" smooth curve to describe the distribution of the collected data.

Using again the data from the study of the armed forces women, estimates of their age distributions produced by kernel smoothing ($h = 10$) are displayed in Figure 10–6. The underlying properties of the age distributions are easily identified and, as the example shows, several distributions can be directly compared on the same set of axes. The primary feature of a kernel-smoothed distribution is that it continuously represents the pattern of a continuous variable. The distribution of these female veterans are continuously displayed from ages 20–70. A histogram produces an unappealing representation of this continuous distribution as a set of discrete rectangles. A continuous description of the age distribution for these women is simply a more realistic representation of the underlying distribution.

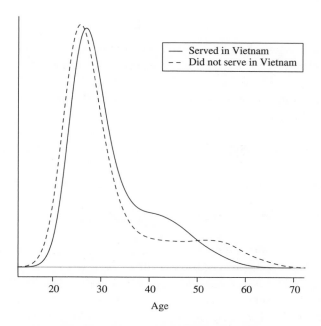

Figure 10–6. Kernel-smoothed estimates of the age distributions of armed forces women who did not serve and served in Vietnam (1956–1973).

SPLINE ESTIMATED CURVES

The term *spline* comes from the name of a flexible strip of plastic or thin metal that enables a draftsmen to easily draw a curve. Much like the draftsmen's tool, a flexible and efficient process called a *spline estimate* allows a statistical curve to be easily created to display the underlying pattern within collected data. Like the two previous smoothing approaches, the spline curve can be viewed as producing a smoothed estimate of the function $f(t)$. This approach to characterizing a pattern within sampled data, as will be seen, utilizes a polynomial function. In principle, any degree polynomial can be used but linear and cubic functions are the focus of the following discussion. A unique feature of a spline-estimated curve is its role in regression analysis as a way to represent assumption-free the occasionally complex relationships between a dependent and an independent variable.

Before describing the spline smoothing process, it is necessary to define a specialized notation. For a sequence of numbers denoted x, the symbol $(x - K)_+$ represents the sequence

$$(x - K)_+ = 0 \quad \text{for} \quad x \leq K \quad \text{and}$$

$$(x - K)_+ = x - K \quad \text{for} \quad x > K.$$

The value represented by K is called a *knot* because it becomes the point at which estimated curves are joined. This somewhat unusual notation directly converts a sequence of values into a sequence of zeros followed by a sequence of "corrected" values determined by the choice of K. For the previous example, "data" labeled y and $K = 5$, then

$$(y - K)_+ = (y - 5)_+ = \{0,\ 0,\ 0,\ 0,\ 0.6,\ 1.2,\ 2.6,\ 3.4,\ 5.2,\ 8.6\}.$$

For the sequence of numbers $x = \{1, 2, 3, \cdots, 20\}$ with a knot at 10 ($K = 10$), then

$$(x - K)_+ = (x - 10)_+ = \{0,0,0,0,0,0,0,0,0,0,1,2,3,4,5,6,7,8,9,10\}.$$

The simplest spline expression is a linear spline consisting of two straight lines. To illustrate, hypothetical observations (denoted y) are generated that randomly deviate from two connected straight lines (Figure 10–7). The two lines that generate the example data are, for $0 \leq x \leq 10$, the line is $Y_x = 10 + 4x$, and for $10 \leq x \leq 20$, the line becomes $Y_x = 70 - 2x$ (Table 10–3 and Figure 10–7). These two lines are connected at the point $x = 10$ (knot $= K = 10$). The linear spline equation describing both lines as a single x/Y-relationship is

$$Y_x = 10 + 4x - 6(x - 10)_+.$$

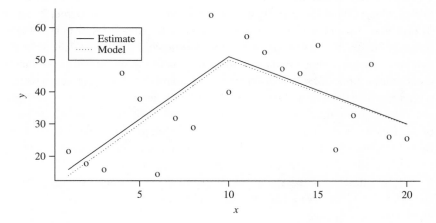

Figure 10–7.   Hypothetical data (circles), theoretical line (Y_x, dotted line), and estimated line ($\hat{y}_x$, solid line).

Table 10–3. Hypothetical data ($n = 20$) generated to illustrate spline estimation in the simplest case, Y_x = exact values and y_x = random values* for $x = 1, 2, \cdots, 20$

	Line 1				Line 2		
x	$(x-10)_+$	Y_x	y_x	x	$(x-10)_+$	Y_x	y_x
1	0	14	21.5	11	1	48	57.3
2	0	18	17.7	12	2	46	52.4
3	0	22	15.8	13	3	44	47.2
4	0	26	45.8	14	4	42	45.8
5	0	30	37.8	15	5	40	54.7
6	0	34	14.4	16	6	38	22.2
7	0	38	31.8	17	7	36	32.7
8	0	42	28.9	18	8	34	48.7
9	0	46	64.0	19	9	32	26.1
10	0	50	40.0	20	10	30	25.6

* = Model: $y_x = Y_x + random\ error$

Table 10–4. Estimates for the model coefficients (a, b, and c) from the hypothetical data (Table 10–3) using a one-knot piecewise linear spline model ($K = 10$)

Variables	Symbols	Estimates	Std. errors	p-Values
Intercept	a	11.988	–	–
First line	b	3.908	1.101	0.002
Second line	c	−6.001	1.858	0.005

LogLikehood $= -1219.11$

For example, the expression produces $Y_7 = 10 + 4(7) - 6(0) = 38$ and $Y_{14} = 10 + 4(14) - 6(14 - 10) = 42$. The model values ($Y_x$) are displayed in Figure 10–7 (dotted line) along with 20 random values (y_x, circles).

The spline expression is a special case of a two-variable linear regression model and is estimated and interpreted as any regression model, using the usual computer software and statistical tools. The general expression, called a *piecewise linear spline model with one knot*, is given by

$$Y_x = a + bx + c(x - K)_+.$$

Estimated values of regression coefficients a, b, and c for this linear spline model based on the observations (y_x, Table 10–3) and the knot $K = 10$ are given in Table 10–4. The estimated piecewise spline equation becomes

$$\hat{y}_x = 11.988 + 3.908x - 6.001(x - 10)_+,$$

and generates the solid line shown in Figure 10–7. To repeat, standard statistical methods are used to estimate the three regression model coefficients $\hat{a} = 11.988$,

Table 10–5.   Rates of autism per 100,000 population observed in Denmark from 1972 to 2000

Year	1972	1974	1976	1978	1980	1982	1984	1986
Rate	0.12	0.11	0.15	0.12	0.12	0.14	0.15	0.27

Year	1988	1990	1992	1994	1996	1998	2000
Rate	0.55	0.61	0.80	1.69	2.05	3.31	3.22

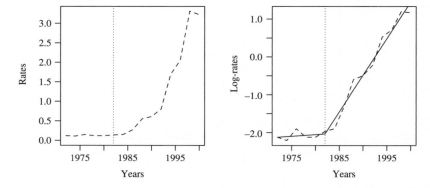

Figure 10–8.   Rates and log-rates of newly diagnosed autism cases in Denmark per 100,000 population during the period 1972–2000.

$\hat{b} = 3.908$, and $\hat{c} = 6.001$. Three example estimated model values are: $\hat{y}_1 = 15.896, \hat{y}_7 = 39.344$, and $\hat{y}_{14} = 42.697$ where the model exact values are: $Y_1 = 14$, $Y_7 = 38$, and $Y_{14} = 42$.

An application of this one-knot linear spline model is illustrated by a description of the autism rates observed in Denmark over a 29-year period (Table 10–5).

Figure 10–8 displays the annual rates (left) and log-rates (right) of newly diagnosed autism cases by year of occurrence. Differences between log-rates are multiplicative differences between rates. For example, a difference of $log(2) = 0.693$ on a log-rate scale means that the difference in the compared rates has doubled. That is, linear changes in the log-rates reflect multiplicative changes in the rates themselves (Chapter 6). As Figure 10–8 shows, Denmark experienced an extreme and essentially linear increase in the log-rates of autism after 1982 (right, dashed line).

Using a piecewise linear spline model with a single knot at $K = 1982$ and the log-rates from the Danish data (Table 10–5), regression techniques produce the estimated line

$$estimated\ log(rate) = \hat{y}_x = \hat{a} + \hat{b}x + (x - 1982)_+$$
$$= -19.513 + 0.009x + 0.185(x - 1982)_+$$

shown in Figure 10–8 (right, solid line). The regression model estimated change in log-rates (slope) during the period 1972–1982 is $\hat{y}_{1982} - \hat{y}_{1972} = -2.122 - (-2.034) = 0.088$ ($e^{0.088} = 1.1$), and the estimated change in log-rates during the period 1982–2000 is $\hat{y}_{2000} - \hat{y}_{1982} = 1.452 - (-2.034) = 3.487$ ($e^{3.487} = 32.7$). An estimated rate of change of 1.1 shows a slight multiplicative increase in autism risk from 1972 to 1982 but, dramatically, the estimated change in rates is close to a 33-fold increase for the following period, 1982–2000.

A one-knot linear spline model can be directly extended to describe several connected straight lines. Again using hypothetical data to illustrate (Table 10–6), a linear spline model made up of four straight lines (based on three knots) is

$$Y_x = b_0 + b_1 x + b_2 (x - K_1)_+ + b_3 (x - K_2)_+ + b_4 (x - K_3)_+.$$

Table 10–6. Hypothetical* data ($n = 80$) generated to illustrate a three-knot spline model

x	y_x	x	y_x	x	y_x	x	y_x
1	30.5	21	−39.3	41	13.5	61	115.5
2	5.1	22	−2.9	42	45.8	62	45.8
3	−14.6	23	−12.4	43	83.8	63	114.6
4	61.4	24	−48.7	44	53.8	64	14.7
5	23.4	25	−61.4	45	41.0	65	117.4
6	−60.7	26	32.8	46	134.7	66	13.7
7	−22.6	27	3.4	47	124.8	67	15.5
8	−45.4	28	17.0	48	126.7	68	28.8
9	45.9	29	73.8	49	130.0	69	106.3
10	−40.1	30	44.2	50	38.2	70	63.7
11	15.9	31	65.1	51	100.8	71	−1.0
12	5.2	32	57.2	52	65.1	72	74.8
13	−6.4	33	74.9	53	27.9	73	92.3
14	−6.6	34	19.7	54	43.3	74	23.3
15	24.0	35	20.2	55	83.8	75	6.9
16	−69.5	36	27.1	56	44.6	76	74.8
17	−33.8	37	84.9	57	35.2	77	−4.2
18	18.1	38	33.3	58	142.9	78	37.8
19	−45.7	39	88.0	59	64.3	79	26.9
20	−43.2	40	87.3	60	32.5	80	−3.3

* = $Y_x = 10 - 2x + 7(x - 20)_+ - 4(x - 40)_+ - 5(x - 60)_+$ and model: $y_x = Y_x + error.$

Specifically, the model is

$$0 \leq x \leq 20: \ Y_x = 10 - 2x,$$
$$20 \leq x \leq 40: \ Y_x = -130 + 5x,$$
$$40 \leq x \leq 60: \ Y_x = 30 + x, \text{ and}$$
$$60 \leq x \leq 80: \ Y_x = 330 - 4x$$

for $x = 1, 2, \cdots, 80$. The knots are: $K_1 = 20$, $K_2 = 40$, and $K_3 = 60$.

Table 10–7 is a detailed description of the underlying mechanics of creating a piecewise linear spline. The hypothetical model consists of four segments (Figure 10–9, dotted line) each describing a different straight line with slopes –2, 5, 1, and –4, respectively (columns 2, 4, 6, and 8, Table 10–7). Furthermore, three terms in the spline expression produce new "intercepts" for each of these segments (columns 3, 5, and 7, Table 10–7). That is, at each knot, one line ends and the next line begins at a new "intercept"; thus, the term *knot*. For the example, at the first knot ($K = 20$), the line $y_x = 10 - 2x$ ends and the new line begins with new "intercept" at –30. The term $-2(x - 20)_+$ is made part of the expression to maintain the new "intercept" at –30 until the next knot ($K = 40$) is reached. The next new "intercept" becomes 70, and it is then maintained by including the term $-5(x - 40)_+$ until the next knot. Finally, the last line begins at knot $K = 60$ and, to maintain the new "intercept" at 90, the term $-1(x - 60)_+$ is included in the spline expression. Each segment is made up of two elements, an element that maintains the new intercept $[b_{i-1}(x - K)_+]$ and an element that creates the values of the next segment $[b_i(x - K)_+]$ (Table 10–7). A detailed expression of the four segments (square brackets) of the three-knot linear spline process is then

$$Y_x = [10 - 2x] + [2(x - 20)_+ + 5(x - 20)_+] + [-5(x - 40)_+ + 1(x - 40)_+]$$
$$+ [-1(x - 60)_+ - 4(x - 60)_+].$$

To make the expression more compact, the like terms are combined and

$$Y_x = 10 - 2x + (2 + 5)(x - 20)_+ + (-5 + 1)(x - 40)_+ + (-1 + -4)(x - 60)_+$$

or

$$Y_x = 10 - 2x + 7(x - 20)_+ - 4(x - 40)_+ - 5(x - 60)_+$$

becomes a three-knot piecewise linear spline model. Using, as noted, conventional regression techniques and spline model "data" y_x values (Table 10–6) produce the estimated coefficients, variances, statistical tests, confidence intervals, and model-generated values in the usual manner (Table 10–8). As always, the independent

Table 10–7. A detailed description of the mechanics of a piecewise three-knot linear spline (knots $= K = 20$, 40, and $= 60$)

	Segment 1	Segment 2		Segment 3		Segment 4		
x	$-2x$	$2(x-20)_+$	$5(x-20)_+$	$-5(x-40)_+$	$1(x-40)_+$	$-1(x-60)_+$	$-4(x-60)_+$	Y_x
0	10	0	0	0	0	0	0	10
1	8	0	0	0	0	0	0	8
2	6	0	0	0	0	0	0	6
3	4	0	0	0	0	0	0	4
—	—	—	—	—	—	—	—	—
20	−30	0	0	0	0	0	0	−30
21	−32	2	5	0	0	0	0	−25
22	−34	4	10	0	0	0	0	−20
23	−36	6	15	0	0	0	0	−15
24	−38	8	20	0	0	0	0	−10
—	—	—	—	—	—	—	—	—
40	−70	40	100	0	0	0	0	70
41	−72	42	105	−5	1	0	0	71
42	−74	44	110	−10	2	0	0	72
43	−76	46	115	−15	3	0	0	73
44	−78	48	120	−20	4	0	0	74
—	—	—	—	—	—	—	—	—
60	−110	80	200	−100	20	0	0	90
61	−112	82	205	−105	21	−1	−4	86
62	−114	84	210	−110	22	−2	−8	82
63	−116	86	215	−115	23	−3	−12	78
64	−118	88	220	−120	24	−4	−16	74
—	—	—	—	—	—	—	—	—
80	−150	120	300	−200	40	−20	−80	10

Note: The piecewise spline represented by Y_x at values x (Figure 10–9) is the sum of the row labeled x and yields the values given in the last column labeled Y_x where $Y_x = 10 - 2x + 7(x - 20)_+ - 4(x - 40)_+ - 5(x - 60)_+$ and $y_x = Y_x + $ *random error*.

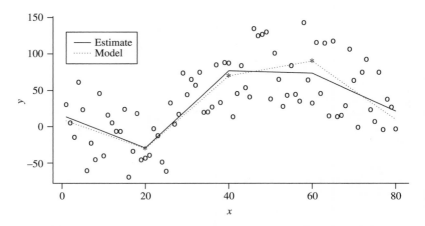

Figure 10–9. The estimated three-knot linear spline from the data (Table 10–6).

Table 10–8.   Estimated coefficients for the three-knot piecewise linear spline regression model from the hypothetical data (Table 10–6)

Variables	Symbols	Estimates	Std. errors	p-Values
Intercept	b_0	15.735	15.918	–
First line	b_1	−2.245	1.134	0.051
Second line	b_2	7.548	1.812	< 0.001
Third line	b_3	−5.465	1.582	< 0.001
Fourth line	b_4	−2.445	1.740	0.164

LogLikehood $= -50,248.0$

variables in a regression model are completely unrestrained (Chapter 5). Spline variables $(x - K_j)_+$ are made up of a sequence of zeros and "corrected" values but, nevertheless, are treated in exactly the same way as any independent variable in a regression model analysis. Therefore, modifications to the estimation process or underlying theory are not necessary. The plot of the hypothetical observations and the estimated line are displayed in Figure 10–9 (knots marked with "*") where

$$\hat{y}_x = \hat{b}_0 + \hat{b}_1 x + \hat{b}_2(x - K_1)_+ + \hat{b}_3(x - K_2)_+ + \hat{b}_4(x - K_3)_+$$
$$= 15.735 - 2.245x + 7.548(x - K_1)_+ - 5.465(x - K_2)_+ - 2.445(x - K_3)_+$$
$$= 15.735 - 2.245x + 7.548(x - 20)_+ - 5.465(x - 40)_+ - 2.445(x - 60)_+ .$$

The values estimated from the spline model $\hat{y}_0 = 15.735$, $\hat{y}_{20} = -29.171$, $\hat{y}_{40} = 76.887$, $\hat{y}_{60} = 73.642$, and $\hat{y}_{80} = 21.473$ produce estimates of the slopes of each of the four line segments (denoted $\hat{B}_i$) where

$$\hat{B}_1 = \frac{\hat{y}_{20} - \hat{y}_0}{20} = \frac{-29.171 - 15.735}{20} = -2.245 = \hat{b}_1,$$

$$\hat{B}_2 = \frac{\hat{y}_{40} - \hat{y}_{20}}{20} = \frac{76.887 - (-29.171)}{20} = 5.303 = \hat{b}_2 + \hat{b}_1,$$

$$\hat{B}_3 = \frac{\hat{y}_{60} - \hat{y}_{40}}{20} = \frac{73.642 - 76.887}{20} = -0.162 = \hat{b}_3 + \hat{b}_2 + \hat{b}_1, \text{ and}$$

$$\hat{B}_4 = \frac{\hat{y}_{80} - \hat{y}_{60}}{20} = \frac{21.473 - 73.642}{20} = -2.608 = \hat{b}_4 + \hat{b}_3 + \hat{b}_2 + \hat{b}_1.$$

The underlying model B_i-values are: $B_1 = -2$, $B_2 = 5$, $B_3 = 1$, and $B_4 = -4$.

Data from central California consisting of vital records and counts of birth defects from the California Births Defects Monitoring Program provide an illustration of a spline model [39]. In 1994, the United States implemented compulsory folic acid fortification in cereal grain products. Manufacturers began fortification with folic acid in 1996 and were mandated to complete the fortification by the end of 1998. Neural tube defects (NTD) data, primarily the occurrences of the birth defects anencephaly and spina bifida, were obtained for the period 1989–2003. The data were collected to compare the trend in prevalence in the prefortification period (1989–1996) to that in the post-fortification period (1998–2003). The data from these three periods are presented in Table 10–9. The Poisson regression model, using a two-knot linear piecewise spline,

$$log(rate) = a + b_1(years) + b_2(years - 1996)_+ + b_3(years - 1998)_+$$

is applied to summarize the pattern of NTD prevalence (Table 10–10, knots are 1996 and 1998). The estimates of the model coefficients (Table 10–11) are then used to describe the prevalence (log-rates) over the before and after periods. Specifically, Figure 10–10 displays the pattern of prevalence based on log-rate estimates from a Poisson regression spline model (Chapter 6).

Estimated from the Poisson model, the slope $\hat{b}_1 = -0.086$, with an associated 95% confidence interval (−0.128, −0.043), indicates a decreasing trend in NTD prevalence observed during the pre-fortification period. The estimated slope for the post-fortification period is $\hat{b}_1 + \hat{b}_2 + \hat{b}_3 = 0.063$. Clearly, the decline in NTD prevalence during the pre-fortification period did not continue during the post-fortification period for these data from the central California.

As usual, the Poisson regression model-estimated coefficients yield estimated numbers of cases. These values then can be compared to the observed values to evaluate the accuracy of the three-line model (Table 10–10). For example, for the year 1989, the model-estimated $log(rate) = -6.792$ makes the estimated rate of NTD births $e^{-6.792} = 112.274$ per 100,000 births. Therefore, the model-estimated

Table 10–9. Neural defects data for the period 1989–2003: years, births*, NTD cases, and rate/100,000 births

Years	Births	NTD	Rate/100,000
1989	55,694	70	125.7
1990	60,869	63	103.5
1991	61,903	50	80.8
1992	61,837	53	85.7
1993	61,348	51	83.1
1994	60,382	34	56.3
1995	58,503	45	76.9
1996	57,180	36	63.0
1997	55,469	40	72.1
1998	56,201	32	56.9
1999	56,010	44	78.6
2000	58,220	34	58.4
2001	59,091	28	47.4
2002	60,973	54	88.6
2003	63,305	56	88.5

* = Births are live births plus fetal deaths

Table 10–10. Poisson spline regression model (two knots): the observed and the estimated numbers of neural tube defects

Years	$(Years - 1996)_+$	$(Years - 1998)_+$	Observed	Estimated
1989	0	0	70	62.53
1990	0	0	63	62.73
1991	0	0	50	58.56
1992	0	0	53	53.69
1993	0	0	51	48.90
1994	0	0	34	44.18
1995	0	0	45	39.29
1996	0	0	36	35.25
1997	1	0	40	33.75
1998	2	0	32	33.75
1999	3	1	44	35.81
2000	4	2	34	39.64
2001	5	3	28	42.84
2002	6	4	54	47.06
2003	7	5	56	52.03

number of NTD births for the year 1989 is 55,694(112.274/100,000) = 62.53. The observed number is 70. Using the classic Pearson goodness-of-fit test statistic applied to compare the 15 observed and the 15 model-estimated counts of NTD

Table 10–11. Poisson spline regression model: estimated model coefficients from NTD data (central California, 1989–2003)

Variables	Terms	Estimates	Std. errors
constant	a	163.566	43.179
years	b_1	−0.086	0.022
$(years - 1996)_+$	b_2	0.073	0.093
$(years - 1998)_+$	b_3	0.076	0.105

LogLikelihood $= -8.269$

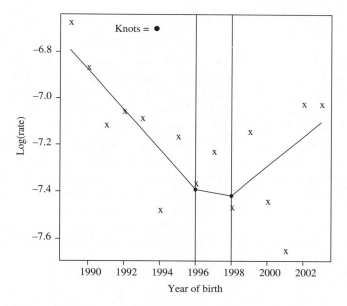

Figure 10–10. NTD log-rates (symbol = x) and the piecewise linear spline model estimate of trend (solid line) during the period 1989–2003 (California).

birth defects (Table 10–10, last two columns) yields the chi-square distributed value of $X^2 = 15.820$ with 11 degrees of freedom (observed values − parameters = $15 - 4 = 11$) and a p-value of $P(X^2 \geq 15.820 | model\ is\ correct) = 0.148$.

Spline estimation similarly creates smooth curves that are not a sequence of connected straight lines. For example, a spline model using three connected cubic polynomials is

$$Y_x = b_0 + b_1 x + b_2 x^2 + b_3 x^3 + b_4 (x - K_1)_+^3 + b_5 (x - K_2)_+^3 + b_6 (x - K_3)_+^3 .$$

Table 10–12.   Estimates of the coefficients for the three-knot cubic spline model from the hypothetical data (Table 10–6)

Variables	Symbols	Estimates	Std. errors
Intercept	b_0	19.631	30.790
x	b_1	−2.600	8.255
x^2	b_2	−0.126	0.591
x^3	b_3	0.008	0.012
$K_1 = 20$	b_4	−0.019	0.016
$K_2 = 40$	b_5	0.017	0.008
$K_3 = 60$	b_6	−0.014	0.014

LogLikehood = −49,998.0

A three-knot cubic spline representation of a pattern can be understood by an analogy based on four pieces of string and five nails. A nail is place at the value of the first observation. Then, a piece of string is tied to the first nail. Then, between the first nail and a second nail at the selected knot, K_1, the string is shaped to best represent the data and tied to the second nail. The only rule is that the string can change directions a maximum of three times. Like the linear spline, the process then starts over. A second string is tied to the second nail and the data are represented by the path of the string, which is then tied to a third nail at the selected knot K_2. The same process is repeated twice more, and the end of the fourth piece of string is tied to the fifth nail placed at the last observation. The string then starts from the first nail (smallest x-value) and passes through the data to the last nail (largest x-value) forming a continuous curve connected at the three in-between knots, producing a single smooth line summarizing the underlying pattern of data. Such spline estimates capture the essence of most relationships. For even extremely complicated relationships (a rare occurrence in human data), all that is needed is more nails (knots). This analogy indicates the reason that spline curves are occasionally called *piecewise polynomial estimates*.

As before, usual regression techniques produces the estimated coefficients. Regression estimation (Table 10–12) produces the cubic spline model components from the data in Table 10–6. Figure 10–11 displays the estimated cubic spline curve and, for the example, estimated values (interpolated) for the selected values $x = 30, 50,$ and 70 are $\hat{y}_{30} = 23.237$, $\hat{y}_{50} = 79.039$, and $\hat{y}_{70} = 53.379$.

The previous sex- and age-specific Hodgkin disease incidence rates for African-American and white SEER populations (top) and spline smoothed rates (bottom) over the life span of 85 years are shown in Figure 10–12. A comparison of the median/mean moving-average estimated curves (Figure 10–2) with the spline estimated curves (Figure 10–12) shows similar patterns. Only in exceptional cases do different smoothing techniques give remarkably different results. However,

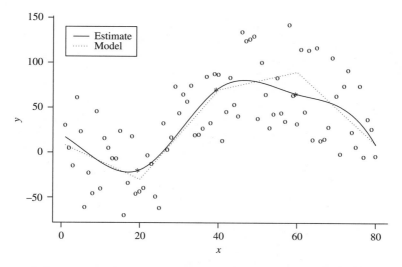

Figure 10–11. A plot of the three-knot cubic spline curve (solid line) estimated from the hypothetical data $\hat{y}_x$ (Table 10–6).

other smoothing techniques are not directly implemented and evaluated with ordinary regression methods.

Another application of spline curve estimation comes from data collected to study weight gain and loss patterns during and after pregnancy. A sample of $n = 1638$ women were weighed a number of times during their pregnancy (kilograms) and during the year after delivery. The data consist of a large number of pairs of weights and days pregnant and days postpartum (about 6.6 weight/time pairs per women over a maximum of 800 days). Figure 10–13 displays the observed pattern of gain and loss for 20 of these women (dashed lines) and a three-knot cubic spline curve (Knots: 270, 284, and 450 days) estimated from the entire data set (solid line).

The same data separated into race/ethnicity groups (white, Hispanic, African-American, and Asian) and summarized by cubic spline curves are displayed in Figure 10–14. The pattern of weight loss after 270 days (delivery) shows increased variability due to the small numbers of race-specific observations over the post-partum year. The variation disappears from the plot when each of the already smoothed spline curves are themselves further smoothed (Figure 10–15). Although these smoother curves no longer directly indicate the influence from random variation, it remains. The estimated curves, smoothed or not, are based on the same data and are subject to the same influences from random variation. Smoothing techniques are designed to reduce the visual influence of extraneous variation. Other techniques are available to rigorously assess the relationships in light of the influence of random variation (Chapter 12).

Age-specific rates

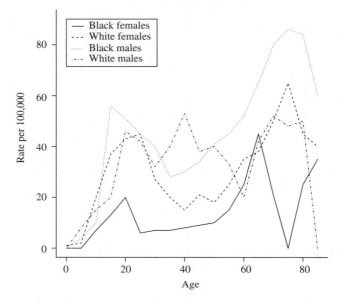

Cubic spline smoothed age-specific rates

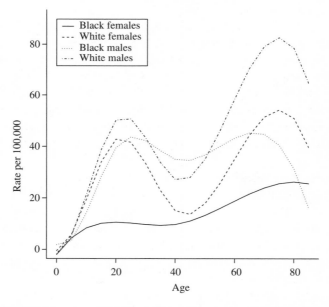

Figure 10–12. The sex- and age-specific incidence rates of Hodgkin disease among African-American and whites for males and females (SEER cancer registry).

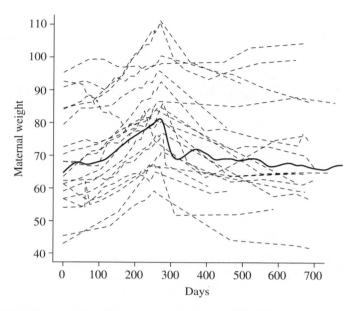

Figure 10–13. A spline-estimated (knots = 270, 284 and 450 days) pattern of weight gain and loss (kilograms) during an 800-day period based on $n = 1638$ pregnant women (the dashed lines are 20 representative study participants).

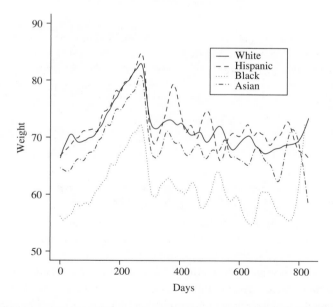

Figure 10–14. A cubic spline-estimated pattern of weight gain and loss (kilograms) during an 800-day period based on $n = 1638$ pregnant women classified into four race/ethnicity groups.

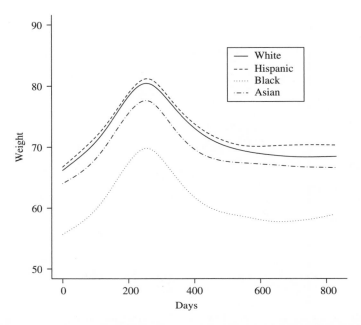

Figure 10–15. A cubic spline-estimated pattern of weight gain and weight loss (kilograms) during an 800-day period based on pregnant women classified into four race/ethnicity groups with additional smoothing (*n* = 1638).

Table 10–13. Spline model-estimated maternal weights at prepregnancy (0 days), delivery (270 days), and 6 months post-partum (450 days) as well as estimated weight gained and retained by race/ethnicity group

	Day = 0	Day = 270	Day = 450	Gained	Retained*	%Gained**	%Retained**
White	66.4	78.0	69.3	13.5	2.9	20.3	4.4
Hispanic	66.7	80.5	74.0	13.8	7.3	20.6	10.9
African-American	56.1	69.0	58.2	13.0	2.1	23.1	3.8
Asian	64.6	76.7	67.1	12.2	2.5	18.9	4.0

* = Weight at 6 months post-partum (day 450) minus prepregnancy weight (day 0)
** = Normalized (divided) by prepregnancy weight

Table 10–13 illustrates one of the many ways spline-estimated curves can produce summary values from sampled data. Maternal weights at three critical times (prepregnancy, delivery, and 6 months post-partum) are interpolated from the estimated spline curves and compared among the four race/ethnicity groups (Figure 10–15).

The choice of knots is an issue in the construction of a spline curve. Occasionally, knots are chosen because they are natural to the data analyzed. For example, the knots for the weight gain/loss curves are traditional and important values: delivery (day 270), 2 weeks post-partum (day 284), and 6 months post partum (day 450). Nonlinear methods exist to estimate "optimum" knots. Computer software that performs spline model estimation often have sophisticated and elegant algorithms for automatically choosing knots. Typically, several alternatives are available. It has been found, however, that in most situations the choice of the knots is not critical [40]. Choosing knots at equally spaced percentiles of the distribution of the independent variable (x_i) is a useful and rarely misleading strategy. This choice guarantees that equally spaced points anchor the estimated spline curve relatively uninfluenced by extreme observations.

Data Analysis with Spline-Estimated Curves: An Example

The previously described natural cubic spline curve is rarely applied to data. Instead, a *restricted cubic spline* curve estimated with a specialized computer algorithm usually takes its place. A restricted cubic spline curve is more efficient, has fewer parameters, and has slightly better properties than a natural cubic spline curve but is not different in principle. The restricted cubic spline, represented by the notation $rcs(x)$, results from an algebraic manipulation of the original spline equation [40].

Using the coronary heart disease (CHD) data from the Western Collaborative Group (WCGS) Study (Chapters 4 and 11, $n = 3153$ study participants), the relationship between CHD risk and body weight is effectively described and evaluated by a three-knot restricted cubic spline logistic regression model. In terms of log-odds, the model is

$$log\text{-}odds = l_i = a + rcs(wt_i)$$

where $rcs(wt_i)$ represents a restricted cubic spline with three knots. Although a spline representation of a variable, such as body weight, is a sophisticated representation of the independent variable, the regression analysis and its interpretation remain essentially unchanged. Of most importance, the curve representing the pattern of CHD–weight risk is entirely determined by the data. The regression analysis estimated curve is displayed for the WCGS data in Figure 10–16. The rate of increase in risk associated with increasing body weight is considerable less for heavy men (*weight* > 175) than lighter men (*weight* < 175), and this pattern is estimated directly from the data. That is, it is entirely assumption-free. The pointwise confidence intervals (dashed lines) give a strong indication that body weight has a nonlinear influence on the log-odds and, therefore, is an important feature of CHD risk.

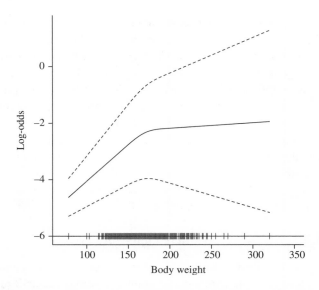

Figure 10–16.   Log-odds risk from body weight estimated with a three-knot restricted cubic spline (WCGS data).

The usual likelihood comparison of the cubic spline logistic regression model to the corresponding linear logistic model provides a formal statistical assessment of the apparent nonlinearity. As always, the possibility exists that this nonlinear curve is an artifact arising from the random variation in the observed data. The standard single-variable logistic regression model

$$log\text{-}odds = l_i = a + b\,wt_i$$

dictates a linear relationship between body weight and CHD log-odds risk. Comparing log-likelihood values generated from the two regression models indicates the importance of the difference between the nonlinear (spline model) and the nested linear model as a description of the pattern of CHD risk associated with body weight. The likelihood ratio chi-square test statistic is

$$X^2 = -2[log(L_{linear}) - log(L_{spline})] = -2[-884.377 - (-882.312)] = 4.132.$$

The probability that the restricted cubic spline model produces the estimated nonlinear pattern (Figure 10–16) by capitalizing only on random variation is $P(X^2 \geq 4.132|linear) = 0.042$ (degrees of freedom = 1).

Adding behavior type to the analysis extends the logistic spline regression model

$$log\text{-}odds = l_i = rcs(wt_i) + bF_i$$

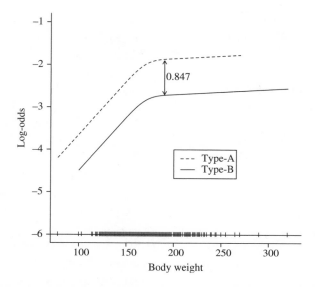

Figure 10–17. Log-odds risk associated with body weight estimated with a three-knot restricted cubic spline model from the WCGS data for type-A and type-B behavior groups.

where $rcs(wt)$ again stands for a three-knot restricted cubic spline representation of the pattern of body weigh and CHD risk (log-odds model). As before, the symbol $F = 0$ indicates type-B individuals and $F = 1$ indicates type-A individuals. The model-estimated behavior type coefficient $\hat{b}$ is 0.847 ($S_{\hat{b}} = 0.140$) and yields a p-value of $P(|Z| \geq 6.028|b = 0) < 0.001$. The spline model-estimated curves are displayed for each behavior type in Figure 10–17. The estimated model coefficient $\hat{b} = 0.847$ is the geometric distance between the log-odds values generated by the two spline-estimated curves and is constant for all body weights, as dictated by the choice of an additive model. The resulting odds ratio $\hat{or} = e^{0.847} = 2.333$ and the 95% confidence interval (1.771, 3.073) reflect the influence of behavior type on coronary risk accounting for influences caused by differences in body weight distributions between type-A and type-B individuals.

The model-dictated additivity is obvious from the plot (the lines are the same distance apart for all body weights). A formal assessment of the postulated additivity is achieved by a comparison of the additive model to a model that allows an interaction between body weight (again, as described by the restricted cubic spline curve) and the binary behavior type variable. Such a logistic regression model is represented by

$$log\text{-}odds = rcs(wt) + bF + c[F \times rcs(wt)].$$

A nonadditive model allows the estimation of a nonlinear relationship between body weight and the likelihood of a CHD event that differs for each behavior type (not equal distances for all body weights). Again, comparing two log-likelihood values provides a formal statistical evaluation of the difference between these two descriptions of the CHD risk (additive vs. nonadditive models). The chi-square likelihood ratio test statistic is

$$X^2 = -2[log(L_{additive}) - log(L_{nonadditive})] = -2[-862.788 - (-861.568)]$$
$$= 2.440.$$

The test statistic X^2 has a chi-square distribution with two degrees of freedom when the nested models differ by chance alone ($c = 0$). The associated p-value $= P(X^2 \geq 2.440|no\ interaction) = 0.295$ provides some assurance that a single odds ratio (additive model) is a useful reflection of the difference in CHD risk between type-A and type-B behavior types adjusted for influences from differing body weight distributions. The body weight and behavior type analysis of CHD risk illustrates that spline representations of a variable easily provide an entirely data-driven and potentially nonlinear description of the independent variables in a regression equation (further discussed in Chapter 11).

11

CASE STUDY: DESCRIPTION AND ANALYSIS

Statistical analysis ideally consists of at least two complementary approaches to understanding the issues reflected by collected data. Descriptive statistics such as means, variances, proportions, ranges, medians, and percentiles provide an intuitive understanding of each of the variables under study. Typical and atypical values become obvious. In addition, graphic representations provide further descriptive insight into the properties of the sampled data. However, descriptive summary statistics and their plots usually yield equivocal conclusions primarily because of the failure to account for the influences of sampling variation. Therefore, statistical tests, confidence intervals, statistical models, and multivariable analytic techniques in conjunction with descriptive methods typically produce intuitively appealing interpretations reinforced by quantitative statistical evaluations. To demonstrate the process of descriptive/graphic methods supported by rigorous statistical analyses, the data from the Western Collaborative Group Study (WCGS, complete description at the end of Chapter 4) relating behavior type to coronary heart disease (CHD) provide a case study. The data were collected to answer the question:

Does lifestyle behavior have an intrinsic (direct) influence on the risk of CHD, or does lifestyle behavior measure only the combined influences of known risk factors (e.g., smoking, cholesterol, etc.) that, in turn, influence the risk of CHD?

Table 11–1. Descriptive statistics for seven WCGS variables relevant to the study of coronary heart disease

Variables	Min.	1st Q.	Medians	Means	3rd Q.	Max.
Age	39.0	42.0	45.0	46.3	50.0	59.0
Weight	78.0	155.0	170.0	170.0	182.0	320.0
Height	60.0	68.0	70.0	69.8	72.0	78.0
Systolic blood pressure	98.0	120.0	126.0	128.6	136.0	212.0
Diastolic blood pressure	58.0	76.0	80.0	82.0	86.0	150.0
Cholesterol levels	103.0	198.0	223.0	226.4	252.0	645.0
Smoking exposure	0.0	0.0	0.0	11.6	20.0	80.0

Q = quartiles

The primary issue is the assessment of the influence of behavior type measures of lifestyle (1588 type-A and 1565 type-B study participants) on the likelihood of a coronary event ($n = 3153$ study participants with 257 coronary events). Table 11–1 contains a few summary statistics describing seven variables relevant to the study of the influence of behavior type on the likelihood of a coronary event (age, weight, height, systolic blood pressure, diastolic blood pressure, cholesterol levels, smoking exposure).

Such descriptions have limited use. They provide a glimpse of the entire distribution (quartiles) but give no hint of the relationships among these variables. For example, systolic and diastolic blood pressure levels are highly correlated, making it impossible to determine their relative influences without further analysis. The typically complex relationships among such variables requires a multivariable approach to begin to identify the role of a specific variable, such as behavior type. In fact, all seven variables were carefully measured and are included in the analysis to assure the best possible description of the specific influence of behavior type on the likelihood of a coronary event.

A table commonly created from multivariable data contains a series of one-at-time comparisons of each risk variable between the two levels of the outcome variable (Table 11–2).

These comparisons do not predict the multivariable relationships. For example, weight and height are correlated, and their influences on the likelihood of a coronary event are not indicated by two separate t-tests. The levels of significance from the pairwise comparisons will typically decrease or sometimes increase in the multivariable analysis depending on the relationships among all risk variables analyzed. Therefore, the magnitude of the differences between individuals with and without a CHD event may be of some descriptive interest but the statistical assessment has no useful interpretation.

Table 11–2. Seven comparisons of the mean values of the risk variables between individuals with (257) and without (2896) a coronary event

Variables	Symbols	CHD	No CHD	t-Tests	p-Values
Age	*age*	48.5	46.1	6.41	< 0.001
Weight	*wt*	174.5	169.6	3.51	0.001
Height	*ht*	69.9	69.8	1.10	0.268
Systolic bp.	*sys*	135.4	128.0	6.58	< 0.001
Diastolic bp.	*dias*	85.3	81.7	5.40	< 0.001
Cholesterol	*chol*	250.1	224.3	8.12	< 0.001
Smoking	*smk*	16.7	11.1	5.45	< 0.001

Table 11–3. Correlation array describing nine CHD risk variables (one dependent variable and eight independent variables)

Variables	*chd*	*age*	*wt*	*ht*	*sys*	*dias*	*chol*	*smk*	*ab*
chd	1.00	0.12	0.06	0.02	0.13	0.10	0.16	0.10	0.11
age	0.12	1.00	−0.03	−0.10	0.17	0.14	0.09	0.00	0.09
wt	0.06	−0.03	1.00	0.53	0.25	0.30	0.01	−0.08	0.04
ht	0.02	−0.10	0.53	1.00	0.02	0.01	−0.09	0.01	0.03
sys	0.13	0.17	0.25	0.02	1.00	0.77	0.12	0.03	0.08
dias	0.10	0.14	0.30	0.01	0.77	1.00	0.13	−0.06	0.06
chol	0.16	0.09	0.01	−0.09	0.12	0.13	1.00	0.10	0.06
smk	0.10	0.00	−0.08	0.01	0.03	−0.06	0.10	1.00	0.09
ab	0.11	0.09	0.04	0.03	0.08	0.06	0.06	0.09	1.00

A next step that is almost always a useful part of sorting out the relative influences of a series of related variables is the calculation of a correlation array (Table 11–3).

The values within a correlation array identify the pairs of variables with strong linear relationships [for example, $correlation(sys, dias) = 0.77$] and the pairs with essentially no linear relationship [for example, $correlation(smk, ht) = 0.01$]. A value denoted r_0 provides a sense of the influence of sampling variation on the values within a correlation array. This critical value is

$$r_0 = \frac{2}{\sqrt{n+2}}, \text{ then } P(|r| > r_0 \mid no\ association) < 0.05 \text{ for } n > 10$$

where r is an estimated correlation coefficient. Comparing the observed correlations to r_0 is roughly equivalent to a t-test of the hypothesis that the underlying correlation coefficient is zero. That is, the absolute value of an estimated correlation coefficient rarely exceeds r_0 by chance alone when no association exists. For the WCGS data, the critical point r_0 is 0.040 where $n = 3153$

observations. For the example, all but one correlation coefficient show a likely nonrandom relationship with the occurrence of a CHD event (Table 11–3, first row). Such comparisons are certainly approximate because making a large number of comparisons substantially increases the number of times the hypothesis of no association will be incorrectly rejected (Chapter 15). The fact that these variables are related further complicates interpretation. Therefore, measures of correlation ultimately have limited interpretations because pairwise relationships are only one step in understanding the interplay of all measured risk factors and the likelihood of an outcome event.

Describing the influences from a risk variable, such as cholesterol, on a binary outcome, such as a CHD event, starts with a plot. The most fundamental plot consists of a series of points distributed along two straight lines (Figure 11–1). This simple plot is not useful. However, the addition of a theoretical statistical structure produces a rich environment, making it possible to extensively explore the relationship between a risk variable and the likelihood of a CHD event. A logistic curve is frequently postulated as a description of the relationship between a risk variable and the probability associated with a binary outcome (Chapters 4 and 5). Specifically, low levels of cholesterol are associated with small probabilities of a CHD event and, as the levels of cholesterol increase, the probability of a CHD event increases in a nonlinear fashion until high levels of cholesterol are associated with probabilities of a CHD event in the neighborhood of 1.0. The

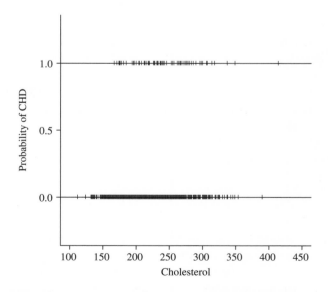

Figure 11–1. Binary CHD data plotted for levels of cholesterol.

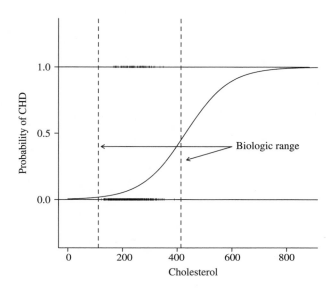

Figure 11–2.   A logistic curve used to describe the influences of cholesterol on the probability of a CHD event.

observed occurrence of a CHD event remains a binary event but the postulated logistic probability of a CHD event reflects the continuous underlying influence of a risk variable. In most applications of logistic probabilities to describe human data, only a portion of the curve is relevant ("biologic range," Figure 11–2). Maximum likelihood estimates produce the best possible estimated logistic curve (Chapter 3). However, no guarantee exists that even the best possible logistic curve accurately represents the underlying pattern of influence. All that can be definitely said is that this " s-shaped" curve never produces values less than zero or more than 1. As with most statistical models, the logistic curve has no physical or biologic justification but is a simple and frequently useful way to summarize the relationships between risk and outcome. Assessing its success or failure to reflect these relationships is a key element of the analysis. Furthermore, the logistic curve is no more than one of a number of possible conjectures.

The adequacy of a logistic model (goodness-of-fit) can be addressed by the familiar process of estimating the CHD–risk relationship based entirely on the data (completely assumption-free) and comparing these values to the corresponding estimates based on a postulated logistic model. Assumption-free estimates are accomplished by grouping the data into a sequence of intervals and directly computing the probability of a coronary event for each interval. For the WCGS data, a table is created to compare ten empirically and theoretically derived CHD probabilities and log-odds values (Table 11–4).

Table 11–4. Cholesterol and the likelihood of CHD: assumption-free and logistic model estimated probabilities and log-odds values

Intervals		<175	175–190	190–203	203–214	Cholesterol levels 214–223	223–234	234–246	246–260	260–280	>280
At-risk		316	315	315	315	316	315	315	315	315	316
cases of CHD		9	11	18	17	14	29	44	27	44	53
mean values		157.1	183.0	197.3	208.5	218.5	228.5	239.6	252.9	269.0	309.3
Data: $P(CHD)$		0.028	0.035	0.057	0.054	0.044	0.095	0.102	0.092	0.140	0.168
log-odds		−3.530	−3.319	−2.803	−2.864	−3.071	−2.251	−2.180	−2.289	−1.818	−1.602
Model: $P(CHD)$		0.032	0.044	0.052	0.059	0.066	0.075	0.085	0.099	0.118	0.186
log-odds		−3.410	−3.087	−2.908	−2.769	−2.644	−2.519	−2.381	−2.214	−2.013	−1.510

* = Estimates for the mean value of each category

Ten empirical probabilities and, therefore, ten log-odds values are directly calculated from the cholesterol categories. For example, individuals with cholesterol levels of less than 175 (mean cholesterol level of 157.1 mg%) had nine coronary events among 316 study participants, yielding the estimated probability of a CHD event of $9/316 = 0.028$ and a log-odds of $log(0.029) = -3.530$ (first cholesterol interval in Table 11–4).

These ten data-generated probabilities are naturally compared to corresponding theoretical probabilities estimated from a logistic regression model. That is, the estimated parametric logistic model

$$log\text{-}odds = \hat{a} + \hat{b}(chol) = -5.372 + 0.0125(chol)$$

and

$$P(CHD|chol) = \frac{1}{1 + e^{-[log\text{-}odds]}} = \frac{1}{1 + e^{-[\hat{a} + \hat{b}(chol)]}}$$
$$= \frac{1}{1 + e^{-[-5.372 + 0.0125(chol)]}}$$

produce model-estimated log-odds values and probabilities of CHD events for any level of cholesterol (*chol*). For example, a cholesterol level of 157.1 (mean level of cholesterol category < 175, first category) produces the estimated log-odds of −3.410, and the estimated probability of a CHD event is $P(CHD|chol = 157.1) = 1/(1 + e^{3.410}) = 0.032$. The degree of correspondence between observed and estimated probabilities of coronary event from each of the ten categories is the first indication of the utility of a logistic model (Figures 11–3).

When a probability is a value from a logistic curve, the corresponding log-odds is a value from a straight line and vice versa (Chapter 4). Straight lines are more intuitive, directly compared and, of most importance, similarities/dissimilarities between data and model values are easily identified. The graphic comparison of the ten observed CHD log-odds and the ten logistic model-estimated CHD log-odds, therefore, indicates the accuracy of the postulated logistic model (Figure 11–4).

These kinds of comparisons made between observed and model-estimated values are useful as long as the sample size is large enough to produce a sequence of intervals containing sufficient numbers of observations to yield stable estimates. Thus, for larger numbers of observations, more categories can be created. Like the single-variable descriptive statistics and the bivariate correlations, these plots are not definitive because the important question is not whether univariate relationships are well represented by a series of logistic models, but rather, the important question is whether the multivariable relationship is well represented by a single logistic model (to be discussed).

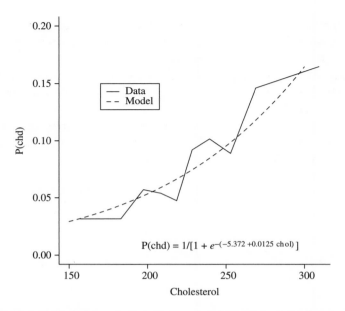

Figure 11–3. CHD–cholesterol relationship estimated directly from the data and from a logistic model, probability of CHD.

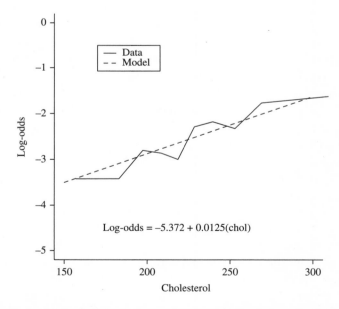

Figure 11–4. CHD–cholesterol relationship estimated directly from the data and the logistic model, log-odds of CHD.

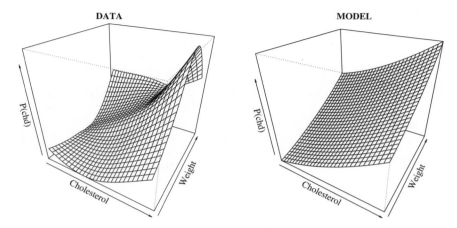

Figure 11–5. Three-dimensional plots of the joint influences of body weight and cholesterol on the probability of CHD, nonparametrically estimated smoothed surface and a model-generated additive surface.

Another step forward in understanding multivariable data is achieved by exploring the joint influence of selected pairs of risk variables. For example, body weight and cholesterol are related to each other, and both variables are related to the probability of a coronary event (Table 11–3). A "three-dimensional" plot (Figure 11–5, left) displays an assumption-free estimate of this bivariate relationship (Chapter 15).   Visually, the plot shows an apparent relationship between the likelihood of CHD and weight that depends on the level of cholesterol (nonadditive relationship). For high levels of cholesterol, the estimated surface is concave and, for low levels, the estimated surface is convex. An additive model requires the relationship between weight and coronary risk to be the same for all levels of cholesterol. The additive logistic model relationship is displayed for comparison (Figure 11–5, right). The failure of the data (left) to reflect the relationship dictated by an additive model (right) is a specific example of an interaction. As almost always, the differences in pattern observed from directly comparing plotted data to postulated model values are complicated by the influences of sampling variation. In fact, interpretation of visual comparisons can be deceptively difficult. A few extreme observations, even a single extreme observation, can produce dramatic features displayed in a plot that are not representative of the relationships under investigation. Therefore, visual descriptions are certainly a useful start but they must be supplemented by a statistical analysis to assess the likelihood that all or some of the apparent features did not arise by chance alone.

Table 11–5. Eight single-variable logistic regression models (one-at-a-time analysis)

Variables	Intercepts ($\hat{a}$)	Slopes ($\hat{b}$)	Std. errors ($S_{\hat{b}}$)	p-Values	Log-likelihoods
Age	−5.939	0.074	0.011	< 0.001	−869.1
Weight	−4.215	0.010	0.003	< 0.001	−884.4
Height	−4.345	0.028	0.026	0.288	−890.0
Systolic bp	−6.022	0.027	0.004	< 0.001	−865.4
Diastolic bp	−5.243	0.034	0.006	< 0.001	−875.6
Cholesterol	−5.372	0.012	0.001	< 0.001	−852.0
Smoking	−2.746	0.024	0.004	< 0.001	−874.7
Behavior (A/B)	−2.934	0.863	0.140	< 0.001	−870.1

For the WCGS data, a single-variable linear logistic model is described by the expression

$$log-odds = log\left[\frac{p}{1-p}\right] = a + bx \quad \text{or} \quad P(CHD|x) = \frac{1}{1 + e^{-(log-odds)}}$$

$$= \frac{1}{1 + e^{-(a + \cdot bx)}}$$

for each risk variable (x). Table 11–5 contains the results from applying a single-variable logistic regression model to estimate the likelihood of a coronary event for each of the eight risk variables (one-at-time).

These results are additionally displayed by model-generated plots of the log-odds (Figure 11–6) and the probabilities of CHD (Figure 11–7) for the seven nonbinary risk variables. The binary behavior type variable produces two estimates, namely the log-odds for type-A and for type-B behavior.

The log-odds plots (straight lines) indicate essentially the same influences from age, weight, systolic blood pressure, diastolic blood pressure, and smoking on likelihood of CHD. However, these variables are related to each other, particularly systolic and diastolic blood pressures (Table 11–3), causing the influence of one risk variable to look much like the other. The similarities continue to be apparent when the estimated probabilities of CHD are plotted from each of the one-at-time analyses (Figure 11–7).

The descriptive statistics, correlation array, plots, and one-at-a-time analyses build a foundation for richer understanding and interpretation of a multivariable model by way of comparisons. Differences between the simple (perhaps naive) analyses and the multivariable logistic model are potentially helpful in identifying and evaluating the extent of the influence of each risk variable. For example, these kinds of comparisons are clearly necessary to assess the confounding and joint confounding influences from the risk variables.

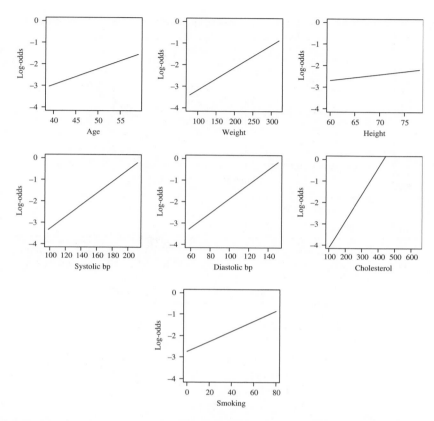

Figure 11–6. Seven separate (one-at-a-time) linear logistic models (age, weight, height, systolic blood pressure, diastolic blood pressure, cholesterol, and smoking exposure), log-odds of CHD.

The additive eight-variable multivariable logistic model for the WCGS data is

$$log\text{-}odds_i = a + b_1 age_i + b_2 weight_i + b_3 height_i + b_4 sys_i$$
$$+ b_5 dias_i + b_6 chol_i + b_7 smk_i + b_8 ab_i$$

or, as always,

$$P(CHD_i | age,\ weight,\ height,\ sys,\ dias,\ chol,\ smk,\ ab)$$

$$= \frac{1}{1 + e^{-log\text{-}odds_i}}$$

$$= \frac{1}{1 + e^{-(a + b_1 age_i + b_2 weight_i + b_3 height_i + b_4 sys_i + b_5 dias_i + b_6 chol_i + b_7 smk_i + b_8 ab_i)}}.$$

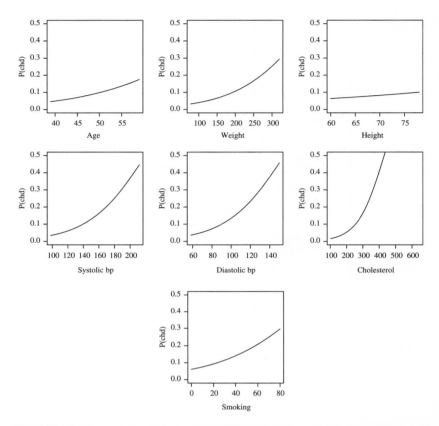

Figure 11–7. Seven separate (one-at-a-time) linear logistic models (age, weight, height, systolic blood pressure, diastolic blood pressure, cholesterol, and smoking exposure), probability CHD.

The maximum likelihood estimates of the eight-variable additive logistic model regression coefficients ($\hat{b}_i$) are given in Table 11–6.

A primary purpose of an additive log-odds model is to produce a separate estimated odds ratio for each variable and a significance probability that indicates whether the observed association is likely to have occurred by chance alone (p-values, Table 11–6).

However, an important first step before interpreting an additive model is to contrast it to a model or models containing interaction terms. The powerful and parsimonious additive model is only a useful statistical tool in the absence of interactions. A logistic model describing CHD risk including all possible two-way interaction terms yields a 36-variable model. One-at-a-time tests (Wald's tests) of each of the additional 28 coefficients measuring the influences of the

Table 11–6. Multivariable linear logistic additive model, estimated regression coefficients

	Symbols	Estimates ($\hat{b}_i$)	Std. errors ($S_{\hat{b}_i}$)	p-Values	Odds ratios
Intercept	a	−13.716	2.315	–	–
Age	age	0.065	0.012	<0.001	1.07
Weight	wt	0.008	0.004	0.048	1.01
Height	ht	0.018	0.033	0.575	1.02
Systolic	sys	0.019	0.006	0.004	1.02
Diastolic	$dias$	−0.002	0.010	0.870	1.00
Cholesterol	$chol$	0.011	0.002	<0.001	1.01
Smoking	smk	0.021	0.004	<0.001	1.02
Behavior (A/B)	ab	0.653	0.145	<0.001	1.92

LogLikelihood = −791.071

pairwise interaction effects (lack of additivity) is not the best way to go about their assessment. The tests are related to each other because the interaction terms are related. The 28 pairwise interaction terms in the 36-variable model consist of different pairwise combinations of the same eight risk variables. Because the estimates are influenced by these relationships (particularly the estimated variances), each test in isolation has relatively little value. In addition, conducting 28 separate statistical tests incurs a substantial likelihood of incorrectly declaring several interaction terms as significant (Chapter 15).

The comparison of the log-likelihood value from the model containing all 28 two-way interaction terms to the log-likelihood value from the nested model with eight additive terms rigorously measures the utility of the simpler model. That is, the critical question becomes: Are the two models sufficiently similar so that the simpler additive model usefully summarizes the relationships under study? Specifically for the CHD data, the nonadditive and the additive model log-likelihood values are:

all two-way interactions included: $LogLikelihood$ =−772.484 and
no two-way interactions included: $LogLikelihood$ =−791.071.

The likelihood ratio test chi-square statistic is

$$X^2 = -2[log(L_{additive}) - log(L_{interaction})]$$
$$= -2[-791.071 - (-772.484)] = 37.175,$$

yielding a p-value of 0.115. The degrees of freedom (28) are, as usual, the degrees of freedom associated with the interaction model (3153 − 37 = 3116) subtracted from the degrees of freedom associated with the additive model $(3153 - 9 = 3144)$. Or, more directly, the degrees of freedom are the difference in the number of parameters used to define the two models, namely 28.

Adding 28 terms to a logistic model undoubtedly produces a noticeable influence. The difference in the log-likelihood values is expected to be roughly equal to the degrees of freedom when the two models differ by chance alone. However, in spite of this expected decrease in the log-likelihood value, no strong statistical evidence emerges of substantial nonadditivity. Nevertheless, it is good idea to inspect several of the stronger interactions.

Using the p-values from the two-way interaction tests (Wald's statistics, not shown) as a guide to the importance (an ad-hoc procedure as noted), the nonadditivity between cholesterol and body weight appears the strongest.

As weight increases, the influence of cholesterol on the likelihood of a CHD event appears to decrease (Figure 11–8). Specifically, for each of three increasing body weight categories (<155, 155–170, and >170 pounds), the model-estimated slope of the line representing the influence of cholesterol on the log-odds likelihood of CHD decreases.

A second notable interaction is between behavior type and body weight (Figure 11–9). Risk (measured by the log-odds) increases at a faster rate in

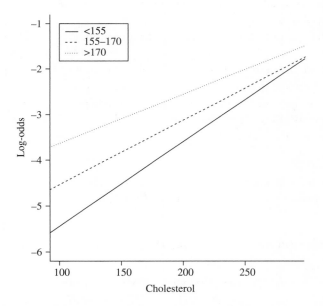

Figure 11–8. Linear logistic model estimated log-odds likelihood of a CHD event associated with cholesterol levels for three body weight categories (<155, 155–170, and >170 pounds), interaction model.

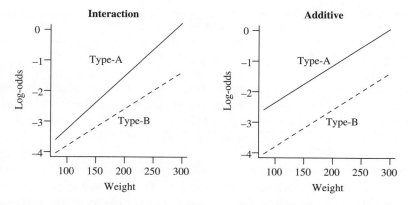

Figure 11–9. Linear logistic model-estimated log-odds likelihood of a CHD event by body weight for type-A and type-B behavior, interaction and additive multivariable models.

type-A individuals than in type-B individuals for the same increase in body weight. However, when assessed as part of the overall question: Are there substantial interactions among the eight risk variables?, there is insufficient evidence to focus on any particular pair of variables in terms of nonadditivity. In addition, tests for the presence/absence of interaction influences suffer from low statistical power (Chapter 4). As before, the failure to identify pairwise interaction influences does not mean that they do not exist. The choice of an additive model typically requires the simplicity of interpretation to be balanced against its potential lack of accuracy. The statistical analysis of interaction influences is part of the decision process but frequently does not supply a definitive answer.

Regression coefficients cannot be directly compared when generated from variables measured in different units. For example, systolic blood pressure ($\hat{b}_4 = 0.019$) and height ($\hat{b}_3 = 0.018$) do not have similar influences in the regression equation because their estimated coefficients are similar. The magnitude of a regression coefficient depends on its units of measurement. If heights were measured in feet rather than inches, for example, the associated regression coefficient would increase by a factor of 12 (new-$\hat{b}_3 = 12(0.018) = 0.216$).

A variety of ways exist to make comparisons among regression coefficients as long as they are measured in the same units. That is, their values are made commensurate. The z-statistics are commensurate because they are unitless. The corresponding p-values and likelihood statistics are also unitless and, therefore, commensurate. A third alternative is created by standardizing the independent variables to have the same units. Each independent variable is divided by its estimated standard deviation, making the variance $= 1.0$ for all variables and, of most importance, they now measure influence in terms of standard deviations. Each

Table 11–7. Regression coefficients, standard deviations, β-values, and ranks for the eight risk variables from the WCGS data

Variables	age	wt	ht	sys	dias	chol	smk	ab
Coefficient ($\hat{b}_i$)	0.065	0.008	0.018	0.019	−0.002	0.011	0.021	0.653
Std. deviation (S_i)	5.525	21.098	2.529	15.012	9.707	43.342	14.471	0.500
β-Value($\hat{\beta}_i$)	0.359	0.162	0.047	0.280	−0.017	0.483	0.301	0.327
Rank	2	6	7	5	8	1	4	3

transformed regression coefficient reflects the change in log-odds for a one standard deviation increase in the corresponding independent variable. A logistic regression analysis using these transformed variables then provides a series of commensurate coefficients, sometimes referred to as β-*values*. For the WCGS data, the eight commensurate regression coefficients based on transformed independent values (β-values) are given in Table 11–7.

The identical values can be directly calculated because the estimated β-value for a specific variable is the estimated coefficient from the analysis in natural units multiplied by the estimated standard deviation of that variable. In symbols, for the ith variable,

$$commensurate\ regression\ coefficient\ from\ standardized\ data = \hat{\beta}_i = \hat{b}_i S_i$$

where S_i represents the estimated standard deviation. For the WCGS data, among these commensurate measures, the β-values indicate that cholesterol is the most important variable in describing the likelihood of a coronary event, followed by smaller but similar contributions from age, systolic blood pressure, smoking, and behavior type, whereas, diastolic blood pressure and height appear to have negligible influences on CHD risk.

A plot of the seven nonbinary variables displays their additive (independent) patterns of influence on the risk of CHD in terms of the log-odds measure of association dictated by the multivariable model (Figure 11–10). The differences between the single one-at-a-time analysis of eight variables (dashed lines) and the single eight-variable analysis (solid lines) indicate the essence of the multivariable analysis. When separated by the additive model, the influence of each of the eight risk variables is substantially reduced. For example, the regression coefficient associated with behavior type decreases from 0.863 (single-variable model) to 0.653 (multivariable model). The parallel reduction in the estimated odds ratio is $e^{0.863} = 2.370$ to $e^{0.653} = 1.921$, after adjustment (additive model) for the presence of the other seven variables. The influences of the other seven variables show similarly differences. Most dramatically, the clearly different influences of systolic and diastolic blood pressure become apparent. Diastolic blood pressure

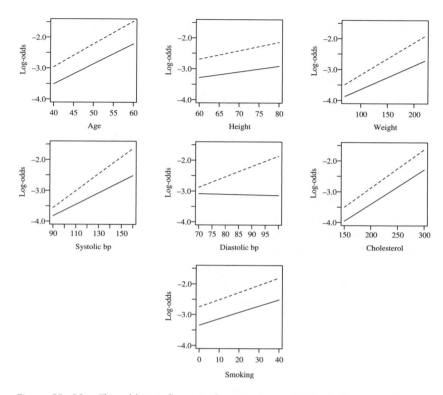

Figure 11–10. The additive influences of seven risk variables based on a multivariable logistic regression model and the same estimates based on one-at-time models (dashed line), log-odds of CHD.

has essentially no adjusted influence on the likelihood of a coronary event. The log-odds are the same for all levels of diastolic blood pressure, a horizontal line (Figure 11–10).

The log-odds relationships between each of the seven risk variables and CHD are linear (Figure 11–10). This linearity (*straight line* $= b_i x$) is a property of the model and not the data. This restrictive assumption is unnecessary. A spline representation of the relationships between each risk variable and the log-odds of a CHD event allows the data alone to dictate additive risk–outcome relationship. Using a spline representation does not eliminate the possibility of a linear pattern; it rather creates a regression model with more sophistication by expanding the possible descriptions of the influences of the risk variables on the likelihood of disease beyond a straight line.

An eight-variable restricted cubic spline additive regression model for the WCGS data is

$$log-odds_i = rcs(age_i) + rcs(wt_i) + rcs(ht_i) + rcs(sys_i)$$
$$+ rcs(dias_i) + rcs(chol_i) + smk_i + ab_i$$

where, as before, $rcs(x)$ denotes the restricted cubic spline representation of the variable x based on quartile knots (Chapter 10).

Thus, the cubic restricted-spline estimates each consist of three coefficients. Behavior type is a binary variable and, therefore, creates a single influence in all situations. Similarly, the number of cigarettes smoked is a discrete variable with an extremely asymmetric distribution (mostly zeros) and is directly analyzed as reported. The estimated logistic model coefficients from the WCGS data (eight variables based on 3153 observations) are given in Table 11–8.

The assessment of the influences of random variation on each estimated spline model representation of a risk variable is not achieved by a single p-value (omitted from the table). Each of the spline variables is made up of three components, and

Table 11–8. Multivariable logistic spline regression model, estimated coefficients

Variables	Estimates	Std. errors
a	−16.601	8.374
age	−0.133	0.087
age_1	1.044	0.437
age_2	−2.207	0.923
wt	0.013	0.016
wt_1	0.016	0.051
wt_2	−0.095	0.165
ht	0.117	0.096
ht_1	−0.335	0.280
ht_2	1.223	1.099
sys	−0.012	0.031
sys_1	0.180	0.152
sys_2	−0.380	0.317
$dias$	0.077	0.044
$dias_1$	−0.275	0.145
$dias_2$	0.878	0.481
$chol$	0.017	0.010
$chol_1$	−0.006	0.027
$chol_2$	0.005	0.085
smk	0.021	0.004
ab	0.675	0.146

LogLikelihood $= -782.493$

it is the combination of these components that is meaningful. Likelihood ratio tests indicate the role of each of the three-component spline variables. The first question is: Does the risk variable make a significant contribution to the regression equation? The answer to this question is addressed by the comparison of two nested models for each variable. The full eight-variable spline model is compared to the model with a specific variable removed. The likelihood ratio comparison of these two nested models measures the extent of the additive influence associated with the removed variable.

A second question becomes: Is there evidence that the risk–outcome relationship is nonlinear? Again the question is addressed by comparing likelihood values from two nested regression models. The full spline model is compared to a model where a specific risk variable is represented as a linear influence (a single term, $b_i x$). The likelihood ratio comparison of these two nested models measures the extent of nonlinearity associated with each variable. The six pairs of these two comparisons are summarized in Table 11–9 for the six continuous WCGS risk variables.

Complementing the likelihood analyses of the multivariable model are the plots of the spline-estimated patterns of risk measured by the log-odds likelihood of a CHD event (Figure 11–11). The influence of age, cholesterol, smoking, and behavior type are clearly evident (p-values < 0.001). In addition, both analyses and plots indicate that only one of the risk variables likely has a nonlinear influence on the log-odds of CHD, namely age (nonlinear: p-value = 0.057).

As with the evaluation of interaction effects, the overall gain in model accuracy achieved by incorporating nonlinear patterns of risk into a logistic model is best assessed with a likelihood ratio test. The log-likelihood value

Table 11–9. Results from the comparison of multivariable spline regression models

	chisq	df	p-Values
Age	32.44	3	< 0.001
nonlinear	5.78	2	0.057
Weight	6.82	3	0.078
nonlinear	2.84	2	0.242
Height	1.57	3	0.665
nonlinear	1.47	2	0.480
Systolic	10.68	3	0.014
nonlinear	1.45	2	0.484
Diastolic	3.75	3	0.290
nonlinear	3.67	2	0.160
Cholesterol	51.00	3	< 0.001
nonlinear	1.49	2	0.475

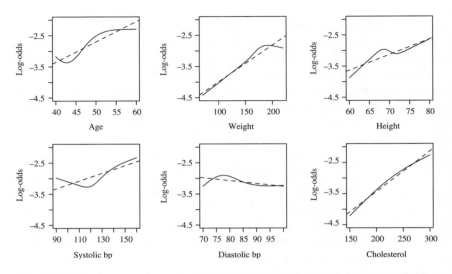

Figure 11–11. Logistic spline regression model including the six risk factors age, weight, height, systolic blood pressure, diastolic blood pressure, and cholesterol, log-odds of CHD (dashed line = linear representation of the risk variables).

from the eight-variable additive logistic model remains $log(L_{linear}) = -791.071$, and the corresponding value for the more sophisticated restricted spline model is $log(L_{spline}) = -782.493$. Thus, the likelihood ratio comparison of these nested models becomes

$$X^2 = -2[log(L_{linear}) - log(L_{spline})] = -2[-791.071 - (-782.493)] = 17.156.$$

The value $X^2 = 17.156$ has a chi-square distribution with 12 degrees of freedom (the additional number of parameters in the spline model) when all eight risk variables have strictly linear influences on the likelihood of a coronary event. In other words, the likelihood ratio test indicates that the difference between these two nested models possibly occurs because the estimation of six spline curves (solid lines in Figure 11–11) capitalizes only on random variation to produce apparent nonlinear influences. The resulting p-value is $P(X^2 \geq 17.156|linear) = 0.144$. It is also worth noting that both the linear and spline models produce similar variable-by-variable assessment in terms of significance probabilities (Table 11–7 compared to Table 11–9). Of central importance, the regression coefficient associated with the influence of behavior type from the linear logistic model is 0.653 (*standard error* = 0.145), and from the logistic spline model, the corresponding coefficient is 0.675 (*standard error* = 0.146). In terms of odds ratios, this difference becomes $e^{0.653} = 1.921$ (linear model) compared to $\hat{or} = e^{0.675} = 1.965$ (spline model).

As always, an additive model and its estimates (Table 11–9) are a useful description of the influence of behavior type on the likelihood of a coronary event, as long as the model adequately represents the relationships among the risk variables. Model accuracy (goodness-of-fit) is always an issue with any analysis based on a theoretical statistical model. As previously mentioned, the logistic model often does not allow a direct comparison of the model-estimated values to the observed binary outcomes with a chi-square statistic (Chapter 5). A graphical comparison, between model and observed log-odds or probabilities, however, is frequently an informative indication of the adequacy of an additive model. A plot of observed and model-estimated values, similar to the earlier cholesterol–CHD analysis, is often an effective approach (Table 11–4 and Figures 11–3 and 11–4). The data are divided into a number of categories based on percentiles of the model-estimated probabilities of a CHD event, much like the chi-square approach described in Chapter 5. As before, these categories must contain sufficient numbers of observations to provide stable estimates and, for the WCGS data, ten categories are again chosen (Table 11–10, about 315 observations per category). Once a series of categories is established, the model log-odds values, the observed log-odds, the model probabilities of a CHD event, and observed probabilities of a CHD event are estimated (Table 11–10).

A formal chi-square evaluation of the goodness-of-fit of a logistic model is not ideal (Chapter 5), but a direct plot of observed and model values (Figures 11–12, log-odds and 11–13, probabilities) displays the correspondence between observed (solid line) and model estimated values (dashed line). Note that the model values are estimated and plotted as a continuous curve.

Table 11–10. The additive spline model-estimated log-odds and probabilities of a CHD event compared to the observed log-odds and probabilities of a CHD event

	Risk levels									
	1	2	3	4	5	6	7	8	9	10
Sample size	316	315	315	315	315	316	315	315	315	316
cases of CHD	0	5	15	12	9	15	31	46	43	81
Model:										
$log-odds$	−4.590	−3.960	−3.534	−3.225	−2.958	−2.711	−2.430	−2.109	−1.719	−1.019
$P(CHD)$	0.010	0.019	0.028	0.038	0.049	0.062	0.081	0.108	0.152	0.267
Data:										
$log-odds$	−	−4.127	−2.996	−3.229	−3.526	−2.999	−2.215	−1.766	−1.845	−1.065
$P(CHD)$	0.000	0.016	0.048	0.038	0.029	0.048	0.098	0.146	0.137	0.256

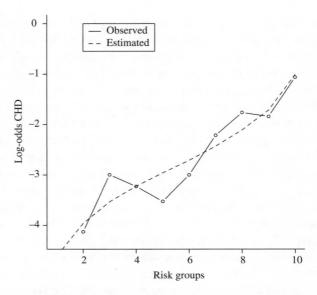

Figure 11–12. The comparison of the observed log-odds (solid line) and spline model-estimated log-odds (dashed line) for ten categories of risk.

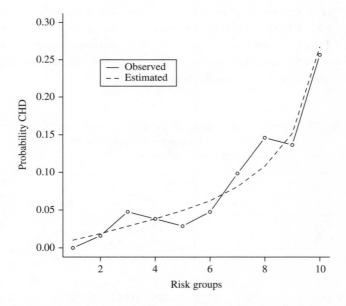

Figure 11–13. The comparison of the observed probabilities (solid line) and spline model-estimated probabilities (dashed line) for ten categories of risk.

For the WCGS logistic spline model, only two of the observed and estimated values deviate noticeably. The values from the third and fifth risk categories are the only questionable deviations among the ten comparisons and appear inconsequential. In terms of expected numbers of CHD events, in the third category the observed number is 15, and the model-predicted value is $315(0.028) = 8.8$ and, for the fifth category, the observed number is 9 and the model predicted values is $315(0.049) = 15.4$ from a total sample of 3153 men.

These two goodness-of-fit plots (Figures 11–12 and 11–13) are based on ten risk categories, so that stable estimates are achieved within each category.

An alternative is to create more risk categories. Then, to compensate for increased variability within categories, a log-odds curve is estimated from the data-generated points using a smoothing technique (Chapters 10 and 15). The results from the WCGS spline model are shown in Figure 11–14. The dashed line is the model-estimated log-odds values, the *x*-symbols are the data-generated log-odds values (50 categories), and the solid line is the *loess estimate* of the log-odds smoothed curve based on these 50 points (Chapter 15). Comparing the model-free log-odds curve to the model-generated log-odds curve is not fundamentally different from the previous direct comparison of data and model values (Figure 11–12) but provides a visually more intuitive plot, particularly for small data sets.

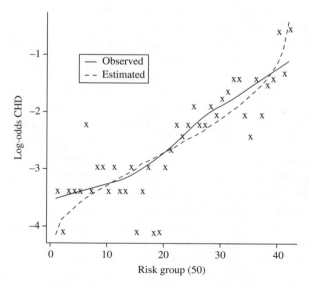

Figure 11–14. The comparison of the observed log-odds (solid line) and spline model-estimated log-odds (dashed line) for 50 categories of risk.

12

LONGITUDINAL DATA ANALYSIS

A longitudinal observation typically consists of a sequence of measurements made on a single subject over a period of time. A longitudinal data set is a collection of these subjects. For example, measures of growth might be recorded on a sample of newborn infants from birth to age 6 months, or weight losses might be measured on a sample of women participating in an experimental diet on a number of occasions, or the levels of exposure to a workplace risk factor might be measured on a sample of workers at four specified and equally spaced times. Each repeated measure adds information about each subject but these observations are almost certainly related. For example, typically, small children tend to remain small and large children tend to remain large regardless of their growth patterns, or a 150-pound woman will likely weigh close to 150 pounds regardless of the success or failure of her diet. For longitudinal data, one observation is usually a good predictor of the next. Cross-sectional variables are frequently measured and included in the data set in addition to the repeated longitudinal measurements. A cross-sectional variable is constant over time. For example, over any time period, a child's sex is the same or a women on a diet is the same height, or a worker's task is the same for all exposure measurements.

Four longitudinal measurements along with two cross-sectional values (labeled A and B) recorded for two subjects labeled "x" and "y" illustrate the structure of longitudinal data and introduce the notation where

Subject	Longitudinal				Cross-sectional	
	Time 1	Time 2	Time 3	Time 4	Variable A	Variable B
Person x	y_{x1}	y_{x2}	y_{x3}	y_{x4}	a_x	b_x
Time	t_{x1}	t_{x2}	t_{x3}	t_{x4}	–	–
Person y	y_{y1}	y_{y2}	y_{y3}	y_{y4}	a_y	b_y
Time	t_{y1}	t_{y2}	t_{y3}	t_{y4}	–	–

Another version of the same two observations is

Subject	Longitudinal		Cross-sectional	
	Measurement	Time	Variable A	Variable B
x	y_{x1}	t_{x1}	a_x	b_x
x	y_{x2}	t_{x2}	a_x	b_x
x	y_{x3}	t_{x3}	a_x	b_x
x	y_{x4}	t_{x4}	a_x	b_x
y	y_{y1}	t_{y1}	a_y	b_y
y	y_{y2}	t_{y2}	a_y	b_y
y	y_{y3}	t_{y3}	a_y	b_y
y	y_{y4}	t_{y4}	a_y	b_y

For both versions, the symbol y_{ij} represents the jth measurement ($j = 1, 2,$ 3, and 4) on the ith subject (subjects x and y) observed at the corresponding time represented by t_{ij} for two subjects with cross-sectional variables, denoted by A and B, with observed values represented by a_x and b_y (subjects x and y).

A property of longitudinal data is called *balanced*. Balanced means that all subjects are measured the same number of times. Longitudinal data are also distinguished by the kind of time interval between measurements. Time intervals are either equally spaced or not. Balanced data with equally spaced time intervals provide the simplest kind of longitudinal data from an analytic and descriptive point of view. The more complicated situations, such as unbalanced data with unevenly spaced time intervals, require more sophisticated estimation procedures. However, the analytic results have essentially the same interpretations. It should be noted that much of human longitudinal data are neither balanced nor collected at equally spaced time intervals. The nature of human data tends to lead to a variable number of measurements per subject and frequently it is difficult to assure that measurements are always made at specified time intervals. A few longitudinal analytic techniques apply only to balanced data with equally spaced time intervals (not to be discussed).

Because longitudinal data, particularly from human populations, are prone to the occurrence of missing values, it is important to distinguish between two kinds of missing values. A value can be missing at random. That is, the reason that a value is missing is unrelated to all other collected variables. For example, a biologic sample might be accidently contaminated or destroyed. Random missing values have the property of being representative of the non-missing values. Thus, accurate estimates of replacement values can be frequently derived from the data at hand. Or, the reason that a value is missing is related to either the outcome variable or other variables in the analysis. This kind of missing value occurs, for example, when individuals measured over a period of time to evaluate a new treatment become too sick to participate in the study or lack symptoms and stop the treatment. Accurate estimates for replacement values are rarely possible because the observed data are little help in estimating these non-representative missing values.

One particularly poor response to missing data is called *list-wise-deletion*. If one or more measurements are missing from an observation, then the entire observation is not considered. When a measurement is missing completely at random, excluding the observation simply reduces the sample size, incurring a loss of statistical power. However, subjects with values missing for reasons related to the outcome variable or other variables in the analysis are far more common. Excluding observations containing these kinds of missing values likely biases the analytic results (said to be nonignorable observations). For example, if older individuals are unable to participate regularly in a study of physical activity, and these older subjects are exclude from the analysis because they have missing data (list-wise-deletion), then subsequent estimates of the effect of physical activity will be influenced disproportionately by younger individuals.

One way to minimize bias incurred from missing values is to use the observed data to predict or impute replacement values. A random missing value, for example, can be replaced by the observed mean of that variable, interpolated from values in the neighborhood of the missing value, or regression analysis techniques can be used to generate a replacement value. In fact, a variety of statistical methods and computer software exist to estimate values to replace random missing values. These kinds of estimated replacement values are not always effective substitutes. However, in the case of random missing longitudinal data, where consecutive measures are generally highly correlated, simple replacement techniques are frequently useful.

Strategies that create replacement values to avoid the potential bias and loss of power incurred from deleting entire observations are often not used because of a hesitancy to "make up" data values. On the other hand, when only a few values are missing, imputed values typically have only small influences on the estimated values, bias likely becomes less of an issue, and valuable data are not lost from the analysis.

WITHIN AND BETWEEN VARIABILITY

An example of longitudinal data comes from the previously described study of elevated levels of noise exposure and the likelihood of hypertension among a cohort of Chinese textile factory workers (Chapter 5). Measurements of extreme noise ($k = 4$) were made on each of 26 specially selected workers ($n = 26$) for each of 4 months (a total of $nk = 26(4) = 104$ measurements). This sample of noise levels (measured in sound pressure level decibels, SPL) produces a 26×4 ($n \times k$) array of balanced and equally spaced longitudinal observations (Table 12–1).

The SPL exposure levels themselves are obviously important in the study of hypertension risk (Chapter 5) but additionally important issues concern the variability among these measurements. For example, interest might be focused on the variation among the $n = 26$ factory workers for each month that the measurements were recorded. Consider the SPL measurements made during the first month (Table 12–1, column 1)

Month one: $y_{11} = 83.59$, $y_{21} = 83.20$, $y_{31} = 88.58$, ... , $y_{26,1} = 86.69$.

The estimated variance from these values is $\hat{\sigma}_1^2 = 22.529$. As usual, this estimate of variability results from dividing the sum of the 26 squared deviations from their mean value $(y_{i1} - \bar{y}_1)^2$ by $n - 1 = 25$ to yield an unbiased estimate of the variance of the population sampled, represented by σ_1^2. Specifically, this estimated variance is

$$\hat{\sigma}_1^2 = \frac{1}{n-1} [\textit{sum of squared deviations}]$$
$$= \frac{1}{n-1} SS_1 = \frac{1}{n-1} \sum (y_{i1} - \bar{y}_1)^2$$
$$= \frac{1}{25} [(83.59 - 84.955)^2 + \cdots + (86.69 - 84.955)^2]$$
$$= \frac{1}{25} (563.213) = 22.529$$

where the mean value for the first month is $\bar{y}_1 = 84.955$. The four estimated variances and their 95% confidence intervals for the monthly SPL measurements are given in Table 12–2. A visual comparison (Figure 12–1) of the estimated variances from the four time periods clearly shows no evidence that the level of variability changes during the 4-month study period. The construction of a confidence interval based on an estimated value follows a general pattern

Table 12–1. Measurements of SPL levels from textile factory workers (rows $= n = 26$) made on 4 consecutive months (columns $= k = 4$)

i	Month 1 y_{i1}	Month 2 y_{i2}	Month 3 y_{i3}	Month 4 y_{i4}	Mean $\bar{y}_i$
1.	83.59	86.17	83.97	85.39	84.780
2.	83.20	83.49	84.08	80.38	82.787
3.	88.58	84.44	88.80	85.54	86.840
4.	81.34	82.61	81.75	81.58	81.820
5.	90.28	90.12	92.32	92.57	91.322
6.	85.70	85.54	86.28	89.02	86.635
7.	87.21	83.10	88.41	84.81	85.882
8.	89.37	89.50	88.20	89.49	89.140
9.	79.42	84.28	82.54	83.34	82.395
10.	82.17	79.89	84.20	82.02	82.070
11.	81.76	82.75	81.89	82.38	82.195
12.	85.68	83.12	82.17	84.96	83.983
13.	73.74	76.45	·74.87	75.76	75.205
14.	82.39	84.58	85.09	83.86	83.980
15.	95.96	94.36	94.20	94.49	94.752
16.	87.07	86.98	89.66	86.25	87.490
17.	85.73	87.49	89.49	86.99	87.425
18.	83.44	80.33	80.89	82.71	81.843
19.	86.35	87.61	88.31	87.27	87.385
20.	86.96	84.59	88.18	87.88	86.903
21.	75.19	75.54	72.81	74.65	74.547
22.	86.90	85.86	85.40	84.37	85.633
23.	80.94	78.76	79.77	80.34	79.953
24.	90.43	89.75	90.23	88.23	89.660
25.	88.75	90.24	89.39	91.48	89.965
26.	86.69	87.17	88.13	88.26	87.562
Mean $\bar{y}_j$	84.955	84.797	85.424	85.155	85.083

Table 12–2. Estimated variances and 95% confidence interval bounds from the textile worker's data ($n = 26$ and $k = 4$) for each of the four monthly measurements of SPL levels

		Estimates		95% Bounds	
	Symbol	SS_j^*	$\hat{\sigma}_j^2$	Lower	Upper
Month 1	σ_1^2	563.213	22.529	13.856	42.929
Month 2	σ_2^2	477.892	19.116	11.757	36.425
Month 3	σ_3^2	623.324	24.933	15.335	47.510
Month 4	σ_4^2	538.264	21.531	13.243	41.027

* = Sum of squares $= SS_j = \Sigma(y_{ij} - \bar{y}_j)^2$ for $i = 1, 2, \cdots, 26$ and $j = 1, 2, 3,$ and 4.

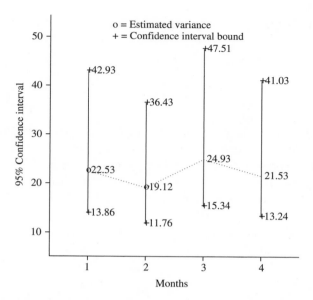

Figure 12–1. Estimated variances of the monthly SPL measurements (circles) and their 95% confidence intervals.

that appears in a number of statistical contexts. The pattern applied to an estimated variance is:

1. Each of n independent values of a variable denoted y_i is known or assumed to be randomly sampled from the same normal distribution, with mean $= \mu$ and variance $= \sigma_Y^2$.
2. The transformed value $z_i = (y_i - \mu)/\sigma_Y$ then has a normal distribution with mean $= 0$ and variance $= 1$.
3. The squared value z_i^2 has a chi-square distribution with one degree of freedom.
4. The sum of these n squared independent z_i-values ($X^2 = \sum z_i^2$) has a chi-square distribution with n degrees of freedom because sums of independent chi-square distributed values have chi-square distributions.
5. When the mean value μ is estimated from the data (denoted $\bar{y}$), the sum

$$X^2 = \sum \hat{z}_i^2 = \frac{1}{\sigma_Y^2} \sum (y_i - \bar{y})^2 = \frac{SS_Y}{\sigma_Y^2} = (n-1)\frac{\hat{\sigma}_Y^2}{\sigma_Y^2}$$

has a chi-square distribution with $n - 1$ degrees of freedom. Once again the chi-square statistic is a measurement of variability.

From the last result, the following is true,

$$P\left[Q_{0.025,n-1} \leq X^2 \leq Q_{0.975,n-1}\right] = P\left[Q_{0.025,n-1} \leq \frac{SS_Y}{\sigma_Y^2} \leq Q_{0.975,n-1}\right]$$

$$= 0.95$$

where Q represents a quantile point (or percentile point) from a chi-square distribution with $n-1$ degrees of freedom. For a 95% confidence interval, the two quantiles represented by Q are $P(X^2 \leq Q_{0.025,n-1}) = 0.025$ (2.5%) and $P(X^2 \leq Q_{0.975,n-1}) = 0.975$ (97.5%). For example, when $n-1 = 25$, these values are 13.120 and 40.646, respectively; thus, $P(13.120 \leq X^2 \leq 40.646) = P(13.120 \leq \frac{SS_Y}{\sigma_Y^2} \leq 40.646) = 0.95$.

Algebraically rearranging the previous expression does not change the probability, 0.95, and

$$P\left[\frac{SS_Y}{Q_{0.975,n-1}} \leq \sigma_Y^2 \leq \frac{SS_Y}{Q_{0.025,n-1}}\right] = P\left[\frac{(n-1)\hat{\sigma}_Y^2}{Q_{0.975,n-1}} \leq \sigma_Y^2 \leq \frac{(n-1)\hat{\sigma}_Y^2}{Q_{0.025,n-1}}\right]$$

$$= 0.95$$

becomes the 95% confidence interval for the variance σ_Y^2, based on its estimate $\hat{\sigma}_Y^2$. Specifically, the confidence interval bounds are

$$A = lower\ bound = \frac{SS_Y}{Q_{0.975,n-1}} \quad \text{and} \quad B = upper\ bound = \frac{SS_Y}{Q_{0.025,n-1}}.$$

For example, the variance estimate $\hat{\sigma}_1^2 = 22.529$ (Table 12–2) produces the 95% confidence interval bounds $A = 563.213/40.646 = 13.856$ and $B = 563.213/13.120 = 42.929$, where again, $Q_{0.025,25} = 13.120$ and $Q_{0.975,25} = 40.646$ are the 2.5th and 97.5th percentiles from a chi-square distribution with 25 degrees of freedom. As with all confidence intervals, the interval describes a range of likely values of the parameter σ^2, based on its estimate $\hat{\sigma}^2$, giving both a sense of the value of the underlying variance and the precision of the estimated value.

The analysis of longitudinal data is in many ways a study of variability. Variability of a longitudinal measured y_{ij} can be viewed as consisting of two components, namely $(y_{ij} - \bar{y}_i)$ and $(\bar{y}_i - \bar{y})$ and $y_{ij} - \bar{y} = (y_{ij} - \bar{y}_i) + (\bar{y}_i - \bar{y})$. In other words, the deviation of a measurement from its overall mean value is the sum of the deviation of the measurement from the i th -subject's mean value plus the deviation of the i th -subject's mean value from the overall mean value. The deviations $y_{ij} - \bar{y}_i$ reflect the variation of the observed values among the k measured values made on each subject, called *within subject variation*. The deviations $\bar{y}_i - \bar{y}$

reflect the variation of the mean values among the n subjects, called *between subject variation*. For example, for the first subject (first row of Table 12–1),

$$y_{ij} - \bar{y} = 83.590 - 85.083$$
$$= within\ subject\ deviation + between\ subject\ deviation$$
$$= (83.590 - 84.780) + (84.780 - 85.083)$$
$$= -1.190 - 0.303 = -1.494.$$

For this first worker, the within deviation measured relative to the worker's own mean value is about four times as large as the between deviation measured relative to the mean value of all 26 workers.

These deviations, summarized over an entire data set, yield the following sums of squared values:

$$SS_{total} = \sum\sum(y_{ij} - \bar{y})^2, SS_{within} = \sum\sum(y_{ij} - \bar{y}_i)^2\ and\ SS_{between} = k\sum(\bar{y}_i - \bar{y})^2$$

where again $i = 1, 2, \cdots, n$ and $j = 1, 2, \cdots, k$. Thus, for the textile worker's data, these sums of squares summarize the total variation ($SS_{total} = 2208.4$), the within subject variation ($SS_{within} = 149.9$), and the between subject variation ($SS_{between} = 2058.5$) among $n \times k = 26 \times 4 = 104$ longitudinal measurements and, furthermore, $SS_{total} = SS_{within} + SS_{between}$ or $2208.405 = 149.923 + 2058.482$. This partition of the total sum of squares into a within sum of squares and a between sum of squares is a fundamental property of data generated from a series of subjects each measured on multiple occasions. In addition, these sums of squares lead to estimates of the variation within subjects (denoted σ^2_{within}) and the variation between subjects (denoted $\sigma^2_{between}$). These two estimated variances play key roles in the analysis of longitudinal data.

Specifically, the total sum of squares estimates the quantity $(nk - 1)\sigma^2_{total}$, the within sum of squares estimates $n(k - 1)\sigma^2_{within}$, and the between sum of squares estimates $(n - 1)(k\sigma^2_{between} + \sigma^2_{within})$ [41]. The within and between variances are estimated from their sums of squares, and their associated degrees of freedom are $n(k - 1)$ and $n - 1$ (Table 12–3). Note that, as with the partitioned sum of squares, the total degrees of freedom also partition into the sum of two corresponding pieces where $nk - 1 = n(k - 1) + n - 1$.

A natural estimate of the within-person variation is

$$\hat{\sigma}^2_{within} = \frac{1}{n(k - 1)}SS_{within}$$

and the estimated between-person variation becomes

$$\hat{\sigma}^2_{between} = \frac{1}{k}\left[\frac{SS_{between}}{n - 1} - \hat{\sigma}^2_{within}\right].$$

Table 12–3. Components of the total variation calculated from the SPL textile worker's data in Table 12–1 (n = number of workers = 26 and k = number of measurements = 4)

Variability	Total $\hat{\sigma}^2_{total}$	Within $\hat{\sigma}^2_{within}$	Between $k\hat{\sigma}^2_{between} + \hat{\sigma}^2_{within}$
Sum of squares (SS)	2208.405	149.923	2058.482
Degrees of freedom (df)	$nk - 1 = 103$	$n(k-1) = 78$	$n - 1 = 25$
SS/df	21.441	1.922	82.339

From the SPL data (Tables 12–1 and 12–3), the within- and between-person variance estimates are

$$\hat{\sigma}^2_{within} = \frac{1}{78}(149.923) = 1.922 \quad \text{and} \quad \hat{\sigma}^2_{between} = \frac{1}{4}\left[\frac{2058.482}{25} - 1.922\right] = 20.104.$$

For the within-subject variance, the 95% confidence interval bounds are

$$A = lower\ bound = \frac{SS_{within}}{Q_{0.975,78}} = \frac{149.923}{104.316} = 1.437$$

and

$$B = upper\ bound = \frac{SS_{within}}{Q_{0.025,78}} = \frac{149.932}{55.466} = 2.703.$$

The approximate 95% confidence interval bounds for the between-subject variance are

$$A = lower\ bound = \frac{1}{k}\left[\frac{SS_{between}}{Q_{0.975,25}} - \hat{\sigma}^2_{within}\right]$$

$$= \frac{1}{4}\left[\frac{2058.482}{40.646} - 1.922\right] = 12.180$$

and

$$B = upper\ bound = \frac{1}{k}\left[\frac{SS_{between}}{Q_{0.025,25}} - \hat{\sigma}^2_{within}\right]$$

$$= \frac{1}{4}\left[\frac{2058.482}{13.120} - 1.922\right] = 38.744.$$

To summarize, the 95% confidence interval for the within-subject variance σ^2_{within} is (1.437, 2.703) based on its estimate $\hat{\sigma}^2_{within} = 1.922$, and the approximate 95% confidence interval for the between-subject variance $\sigma^2_{between}$ is (12.180, 38.744) based on its estimate $\hat{\sigma}^2_{between} = 20.104$.

A SIMPLE EXAMPLE

As emphasized, a defining characteristic of a longitudinal data analysis is the clear separation of the variation within the study subjects from the variation between study subjects. A simple example illustrates this property in the context of a regression analysis using nine fictional observations. The data consist of three measurements (y) made on separate occasions (t) on each of three subjects, a total of nine pairs of values. These data are:

	Subject 1			Subject 2			Subject 3		
Times (t)	1	2	3	1	2	3	1	2	3
Measurements (y)	4.7	5.4	8.8	5.4	10.5	10.9	8.3	11.7	11.7

First, ignoring the fact that same subject is measured three times, the nine values and standard linear regression estimates produce a summary line with an estimated intercept of $\hat{a} = 4.267$ and slope of $\hat{b} = 2.167$ (first two rows in Table 12–4), characterizing the change in y over time t. A plot of the estimated line $\hat{y} = 4.267 + 2.167t$ and the data are displayed in Figure 12–2 (left). The "unexplained" variability in the measurements y is estimated as $S^2_{Y|t} = 35.773/7 = 5.110$. A test of linear trend based on the conjecture that $b = 0$ yields the test statistic $z = 2.167/0.923 = 2.348$, producing a p-value of 0.051.

Taking into account the between-subject variation produces the identical estimated summary line (solid line in both plots) but the "unexplained" variability is substantially reduced. Three subject-specific regression analyses each produce estimated intercepts and slopes (Table 12–4 and Figure 12–2, right) and are not influenced by the variation among the three measured subjects. The considerably

Table 12–4. Estimates from the example of two regression analyses based on nine hypothetical observations (three subjects measured on three occasions)

Combined	$\hat{a}$	$\hat{b}$	$\sum(y_{ij} - \hat{y}_{ij})^2$
Subjects ignored	4.267	2.167	35.773
Std. error	1.994	0.993	
Separate	$\hat{a}_i$	$\hat{b}_i$	$\sum(y_{ij} - \hat{y}_{ij})^2$
Subject 1	2.200	2.050	1.215
Subject 2	3.433	2.750	3.682
Subject 3	7.167	1.700	1.927
Mean model	4.267	2.167	6.823
Std. error	–	0.616	

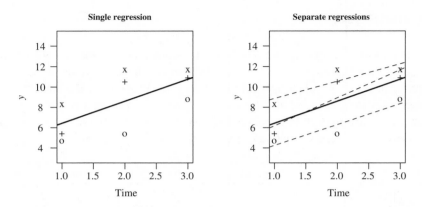

Figure 12–2. Regression lines estimated from nine hypothetical observations (three subjects measured on three occasions).

closer correspondence of the three estimated lines to the observations is apparent from the plot (dashed lines). Formally, the sum of the squared deviations of the observed values from the estimated values is 6.823, as compared to the first analysis, in which the value of the same summary statistic is 35.773 (Table 12–4). The "unexplained" variability in the measurements y is now estimated as $S^2_{Y|t} = 6.823/3 = 2.274$. Accounting for the differences among individuals clearly increases the accuracy of the model values to predict the observed values. As a result, the estimated variance of the slope is reduced and the test of the linear trend ($b = 0$) becomes far more powerful, yielding the test statistic $z = 2.167/0.616 = 3.518$ and a p-value less than 0.001. The estimated mean line (mean of the intercepts and slopes from the three separate regression analyses) is identical to the line estimated from the analysis that completely ignores the variation among the subjects (solid lines, Figure 12–2). Similar to many statistical techniques, the second analysis consists of three strata-specific estimates combined to estimate a common summary (a regression line), while eliminating influences from extraneous variation between subjects.

Two elements of this example that analogously occur in longitudinal analyses involving far more complex data and statistical issues are:

1. Models including and excluding the influence of subject-to-subject variability produce similar summary mean estimates and
2. Eliminating for the subject-to-subject variation improves the accuracy of the model by reducing the variance of the estimated model parameters, increasing statistical power.

More complex data clearly require more sophisticated models and estimation techniques, but the two properties illustrated by this example remain a fundamental part of longitudinal data analysis.

ELEMENTARY LONGITUDINAL MODELS: POLYNOMIAL MODELS

A traditional approach to identify and analyze patterns associated with longitudinal data employs conventional polynomial models. This approach was among the first used to analyze longitudinal data. To illustrate, a sequence of four elementary polynomial regression models are considered, namely

1. $y_{ij} = b_0 + b_1 t_{ij} + b_2 F_i,$
2. $y_{ij} = b_0 + b_1 t_{ij} + b_2 t_{ij}^2,$
3. $y_{ij} = b_0 + b_1 t_{ij} + b_2 t_{ij}^2 + b_3 F_i,$ and
4. $y_{ij} = b_0 + b_1 t_{ij} + b_2 t_{ij}^2 + b_3 F_i + b_4(t_{ij} \times F_i) + b_5(t_{ij}^2 \times F_i).$

The symbol F represents a binary cross-sectional variable that indicates members of two groups of longitudinal observations ($F = 0$ for one group and $F = 1$ for the other). As before, the value t_{ij} represents the time that the j th measurement was made on the i th individual, denoted again as y_{ij}. Figure 12–3 displays examples of these four models (two straight lines, a single quadratic curve, two additive quadratic curves [constant distanced apart], and two nonadditive quadratic curves). Of course, many other ways exist to represent the pattern of observations y_{ij} over times t_{ij}.

Highly unbalanced data with unevenly spaced time intervals present special problems for the estimation but not the interpretation of the model parameters. Computer software to estimate model parameters from longitudinal data is available from most statistical analysis systems, to name the most popular, SAS, Stata, SPLUS, SPSS, and R. In addition, it is a simple matter to include cross-sectional variables in such longitudinal models to explore their additional influences on the pattern of response (examples follow).

Occasionally, the time variable is defined so that a value centered at zero has a useful interpretation, sometimes called *centering a variable*. The time variable for the example polynomial models is centered (Figure 12–3). For some longitudinal data sets, centering a variable also reduces the correlation between the time measure and the response variable, thus increasing the precision of the estimated model parameters.

Data from a study of weight gained during pregnancy illustrate the application of a polynomial model approach to describing longitudinal data. Women routinely

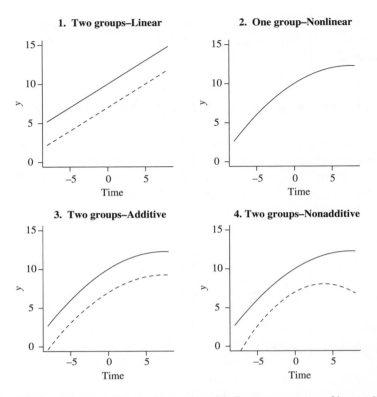

Figure 12–3. Examples of four polynomial models illustrating patterns of longitudinal measurements over time.

weighed during prenatal visits produce longitudinal weight and time measurements over their pregnancy. These $n = 110$ mothers, measured more than 15 times at different intervals during their first pregnancy, are separated into two groups by their pre-pregnancy body mass index ($F = 0$ for $< 29 =$ normal and $F = 1$ for $\geq 29 =$ obese).

A good place to start is a linear representation summarizing the pattern of weight gained (model 1) where, in symbols, the longitudinal model is

$$y_{ij} = b_0 + b_1 t_{ij} + b_2 F_i .$$

Applying this simple and linear longitudinal model to the weight-gained data produces the parameter estimates (Table 12–5) and provides a comparison of weight gained between normal weight and obese women. A time variable of zero ($t_{ij} = 0$) indicates the start of pregnancy.

Table 12–5. Parameter estimates for an additive and linear model describing weight gained during pregnancy by $n = 110$ pregnant mothers separated into two body mass index groups (BMI ≤ 29 = normal and BMI ≥ 29 = obese)

Variables	Symbols	Estimates	Std. errors	p-Values
Intercept	b_0	64.061	1.109	–
Time (t)	b_1	0.069	0.002	<0.001
BMI	b_2	20.534	0.783	<0.001

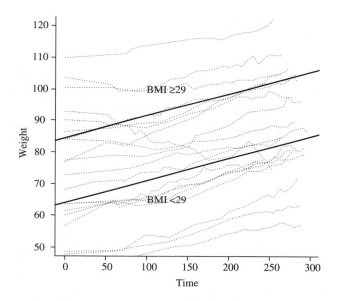

Figure 12–4. Pattern of weight gained during pregnancy for a sample of 20 representative mothers (dotted lines) and the estimated mean model for two BMI groups based on the entire sample of $n = 110$ mothers (a total of 1870 weight measurements), additive linear longitudinal model.

The estimated mean lines (summary) for the two BMI groups are shown in Figure 12–4. The complete data on 20 representative mothers are also included (dotted lines). The estimated "distance" between these two groups is $\hat{b}_2 = 20.534$. Thus, based on the additive linear model, the estimated difference in weight gained between the two BMI groups is 20.534 kilograms, regardless of the duration of pregnancy.

An additive longitudinal model dictates a linear pattern of weight gained that is identical for both BMI groups. To assess this requirement of a constant

Table 12–6. Parameter estimates for the nonadditive and linear model describing weight gained during pregnancy by $n = 110$ mothers

Variables	Symbols	Estimates	Std. errors	p-Values
Intercept	b_0	63.075	1.133	–
Time (t)	b_1	0.074	0.002	–
BMI	b_2	24.229	1.202	–
BMI × time	b_3	−0.020	0.005	<0.001

difference between BMI groups, the corresponding nonadditive but linear model (model 2)

$$y_{ij} = b_0 + b_1 t_{ij} + b_2 F_i + b_3 (t_{ij} \times F_i)$$

is proposed, where the model coefficient b_3 reflects the extent of nonadditivity (Table 12–6). The estimated coefficient $\hat{b}_3$ provides strong evidence that a linear pattern of increasing weight within the two BMI groups do not have the same slopes. Formally, the test of the estimated "interaction" coefficient $\hat{b}_3$ is

$$X^2 = \left[\frac{\hat{b}_3 - 0}{S_{\hat{b}_3}}\right]^2 = \left[\frac{-0.020 - 0}{0.0049}\right]^2 = 16.349$$

and the chi-square distributed test-statistic X^2 has an associated significance probability of less than 0.001 (p-value < 0.001). For longitudinal data analyses, the likelihood ratio test potentially gives unreliable results. The nonadditive model is displayed in Figure 12–5, where the estimated slope of the line summarizing weight gained pattern in the low BMI group is greater than the slope estimated for the high BMI group ($\hat{b}_{low} = \hat{b}_1 = 0.074$ and $\hat{b}_{high} = \hat{b}_1 + \hat{b}_2 = 0.074 - 0.020 = 0.054$).

Both the natural course of pregnancy and the plotted data (Figures 12–4 and 12–5) suggest a nonlinear relationship between gestation (days) and maternal weight gained (kilograms). An additive longitudinal model with a quadratic term included to account for an accelerating rate of weight gained during the later part of pregnancy (model 3) is

$$y_{ij} = b_0 + b_1 t_{ij} + b_2 t_{ij}^2 + b_3 F_i$$

where, as before, F is a cross-sectional binary variable, where $F = 0$ for a BMI <29 and $F = 1$ for a BMI ≥29. The estimated parameters are given in Table 12–7.

Little doubt exists that a nonlinear (quadratic) curve improves the representation of the weight gained over time. Formally, the chi-square assessment of the

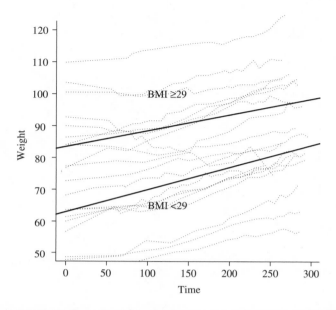

Figure 12–5. Pattern of weight gained during pregnancy for a sample of 20 representative mothers (dotted lines) and the estimated mean model for two BMI groups based on the entire sample of $n = 110$ mothers, nonadditive linear longitudinal model.

Table 12–7. Parameter estimates for an additive and nonlinear longitudinal model (t and t^2) describing weight gained during pregnancy by $n = 110$ mothers

Variables	Symbols	Estimates	Std. errors	p-Values
Intercept	b_0	67.580	1.186	–
Time (t)	b_1	0.003	0.008	–
Time (t^2)	b_2	0.00021	0.00003	<0.001
BMI	b_3	20.401	0.769	<0.001

estimated coefficient $\hat{b}_2$

$$X^2 = \left[\frac{\hat{b}_2 - 0}{S_{\hat{b}_2}}\right]^2 = \left[\frac{0.00021 - 0}{0.000025}\right]^2 = 70.680,$$

yields a p-value < 0.001 (degrees of freedom $= 1$) indicating that the observed nonlinearity of the weight-gained curve is almost certainly not a result of random variation. The estimated mean model displays two curves (Figure 12–6). As always, additivity guarantees that the difference between the two groups ($\hat{b}_3 = 20.401$ kilograms) is identical at any time t.

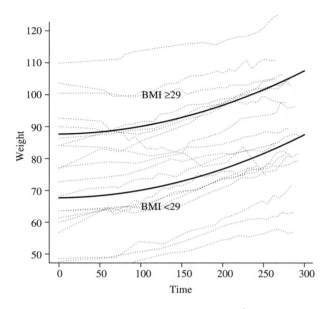

Figure 12–6. Additive quadratic regression model (t and t^2) describing weight gained during pregnancy by $n = 110$ mothers.

An estimate such as the difference of 20.401 kilograms usefully summarizes the difference between BMI groups with a single value only when the time–gain relationship is the same in both groups (no interaction). Therefore, the estimation should be supported by a comparison of additive and nonadditive (interaction) models.

A relevant nonadditive model (model 4) is

$$y_{ij} = b_0 + b_1 t_{ij} + b_2 t_{ij}^2 + b_3 F_i + b_4(F_i \times t_{ij}) + b_5(F_i \times t_{ij}^2).$$

The estimates for the six model parameters are presented in Table 12–8. (displayed in Figure 12–7). The primary focus is on the two interaction terms ($\hat{b}_4$ and $\hat{b}_5$), where the chi-square statistics are 15.503 and 9.458, each with one degree of freedom. These extremely large chi-square values with both p-values less than 0.003 indicate that it is unlikely that weight-gained patterns within the BMI groups are usefully described by an additive quadratic model. Therefore, a quadratic pattern of weight gain likely differs between the two BMI groups.

Table 12–8. Parameter estimates for a nonadditive longitudinal model describing weight gained during pregnancy ($n = 110$ mothers)

Variables	Symbols	Estimates	Std. errors	p-Values
Intercept	b_0	65.994	1.230	–
Time (t)	b_1	0.023	0.009	–
Time (t^2)	b_2	0.00016	0.00003	–
BMI	b_3	26.352	1.435	–
BMI × time	b_4	−0.074	0.019	<0.001
BMI × time^2	b_5	0.0002	0.000060	0.002

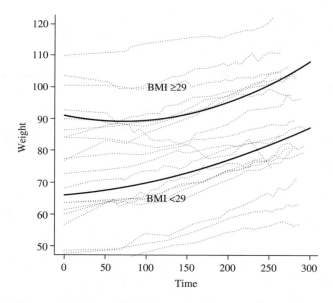

Figure 12–7. Nonadditive quadratic regression model describing weight gained during pregnancy by $n = 110$ mothers.

ELEMENTARY LONGITUDINAL MODELS: SPLINE MODELS

Similar to polynomial models, spline representations of the pattern of measurements over time also produce valuable descriptions of longitudinal data. Four basic longitudinal models based on piecewise linear spline representations of the time–outcome relationship are:

1. $y_{ij} = b_0 + b_1 t_{ij} + b_2 F_i$
2. $y_{ij} = b_0 + b_1 t_{ij} + b_2 (t_{ij} - K)_+$
3. $y_{ij} = b_0 + b_1 t_{ij} + b_2 (t_{ij} - K)_+ + b_3 F_i$
4. $y_{ij} = b_0 + b_1 t_{ij} + b_2 (t_{ij} - K)_+ + b_3 F_i + b_4 t_{ij} \times F_i + b_5 (t_{ij} - K)_+ \times F_i$

The symbol F represents again a cross-sectional binary variable identifying members of two groups ($F = 0$ for one group and $F = 1$ for the other). For these piecewise linear spline models, a single knot is represented by K. Furthermore, the models, as illustrated in Figure 12–8, can indicate a "before/after" kind of structure (centered by the knot). The application of a spline representation of a variable measured over time in a longitudinal model is fundamentally the same as the applications described for the polynomial models.

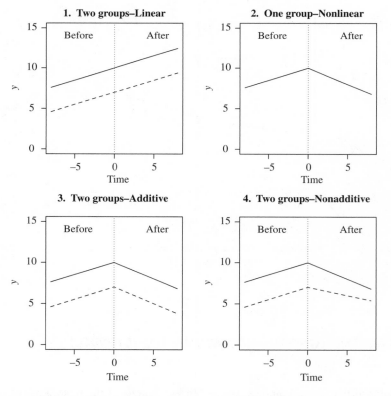

Figure 12–8. Examples of four piecewise linear spline models displaying possible before/after patterns of a longitudinal variable (y_{ij}) over time (t_{ij}) with single knot $K = 0$.

Table 12–9. Estimated parameters for the piecewise linear spline (knot $= K = 30$ days) applied to the weight loss data from $n = 344$ mothers of newborn infants measured longitudinally for one year postpartum

Variables	Symbols	Estimates	Std. errors	p-Values
Intercept	b_0	83.937	0.822	–
t_{ij}	b_1	−0.423	0.009	<0.001
$(t_{ij} - 30)_+$	b_2	0.417	0.010	<0.001

Data on weight retention after pregnancy among four race/ethnicity groups illustrate the application of piecewise linear spline variables. Applying the longitudinal/spline model

$$y_{ij} = b_0 + b_1 t_{ij} + b_2(t_{ij} - 30)_+$$

to $n = 344$ mothers of newborns infants, measured on average 7.1 times at different time intervals after delivery, yields a simple description of the pattern of weight loss (in kilograms) during their first postpartum year (model 2). The natural value (knot) of $K = 30$ days postpartum is chosen for this piecewise linear spline (Chapter 10). The estimated model parameters b_0, b_1, and b_2 are given in Table 12–9, and the model-estimated pattern of weight retention is displayed in Figure 12–9 (solid line = estimated mean pattern of weight loss).

Again using a piecewise linear spline and an additive model, the pattern of postpartum weigh lost is effectively compared among four race/ethnicity groups (white, Hispanic, African-American, and Asian). An extension of the piecewise linear spline regression model is

$$y_{ij} = b_0 + b_1 t_{ij} + b_2(t_{ij} - 30)_+ + c_1 z_{i1} + c_2 z_{i2} + c_3 z_{i3}$$

where the added z-variables are components of a design variable (a nominal and cross-sectional variable) that allows influences from the differences among four race/ethnicity groups to be incorporated into the model.

The parameter estimates (Table 12–10) produce the plot based on the estimated mean model that displays a separate (additive) weight loss pattern for each of the four race/ethnicity groups (Figure 12–10).

The additive model, as always, produces parallel lines and, in this case, the parallel lines are linear piecewise splines. As required, the model-estimated differences in retained weight among the four race/ethnicity groups are the same regardless of the time chosen for comparison (adjusted). The differences at all times are then estimated by the coefficients $\hat{c}_1$, $\hat{c}_2$, and $\hat{c}_3$ for three race/ethnicity groups relative to the white mothers. Consider the postpartum t_{ij} time of 150 days,

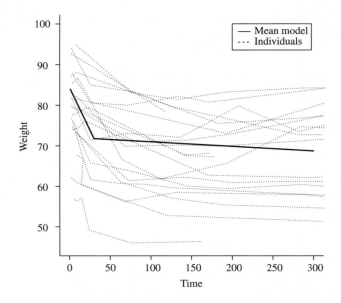

Figure 12–9. Weight retention patterns: 20 representative mothers (dotted lines) and the estimated mean piecewise linear spline model (solid line) with a single knot $= K = 30$ days based on $n = 334$ women.

Table 12–10. Estimated parameters for the piecewise additive and linear spline model (knot $= K = 30$ days) applied to the weight loss of mothers measured sequentially for 1 year postpartum by race/ethnicity ($n = 344$)

Variables	Symbols	Estimates	Std. errors	p-Values
Intercept	b_0	85.150	0.993	–
t_{ij}	b_1	–0.423	0.009	< 0.001
$(t_{ij} - 30)_+$	b_2	0.417	0.010	< 0.001
Hispanic	c_1	2.679	2.484	0.281
African-American	c_2	–12.129	2.598	< 0.001
Asian	c_3	–1.748	2.263	0.440

then for white mothers ($z_{i1} = z_{i2} = z_{i3} = 0$), the model-estimated maternal mean weight (white) is $85.150 - 0.423(150) + 0.417(150) = 71.400$ then, estimated maternal mean weight (Hispanic) $= 71.400 + 2.679 = 74.079$, estimated maternal mean weight (African-American) $= 71.400 - 12.129 = 59.271$, and estimated maternal mean weight (Asian) $= 71.400 - 1.748 = 69.652$.

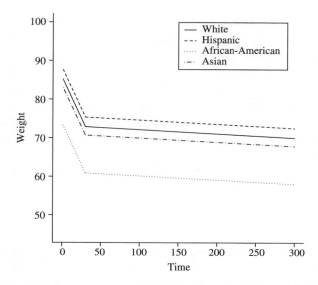

Figure 12–10.   Weight retention patterns: the weight loss of mothers described by a piecewise additive and linear spline model with knot $= K = 30$ days for four race/ethnicity groups ($n = 330$).

RANDOM INTERCEPT MODEL

Not surprisingly, the way data are collected dictates the appropriate statistical model and influences the method of analysis. For example, a study of children's growth could begin by collecting a sample of 6-year-olds, a sample of 8-year-olds, and a sample of 10-year-olds. Recording their weight gained over time then creates a longitudinal data set. Another approach is to randomly sample children between the ages 6 and 10 years old and record their weight gained over time. These data also create a longitudinal data set in which each child begins the study at a random age between 6 and 10 years. The distribution of their ages is representative of the population sampled. The following describes a statistical model designed for the analysis of this kind of longitudinal data called a *random intercept model*.

Many statistical models require that the data consist of observations that are unrelated (statistical independence). As noted, this requirement is almost never realistic when the data are collected in a longitudinal manner because repeated measurements made on the same subject are almost certainly related (correlated). A random intercept model fully utilizes longitudinal data and accounts for this correlation.

In the context of longitudinal data analysis, the word "mixed" has a technical meaning. A mixed model contains two kinds of components, fixed and random.

Parametric model components postulate a fixed statistical structure that can range from simple to complex. These mathematically defined relationships, used in many analytic contexts, are also commonly applied to longitudinal data and are called *fixed effects*. A defining feature of longitudinal data analysis is the opportunity to enrich the description of these fixed relationships by estimating and accounting for influences of sampling variation, called *random effects*.

Frequently, an analysis of longitudinal data using a random intercept model starts with a linear regression mixed model applied to a series of observations y_{ij} measured at times t_{ij} (again the ith subject measured on the jth occasion). Three versions of this model reveal the roles of the fixed and random components. A simple random intercept linear regression model represented by

$$y_{ij} = a + bt_{ij} + E_{ij}$$

has the same form as the typical single-variable fixed effects model, in that the intercept and slope parameters a and b are fixed values (Chapter 2). The difference lies in the structure of the random error term, denoted E_{ij}. A second version of the same model is

$$y_{ij} = a + bt_{ij} + \tau_i + e_{ij}, \quad \text{where the error term} = E_{ij} = \tau_i + e_{ij}.$$

This version of a regression model explicitly divides the influences of sampling variation into two sources; one associated with each individual sampled (the ith-subject,) denoted τ_i) and one associated with measurements made on the same individual (within the ith subject on the jth occasion, denoted e_{ij}). The variability within all individuals sampled is formally assumed to be the same. More technically, the distribution of the error term e_{ij} is assumed to have a mean value of zero and a variance denoted as $variance(e_{ij}) = \sigma_w^2$ for all individuals sampled. A third version of this model is

$$y_{ij} = a_i + bt_{ij} + e_{ij}, \quad \text{where the intercept} = a_i = a + \tau_i$$

and clearly shows the reason for the name "random intercept model." In this context, the intercept represents a randomly sampled value from a distribution with a mean value represented by a and a variance represented by $variance(a_i) = \sigma_b^2$. The intercept term a_i (or τ_i) allows the model to account for variation caused by the differences among the study subjects. For example, the differences associated with age among the children sampled to study growth. Furthermore, the measurements within each individual are assumed to be unrelated to each other and unrelated to the intercept values a_i. Technically, the model requires

$$covariance(e_{ij}, e_{ik}) = 0 \quad \text{and} \quad covariance(e_{ij}, a_i) = 0.$$

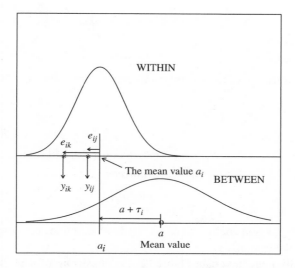

Figure 12–11. A schematic view of the data structure generating a random intercept model.

Thus, the correlation between measurements on the same individual occurs only because these measurements are random deviations from the same value, namely a_i. The model coefficient b represents a nonrandom part of the description of the outcome y_{ij} (a linear fixed effect). That is, the regression coefficient b represents a single constant underlying parameter value.

Figure 12–11 is a schematic representation of a random intercept model. The distribution of the sampled population (labeled BETWEEN) is depicted as a normal distribution (a frequent assumption) that produces a randomly sampled subject with intercept value represented by the value a_i $(a + \tau_i)$. Two measurements on the ith subject yield the within-subject measures $a_i + e_{ij}$ and $a_i + e_{ik}$, depicted again as sampled from a normal distribution (labeled WITHIN). Thus, the jth and k^{th} observations for the ith person sampled, denoted y_{ij} and y_{ik}, conform to a random intercept model. The random elements, a_i and e_{ij}, respectively, account for the sources of the between- and within-variation associated with the jth measurement on the ith individual. The diagram shows a sample of two measurements on a single subject. In fact, longitudinal data typically consists of n subjects each measured k times sequentially over a period of time.

Two technical consequences of a random intercept model are:

1. The variance of an observation is

$$variance(y_{ij}) = variance(a_i + bt_{ij} + e_{ij})$$
$$= variance(a_i + e_{ij})$$

$$= variance(a_i) + variance(e_{ij})$$
$$= \sigma_b^2 + \sigma_w^2.$$

2. The covariance of two observations on the same subject at different times is

$$
\begin{aligned}
covariance(y_{ij}, \ y_{ik}) &= covariance(a_i + bt_{ij} + e_{ij}, \ a_i + bt_{ik} + e_{ik}) \\
&= covariance(a_i + e_{ij}, \ a_i + e_{ik}) \\
&= covariance(a_i, \ a_i) + covariance(e_{ij}, \ e_{ik}) \\
&= variance(a_i) = \sigma_b^2.
\end{aligned}
$$

Because the regression coefficient b is a fixed value, it does not contribute to the variability of the response y_{ij}.

Artificially generated data (Table 12–11) consisting of $n = 20$ individuals each measured $k = 5$ times introduce the properties of a random intercept model. The intercept values a_i are a random sample of 20 observations from a normal distribution with mean value $= a = 8$ and variance of $variance(a_i) = \sigma_b^2 = 9$. In addition, each of these 20 individuals is measured five times, where the within-subject variation is $variance(e_{ij}) = \sigma_w^2 = 25$ associated with all $nk = 20(5) = 100$ measurements. The regression coefficient is the fixed value $b = 4.0$. The random intercept regression model then becomes

$$y_{ij} = 8 + 4t_{ij} + \tau_i + e_{ij} = a_i + 4t_{ij} + e_{ij}.$$

The estimated $k \times k$ variance/covariance array associated with a random intercept model (see section at the end of the chapter for a description of the mechanics of a variance/covariance array) is represented by

$$
V = \left\{
\begin{array}{ccccc}
v_b^2 + v_w^2 & v_b^2 & v_b^2 & -- & v_b^2 \\
v_b^2 & v_b^2 + v_w^2 & v_b^2 & -- & v_b^2 \\
v_b^2 & v_b^2 & v_b^2 + v_w^2 & -- & v_b^2 \\
-- & -- & -- & -- & -- \\
-- & -- & -- & -- & -- \\
v_b^2 & v_b^2 & v_b^2 & -- & v_b^2 + v_w^2
\end{array}
\right\}
$$

and is estimated from the data (Table 12–11) by the 5×5 symmetric variance/covariance array based on the sample of five measurements made on each of the 20 subjects. The symbol $v_b^2 + v_w^2$ represents the estimated variance of

Table 12–11. Artificial data generated from a random intercept model
($n = 20$ and $k = 5$), where $\sigma_b^2 = 9$ and $\sigma_w^2 = 25$

	Time 1	Time 2	Time 3	Time 4	Time 5
1.	19.1	23.0	20.2	35.0	24.3
2.	0.2	17.0	17.0	21.4	33.6
3.	11.1	22.5	22.1	26.6	30.1
4.	11.9	17.1	18.4	20.9	30.6
5.	12.6	18.0	16.7	29.1	38.6
6.	11.8	9.6	22.3	20.4	27.9
7.	10.3	14.0	10.6	13.2	22.3
8.	21.0	21.6	29.9	29.3	26.5
9.	6.5	22.4	24.2	28.0	28.6
10.	11.6	12.4	22.7	17.1	9.5
11.	14.4	17.9	16.2	13.5	34.2
12.	8.4	10.8	18.4	19.2	25.8
13.	12.4	6.9	10.7	22.0	17.6
14.	12.2	19.5	24.4	17.0	34.3
15.	8.7	17.5	21.0	30.8	28.3
16.	8.6	13.6	9.5	16.2	23.7
17.	3.9	10.7	15.7	18.3	22.9
18.	8.9	19.0	17.2	39.9	25.2
19.	12.1	13.4	15.8	19.6	27.2
20.	10.8	7.2	13.6	22.5	22.4

y_{ij} $(\sigma_b^2 + \sigma_w^2)$, and the symbol v_b^2 represents the estimated variance between subjects (σ_b^2). Specifically, the estimated variance/covariance array is

$$
V = variance(Y) = \left\{
\begin{array}{rrrrr}
20.82 & 6.05 & 7.96 & 6.63 & -1.15 \\
6.05 & 25.31 & 14.74 & 18.27 & 16.02 \\
7.96 & 14.74 & 26.67 & 12.96 & 5.98 \\
6.63 & 18.27 & 12.96 & 51.54 & 5.69 \\
-1.15 & 16.02 & 5.98 & 5.69 & 41.40
\end{array}
\right\}
$$

The array V contains five variances and ten different covariances estimated in the usual way from the data (Table 12–11). The random intercept model requires that the five variances ($\sigma_b^2 + \sigma_w^2 = 34$) be equal and the ten covariances ($\sigma_b^2 = 9$) be equal. Therefore, the differences among the variances (diagonal values) and covariances (nondiagonal values) observed in the estimated 5×5 variance/covariance array V are due to sampling variation.

Estimates of the within- and between-variances can be calculated directly from the estimated variance/covariance array V for a balanced longitudinal data set, such as the observations in Table 12–11. The main diagonal of the array contains estimates of the variance of the observations y_{ij} (denoted v_{ii}). Thus, each of the five observed values v_{ii} estimate the same quantity, namely $\sigma_b^2 + \sigma_w^2$. Similarly, each of the ten nondiagonal values (denoted v_{ij}) estimates the common between variance, namely σ_b^2.

For the fictional data, the estimated variance/covariance array V simply yields estimates of the between- and within-subject variation (denoted $\hat{\sigma}_b^2$ and $\hat{\sigma}_w^2$). Two mean values from the array V yields estimates of the constant variance and covariance and are

$$\bar{v}_{ii} = \frac{1}{k} \sum v_{ii} = \frac{20.82 + 25.31 + \cdots + 41.40}{5} = \frac{165.352}{5} = 33.070$$

where $i = 1, 2, \cdots, k = 5$ and

$$\bar{v}_{ij} = \frac{1}{k(k-1)/2} \sum v_{ij} = \frac{6.05 + 7.96 + \cdots + 5.69}{10} = \frac{92.785}{10} = 9.278$$

where $i > j = 1, 2, \cdots, k(k-1)/2 = 10$. Intuitive estimates of the underlying variability between subjects and within subjects then become

$$\hat{\sigma}_b^2 = \bar{v}_{ij} = 9.278$$

and

$$\hat{\sigma}_w^2 = \bar{v}_{ii} - \bar{v}_{ij} = 33.070 - 9.278 = 23.792.$$

A summary quantity called the *intraclass correlation coefficient* (denoted ρ) estimated from these two variance estimates is

$$\hat{\rho} = \frac{\hat{\sigma}_b^2}{\hat{\sigma}_b^2 + \hat{\sigma}_w^2} = \frac{9.278}{9.278 + 23.792} = 0.281.$$

As the name suggests, the intraclass correlation coefficient reflects the relative degree of "closeness" of the n patterns consisting of k measures made on each subject. More specifically, when the within-subject variation is zero ($\sigma_w^2 = 0$), the estimated intraclass correlation will be in the neighborhood of 1 ($\hat{\rho} \approx 1.0$). On the other hand, if no difference exists among the subjects ($\tau_i = 0$ or $\sigma_b^2 = 0$), then the estimate $\hat{\rho}$ will be in the neighborhood of zero. The longitudinal observations are then a sample from a single distribution. Figure 12–12 displays four examples of an intraclass correlation coefficient calculated from data sets made-up of five subjects measured 20 times. The plots demonstrate that, as the intraclass coefficient increases, the similarity in the pattern among the longitudinal measurements increases. The plots also demonstrate that the intraclass correlation

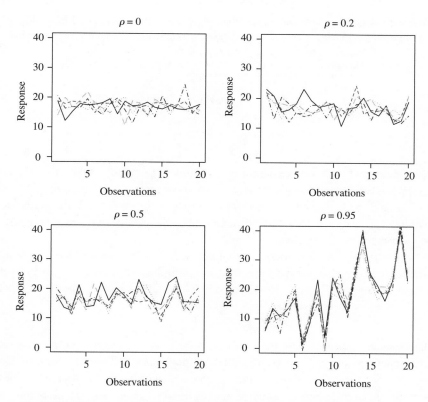

Figure 12–12.   Examples of four sets of longitudinal data with different intraclass correlation coefficients.

Table 12–12.   Estimates from the data generated to illustrate the properties of a random intercept regression model (values of the model parameters are in parentheses)

Variables	Symbols	Estimates	Std. errors	p-Values
Intercept	a	7.207 (8)	1.320	–
Time (t)	b	3.901 (4)	0.340	<0.001

$$\hat{\sigma}_b^2 = 9.412 \ (9), \ \hat{\sigma}_w^2 = 23.126 \ (25), \ \text{and} \ \hat{\rho} = 0.265 \ (0.26)$$

coefficient is a relative measure in the sense that, as the within-subject variance changes, the variance associated with the observations also changes.

Table 12–12 contains the estimated values from the artificial data (Table 12–11) as if the parameter estimates were unknown.   The estimates of the between- and within-variances differ slightly from the previous estimates because they

Table 12–13. Parameter estimates of the random intercept regression model applied to data describing weight gained during pregnancy by $n = 49$ small mothers, linear model

Variables	Symbols	Estimates	Std. errors	p-Values
Intercept	a	44.266	0.646	–
Time	b	0.066	0.001	<0.001

$$\hat{\sigma}_b^2 = 17.872, \ \hat{\sigma}_w^2 = 5.639, \text{ and } \hat{\rho} = 0.760$$

were estimated with a more commonly used method called *restricted maximum likelihood estimation*. Such estimates are an improvement over the slightly biased maximum likelihood estimates and are sometimes referred to as REML estimates. The complexity of the REML estimation process usually requires a computer algorithm for most analyses.

Data describing the pattern of weight gained during pregnancy by $n = 49$ small mothers (prepregnancy weight less than 50 kilograms) illustrate an application of a random intercept linear regression model. To start, the simplest possible random intercept regression model is

$$y_{ij} = a_i + bt_{ij}.$$

The symbol y_{ij} represents the mother's weight measured at time t_{ij} days of pregnancy, where $t_{ij} = 0$ is the start of pregnancy. The estimates of the model parameters for these highly irregularly measured longitudinal values require specific computer software but again present no special problems in the interpretation of the summary values. The estimated model parameters (Table 12–13) produce the mean regression line displayed in Figure 12–13 (solid line = mean linear model and dotted lines = individual data). The intercept $\hat{a} = 44.266$ is the estimated mean of the distribution of the prepregnancy weights ($t_{ij} = 0$). In addition, the estimated variance within these individuals is $\hat{\sigma}_{within}^2 = 5.639$ and the between-variance is $\hat{\sigma}_{between}^2 = 17.872$. The intraclass correlation coefficient $\hat{\rho} = 0.760$ reflects the degree of consistency in the pattern of weight gained among these small mothers (Figure 12–13) as a value between zero (no pattern) and 1 (a single pattern). The rate of weight gained (b) is estimated as 0.066 kilograms per day, or about 6 kilograms each trimester, or about 18 kilograms for the entire pregnancy. Of course, this estimate depends on a model that requires weight gained during pregnancy to be strictly linear.

The question of linearity is directly addressed. The plot (Figure 12–13, dotted lines) visually indicates that substantial numbers of mothers appear to have nonlinear patterns of weight gained during pregnancy. Postulating a random intercept model with a quadratic component

$$y_{ij} = a_i + bt_{ij} + ct_{ij}^2$$

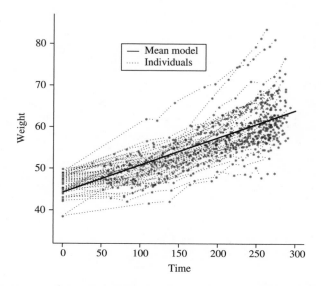

Figure 12–13. Data (dotted lines) and the estimated mean model (solid line) describing the weight gained during pregnancy by $n = 49$ small mothers, random intercept linear model.

Table 12–14. Parameter estimates of the random intercept regression model applied to the description of weight gained during pregnancy of $n = 49$ small mothers, quadratic model

Variables	Symbols	Estimates	Std. errors	p-Values
Intercept	a	45.993	0.671	–
Time (t)	b	0.030	0.004	–*
Time (t^2)	c	0.00012	0.00001	<0.001

$$\hat{\sigma}_b^2 = 17.907, \ \hat{\sigma}_w^2 = 4.974, \text{ and } \hat{\rho} = 0.783$$

* = the coefficient b directly reflects a linear influence only when $c = 0$

likely improves the model accuracy. The parameter estimates (Table 12–14) produce the estimated regression line (Figure 12–14, solid line = mean quadratic model).

The expected improvement in fit achieved by adding a quadratic term to the previous linear model is visually clear and is formally measured by the model coefficient c. The nonlinear influence assessed with the usual chi-square test statistic is specifically,

$$X^2 = \left[\frac{\hat{c} - 0}{S_{\hat{c}}}\right]^2 = \left[\frac{0.00012 - 0}{0.000013}\right]^2 = 80.048.$$

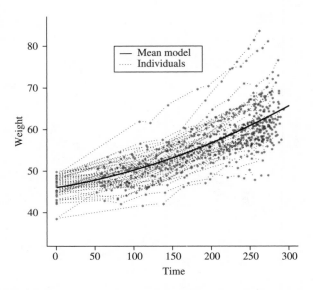

Figure 12–14. Data (dotted lines) and the estimated mean model (solid line) describing the weight gained during pregnancy by $n = 49$ small mothers, quadratic random intercept model.

The corresponding p-value is less than 0.001 (degrees of freedom $= 1$), leaving little doubt that adding a quadratic term to the model substantially improves the previous linear model.

One of the primary purposes for exploring these data is to assess the influence of maternal age (*age*) on the weight-gained pattern during pregnancy. This cross-sectional variable directly added to the random intercept regression model produces the expression

$$y_{ij} = a_i + bt_{ij} + ct_{ij}^2 + d\,age_i.$$

The parameter estimates from this mixed-effects random intercept model are summarized in Table 12–15.

Maternal age appears remarkably unrelated to the weight-gained pattern (p-value $= 0.998$). However, including two additional and important cross-sectional variables produce a more detailed picture. The same random intercept model including the cross-sectional variables infant birth weight (*bwt*) and maternal height (*ht*) is

$$y_{ij} = a_i + bt_{ij} + ct_{ij}^2 + d_1 age_i + d_2 bwt_i + d_3 ht_i.$$

The parameter estimates are given in Table 12–16.

Table 12–15. Parameter estimates of the random intercept model applied to the description of the weight gained during pregnancy of $n = 49$ small mothers, quadratic model including maternal age

Variables	Symbols	Estimates	Std. errors	p-Values
Intercept	a	46.030	2.691	–
Time (t)	b	0.030	0.004	–
Time (t^2)	c	0.00012	0.000013	< 0.001
Age	d	−0.0015	0.106	0.998

$$\hat{\sigma}_b^2 = 18.296, \ \hat{\sigma}_w^2 = 4.974, \text{ and } \hat{\rho} = 0.786$$

Table 12–16. Parameter estimates of the random intercept model applied to the description of the weight gained during pregnancy of $n = 49$ small mothers, quadratic model including maternal age, height, and infant birth weight

Variables	Symbols	Estimates	Std. errors	p-Values
Intercept	a	−3.914	18.600	–
Time (t)	b	0.030	0.004	–
Time (t^2)	c	0.00012	0.000013	< 0.001
Age	d_1	0.097	0.107	0.368
Bwt	d_2	0.692	1.402	0.622
Height	d_3	0.289	0.111	0.010

$$\hat{\sigma}_b^2 = 16.396, \ \hat{\sigma}_w^2 = 4.974, \text{ and } \hat{\rho} = 0.767$$

RANDOM INTERCEPT AND RANDOM SLOPE REGRESSION MODEL

A natural extension of the random intercept model is created when the slope, like the intercept, is considered as a random selection from a distribution of possible slopes. Specifically, an expression for a basic random intercept/slope linear regression model is

$$y_{ij} = a + bt_{ij} + \tau_i + \gamma_i t_{ij} + e_{ij}$$

or, equivalently,

$$y_{ij} = a_i + b_i t_{ij} + e_{ij}$$

where the intercepts a_i are again $a_i = a + \tau_i$ and the slopes b_i are $b_i = b + \gamma_i$ and $i = 1, 2, \cdots, n =$ number of subjects. Parallel to the random intercept a_i, the slope b_i is treated as a randomly sampled value from a distribution with mean value represented by b and variance represented by $variance(b_i) = variance(\gamma_i) = \sigma_\gamma^2$. That is, the measured values for the ith subject (y_{ij}) are random deviations from a specific straight line ($a_i + b_i t_{ij}$). This regression model accounts for three sources

Table 12–17. Parameter estimates of the random intercept/slope regression model applied to the description of weight gained during pregnancy of $n = 49$ small mothers, linear model

Variables	Symbols	Estimates	Std. errors	p-Values
Intercept	a	44.254	0.429	–
Time (t)	b	0.066	0.003	<0.001

$$\hat{\sigma}_b^2 = 7.993,\ \hat{\sigma}_w^2 = 2.175,\ \hat{\sigma}_\gamma^2 = 0.0005,\ \text{and}\ \hat{\rho} = 0.786$$

Table 12–18. Parameter estimates of the random intercept/slope regression model applied to the description of weight gained during pregnancy of $n = 49$ small mothers, quadratic model

Variables	Symbols	Estimates	Std. errors	p-Values
Intercept	a	46.033	0.443	–
Time (t)	b	0.030	0.004	–
Time (t^2)	c	0.00012	0.00001	<0.001

$$\hat{\sigma}_b^2 = 8.443,\ \hat{\sigma}_w^2 = 1.392,\ \hat{\sigma}_\gamma^2 = 0.0005,\ \text{and}\ \hat{\rho} = 0.858$$

of variation (among individuals, among slopes, and within individuals, τ_i, γ_i, and e_{ij}, respectively).

The following regression analyses (Tables 12–13 to 12–16) illustrate the application of the random intercept/slope models. The parameter estimates of a linear regression model applied to the longitudinal data again describe the weight gained during pregnancy of $n = 49$ exceptionally small mothers (Table 12–17).

Like the previous random intercept model, a nonlinear representation of the influence of time (t_{ij}) clearly improves the model fit. A nonlinear (quadratic term added) random intercept/slope model is

$$y_{ij} = a_i + b_i t_{ij} + c_i t_{ij}^2 + e_{ij},$$

and the parameter estimates of this model are given in Table 12–18.

The fundamental difference in the results from the random intercept model and the random intercept/slope model is a substantial reduction of the between and within variances (σ_b^2 and σ_w^2). The intraclass correlation coefficient increases from 0.783 to 0.858. That is, a substantial improvement in accuracy (goodness-of-fit) occurs (Table 12–14 compared to Table 12–18). The estimates of the mean model parameters, however, are similar to those of the previous random intercept models (Table 12–14).

Table 12–19. Parameter estimates of the random intercept/slope regression model applied to the description of weight gained during pregnancy of $n = 49$ small mothers, quadratic model including maternal age, height, and infant birth weight

Variables	Symbols	Estimates	Std. errors	p-Values
Intercept	a	18.332	12.331	–
Time (t)	b	0.029	0.004	–
Time (t^2)	c	0.00012	0.00001	< 0.001
Age	d_1	0.162	0.071	0.023
Bwt	d_2	0.294	0.926	0.751
Height	d_3	0.145	0.073	0.048

$$\hat{\sigma}_b^2 = 7.913,\ \hat{\sigma}_w^2 = 1.392,\ \hat{\sigma}_\gamma^2 = 0.0005,\ \text{and}\ \hat{\rho} = 0.850$$

Finally, a random quadratic intercept/slope model including the three cross-sectional variables (age, height, and infant birth weight) is

$$y_{ij} = a_i + b_i t_{ij} + c_i t_{ij}^2 + d_1 age_i + d_2 bwt_i + d_3 ht_i.$$

The parameter estimates are given in Table 12–19.

MECHANICS OF A VARIANCE/COVARIANCE ARRAY

Data. Size = number of rows (n) × number of columns (k) or $n \times k$:

$$Y = \begin{Bmatrix} y_{11} & y_{12} & y_{13} & -- & y_{1k} \\ y_{21} & y_{22} & y_{23} & -- & y_{2k} \\ y_{31} & y_{32} & y_{33} & -- & y_{3k} \\ -- & -- & -- & -- & -- \\ -- & -- & -- & -- & -- \\ y_{n1} & y_{n2} & y_{n3} & -- & y_{nk} \end{Bmatrix}$$

For the jth column, the estimated variance is

$$variance(y_j) = v_j^2 = \frac{1}{n-1}\sum(y_{ij} - \bar{y}_j)^2 \quad i = 1, 2, \cdots, n,$$

and the estimated covariance between the jth and the lth columns is

$$covariance(y_j, y_l) = v_{jl} = \frac{1}{n-1}\sum(y_{ij} - \bar{y}_j)(y_{il} - \bar{y}_l)$$
$$j \text{ and } l = 1, 2, \cdots, k \ (j \neq l)$$

where $y_j = \{y_{1j}, y_{2j}, y_{3j}, \cdots, y_{nj}\}$ and $y_l = \{y_{1l}, y_{2l}, y_{3l}, \cdots, y_{nl}\}$.

Variance/covariance array. Size $= k \times k$:

$$
\Sigma = \left\{
\begin{array}{ccccc}
\sigma_1^2 & \sigma_{12} & \sigma_{13} & -- & \sigma_{1k} \\
\sigma_{12} & \sigma_2^2 & \sigma_{23} & -- & \sigma_{2k} \\
\sigma_{13} & \sigma_{23} & \sigma_3^2 & -- & \sigma_{3k} \\
-- & -- & -- & -- & -- \\
-- & -- & -- & -- & -- \\
\sigma_{1k} & \sigma_{2k} & \sigma_{3k} & -- & \sigma_k^2
\end{array}
\right\}
$$

Estimated variance/covariance array. Size $= k \times k$:

$$
V = \left\{
\begin{array}{ccccc}
v_1^2 & v_{12} & v_{13} & -- & v_{1k} \\
v_{12} & v_2^2 & v_{23} & -- & v_{2k} \\
v_{13} & v_{23} & v_3^2 & -- & v_{3k} \\
-- & -- & -- & -- & -- \\
-- & -- & -- & -- & -- \\
v_{1k} & v_{2k} & v_{3k} & -- & v_k^2
\end{array}
\right\}
$$

A numerical example. Size $= 4 \times 3$:

$$
Y = \left\{
\begin{array}{ccc}
1 & 2 & 3 \\
2 & 5 & 6 \\
3 & 6 & 8 \\
4 & 7 & 9
\end{array}
\right\}
$$

For example, the estimated variance associated with the first column is

$$
v_1^2 = \frac{1}{3}\left[(1-2.5)^2 + (2-2.5)^2 + (3-2.5)^2 + (4-2.5)^2\right] = 1.67,
$$

and the estimated covariance v_{12} (columns 1 and 2) is

$$
v_{12} = \frac{1}{3}\left[(1-2.5)(2-5) + (2-2.5)(5-5) + (3-2.5)(6-5) + (4-2.5)(7-5)\right]
$$
$$
= 2.67
$$

where $y_1 = \{1, 2, 3, 4\}$ and $y_2 = \{2, 5, 6, 7\}$.

Estimated variance/covariance array. Size $= 3 \times 3$:

$$
\text{estimated variance of } Y = V = \left\{
\begin{array}{ccc}
1.67 & 2.67 & 3.33 \\
2.67 & 4.67 & 5.66 \\
3.33 & 5.67 & 7.00
\end{array}
\right\}
$$

13

ANALYSIS OF MULTIVARIATE TABLES

ANALYSIS OF ORDINAL DATA

An important statistical decision, not often emphasized, is the choice of a measurement scale for the variables to be analyzed. For example, risk from cigarette smoking is typically measured in number of cigarettes smoked per day. This choice of scale implies a linear relationship and, at best, measures exposure and not dose. The influence of maternal weight gain on the likelihood of a low-birth-weight infant is usually measured directly in pounds or kilograms, making the influence of a gain of 10 pounds the same for a 100-pound or a 200-pound mother. In the study of nutrition, individuals are asked to remember what they have eaten, and their responses are converted into numerical nutritional intake values and, like smoking exposure and weight gain, frequently entered directly into a statistical model, thus implying an accurate and linear scale. Such scales automatically create a variable where an increase at low levels has the same influence as the same increase at high the levels (linear). In addition, little attention is typically given to the choice between additive or multiplicative influences. Variables are measured by multiplicative scales for no apparent reason. For example, type-A behavior doubles the risk of a coronary heart disease (CHD) event (Chapter 4), and perinatal death rates among African-Americans infants are 75% those of white infants (Chapter 6).

Tradition appears the main reason that rates are usually reported in terms of ratios or in terms of logarithms of rates. Perhaps the least rigorous scale is produced by questionnaire respondents who are asked to reply to a statement by indicating a numeric value from "I completely disagree" to " I completely agree," producing a separate and unknown scale for each respondent.

One alternative to adopting scaled measures directly into the analysis begins with creating a series of categories that reflect ordering but do not require a specific scale. Such variables are called *ordinal variables*. An analysis involving nutritional intake, for example, would be less powerful but not subject to the use of an arbitrary and perhaps misleading numeric scale if the nutritional measurements were simply classified as low, medium, and high. Other variables have only ordinal values. For example, the classification of accident injuries is only sensible with an ordinal scale (none, slight, moderate, severe, and death). Ordinal variables lack sensitivity and are not fully efficient. However, creating an ordinal scale can provide an effective alternative to choosing a specific numeric scale that potentially produces ambiguous or, perhaps, even misleading results. As an introduction, the following describes a few statistical methods created to analyze ordinal variables.

WILCOXON (MANN-WHITNEY) RANK SUM TEST

Ranked values are ordinal data and provide a scale-free approach in a variety of situations. The distribution of the original observations is no longer an issue. The Wilcoxon rank sum test is designed to identify differences between two samples of ranked observations and provides an alternative to the classic Student's t-test. This statistical test, because it is based on ranked data, produces a scale-free analysis. The Wilcoxon test is slightly less efficient (lower statistical power) than a parallel t-test but does not require the knowledge or assumption that the data are numeric values sampled from normal distributions with the same variance.

To compare two groups (designated as group 1 and group 2 for convenience), the Wilcoxon test-statistic is the sum of the ranks (denoted R_i) of the observations contained in group 1 (or group 2), where the observations are ranked from the smallest to the largest regardless of group membership. When only random differences exist between the compared groups, this sum of ranks (denoted W) is likely to be approximately proportional to the number of observations in the group. That is, the sum of the ranks of the values from group 1 should be in the neighborhood of $n_1(N+1)/2$, where the quantity $(N+1)/2$ is the mean rank, n_1 represents the number of observations in group 1, and $N = n_1 + n_2$ is

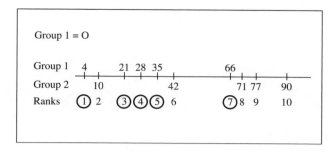

Figure 13–1. A visual display of the calculation of the Wilcoxon test statistic to measure a scale-free "distance" between two samples of data.

the total number of observations (n_2 represents the number of observations in group 2). When two groups systematically differ, the sum of the ranks of the observations contained in group 1 are likely to be substantially smaller or larger than $n_1(N+1)/2$. For an example, consider the

- data from group 1: 4, 35, 21, 28 and 66 $n_1 = 5$ and
- data from group 2: 10, 42, 71, 77 and 90 $n_2 = 5$.

The sum of the ranks associated with group 1 is $W = \sum R_i = 1+3+4+5+7 = 20$ (Figure 13–1). When no systematic difference exists between groups 1 and 2, the test statistic W differs from the value of $n_1(N+1)/2 = 5(11)/2 = 27.5$ by chance alone.

A seemingly different approach to the same two-sample comparison is called the *Mann-Whitney test*. The Mann-Whitney approach utilizes a test statistic created by counting the number of observations in one group that are smaller than each observation in the other group (denoted u_i). For the example, there are two observations in group 2 (10 and 42) that are less than the fifth largest value (66) in group 1, yielding the Mann-Whitney count of $u_5 = 2$. The Mann-Whitney test statistic is the sum of these u_i-values (denoted $U = \sum u_i$ where $i = 1, 2, \cdots,$ n_1). Like the Wilcoxon test statistic, the count U reflects the lack of similarity of the compared groups and becomes extreme when the groups systematically differ. For the example data, the $n = 10$ observations, yield $U = \sum u_i = 0+1+1+ 1+2 = 5$.

A table can be used to create the counts u_i, where the rows are the ordered values from group 2, the columns are the ordered values from group 1, and the cells of the table contain a one if the value in group 2 is less than the value in group 1 and a zero otherwise. The value U is the total number of ones among the $n_1 n_2$ values in the table. Such a table constructed from the example data is

		Group 1				
		4	21	28	35	60
	10	0	1	1	1	1
	42	0	0	0	0	0
Group 2	71	0	0	0	0	0
	77	0	0	0	0	0
	90	0	0	0	0	0
	u_i	0	1	1	1	2

The Wilcoxon and Mann-Whitney test statistics (W and U) produce the identical statistical analysis because they only differ by a constant value. Specifically, $W = U + n_1(n_1 + 1)/2$, where n_1 is the fixed sample size of group 1. For the example, when $W = 20$, then $U = 5$ because $n_1(n_1 + 1)/2 = 5(6)/2 = 15$.

The rank of the ith observation from group 1 is the sum of two values. It is the rank of the observations within group 1 (namely, i) plus the number of observations less than the ith observation from group 2 (u_i). In symbols, the rank of the ith observation in group 1 is $R_i = i + u_i$. The Wilcoxon sum of these ranks is

$$W = \sum R_i = \sum (u_i + i) = \sum u_i + \sum i = U + \frac{n_1(n_1 + 1)}{2} \qquad i = 1, 2, \cdots, n_1.$$

Specifically, for the example data,

Group 1	R_i	i	u_i
4	1	1	0
21	3	2	1
28	4	3	1
35	5	4	1
66	7	5	2
Sum	20	15	5

In terms of describing differences between two groups, the test statistic U has a useful and intuitive interpretation. Among the $n_1 n_2$ total number of possible pairs of observations from two samples, the value U is the total number of pairs where the value from group 2 is less than a value from group 1. The value $\hat{P} = U/(n_1 n_2)$ then becomes an estimate of the probability that a value selected randomly from group 2 is less than a value selected randomly from group 1. For the example data, this estimate is $\hat{P} = U/n_1 n_2 = 5/25 = 0.2$. Figure 13–2 schematically displays the logic of the test statistic $\hat{P}$.

A Mann-Whitney estimated probability $\hat{P}$ near 0.5 provides no evidence of an association. That is, a randomly chosen value from group 1 is equally likely to be smaller or larger than a randomly chosen value from group 2. However, as the

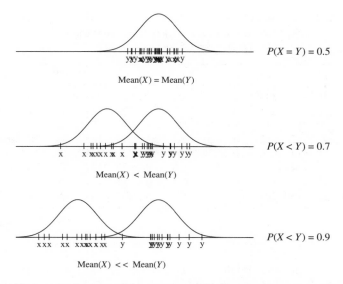

Figure 13–2. A visual display of the property of the Mann-Whitney test statistic used to measure the "distance" between two samples of data.

value $\hat{P}$ increasingly differs from 0.5, evidence increases that the compared groups systematically differ (Figure 13–2). Furthermore, this interpretation remains useful when the difference between the two compared groups is measured by a variable that is not numeric but has a meaningful ordering (an ordinal variable). The Mann-Whitney test statistic also plays a key role in an important approach to assessing the accuracy of a classification procedure (Chapter 14).

Approximate statistical tests based on the normal distribution exist to evaluate the influence of sampling variation on the test statistics W, U, and $\hat{P}$ when neither n_1 and n_2 are small (both greater than ten observations). That is, the data are ordinal but the distribution of the test statistic has an approximate normal distribution. Specifically, when only random differences exist between the two groups compared ($P = 0.5$), the Mann-Whitney estimated probability $\hat{P}$ has an approximate normal distribution with variance estimated by the expression

$$variance(\hat{P}) = \frac{1}{12n_1} + \frac{1}{12n_2},$$

and the test statistic

$$z = \frac{\hat{P} - 0.5}{\sqrt{\dfrac{1}{12n_1} + \dfrac{1}{12n_2}}}$$

Table 13–1. Cholesterol levels of 40 study participants whose weight is more than 225 pounds classified by A/B-behavior type (WCGS data, Chapters 4 and 11)

	Chol	A/B		Chol	A/B		Chol	A/B		Chol	A/B		Chol	A/B
1	344	B	9	246	B	17	224	A	25	242	B	33	252	A
2	233	A	10	224	B	18	239	A	26	252	B	34	202	A
3	291	A	11	212	B	19	239	A	27	153	B	35	218	A
4	312	A	12	188	B	20	254	A	28	183	B	36	202	B
5	185	B	13	250	B	21	169	B	29	234	A	37	212	A
6	250	A	14	197	A	22	226	B	30	137	B	38	325	A
7	263	B	15	148	B	23	175	B	31	181	A	39	194	B
8	246	A	16	268	A	24	276	A	32	248	A	40	213	B

has an approximate standard normal distribution. This test statistic addresses the question: Do systematic differences likely exist between the two compared groups? Parallel statistical tests based on W and U produce the same results (p-values).

The Mann-Whitney procedure is symmetric in the sense that the same test statistic can be constructed based on the probability that a randomly selected individual from group 2 has a larger value than a randomly selected individual from group 1. For the example, the value $\hat{Q} = 20/25 = 0.80 = 1 - \hat{P}$. However, no difference occurs in the analysis.

Data on levels of cholesterol and behavior type for the 40 heaviest Western Collaborative Group Study (WCGS) participants illustrate the application of the Mann-Whitney (Wilcoxon) test (Table 13–1, WCGS data repeated from Table 8–6 and described in Chapters 4 and 11). The mean cholesterol level of the type-A men is 245.050 and of type-B is 210.300, making the difference 34.750. As always, the question arises: Is this difference likely by chance? A Student's t-test yields a test statistic of $T = 2.562$ with an associated p-value of $P(T \geq 2.562 | no\ difference) = 0.007$.

As described, the Wilcoxon test begins by replacing the N observed values with their ranks, making it scale-free. Regardless of the values of the original sampled data, the "data" are now the ranks $1, 2, 3, \cdots, N$. The test statistic becomes the sum of the ranks associated with one of the two groups (again denoted W). For the WCGS data, the sum of the ranks of the 20 type-A individuals is $W = \sum R_i = 503$. When no difference exists between type-A and type-B individuals in levels of cholesterol, the expected value of W is $n_1(N+1)/2 = 20(41)/2 = 410$. The variance of the test statistic W is given by the expression

$$variance(W) = \frac{n_1 n_2 (N+1)}{12},$$

where n_1 is the number of type-A individuals and n_2 is the number of type-B individuals ($N = n_1 + n_2 = 20 + 20 = 40$). The specific test statistic becomes

$$z = \frac{W - n_1(N+1)/2}{\sqrt{variance(W)}} = \frac{503 - 410}{\sqrt{1366.67}} = 2.516$$

where z has an approximate standard normal distribution when no type-A/type-B difference exists in cholesterol levels. The p-value is $P(W \geq 410 | no\ difference) = P(|Z| \geq 2.516 | no\ difference) = 0.006$. For the parallel t-test, the p-value is 0.007.

The Mann-Whitney test-statistic ($\hat{P}$) equally reflects differences in cholesterol levels and has the further interpretation as the probability that an individual selected at random from the type-B group will have a lower cholesterol value than a randomly selected individual from the type-A group. This probability is estimated by

$$\hat{P} = \frac{U}{n_1 n_2} = \frac{293}{20(20)} = 0.733$$

where

$$U = W - \frac{n_1(n_1+1)}{2} = 503 - 210 = 293.$$

In symbols,

$$P(cholesterol\ value\ of\ a\ type\text{-}B < cholesterol\ value\ of\ a\ random\ type\text{-}A)$$
$$= 0.733.$$

As noted, the Mann-Whitney approach based on the measure $\hat{P}$ yields the identical analytic result as the Wilcoxon rank test. The test statistic is

$$z = \frac{\hat{P} - 0.5}{\sqrt{variance(\hat{P})}} = \frac{0.733 - 0.5}{\sqrt{0.00854}} = 2.516$$

and, as before, the p-value is 0.006. Note that $variance(\hat{P}) = variance(W)/(n_1 n_2)^2$ because $\hat{P} = W/(n_1 n_2)$.

The Mann-Whitney estimated probability $\hat{P}$ applies to a $2 \times k$ table and again effectively identifies possible differences between two compared groups without specifying a specific scale. Consider the answer to a question from a health attitudes survey: Do you think that exercise increases the length of your life? The yes/no responses from a sample of 165 individuals surveyed are also classified by the amount of physical exercise (none, occasional, moderate, and strenuous; an ordinal variable) reported by the respondent (Table 13–2).

Table 13–2.   Responses ($n = 165$) to a question on life expectancy
and reported physical activity (an ordinal variable)

	None	Occasional	Moderate	Strenuous	**Total**
Yes	7	7	8	20	42
No	25	34	32	32	123
Total	32	41	40	52	165

The Mann-Whitney statistic $\hat{P}$ is an estimate of the probability that a random person in group 2 (the no-group) reports a lower level of exercise than a random person in group 1 (the yes-group). This estimate is, as before, the count of the total number of individuals in the no-group who reported lower levels of exercise than each member of the yes-group, divided by the total number possible pairs. In addition, individuals at the same level (same exercise category) are assumed to be uniformly distributed within that category. Consequently, within that category, half the no-individuals are assumed to be below the yes-individuals and, necessarily, half above the yes-individuals. In the context of a $2 \times k$ table, the Mann-Whitney statistic $\hat{P}$ is sometimes called a *ridit value*.

Mechanically, for each level of physical activity, the Mann-Whitney u_i values are the counts of individuals in the no-group in categories to the left of each of the yes-group individuals plus one-half the counts of individuals in the same category ("tied"). For example, in the moderate physical activity category, there are $25 + 34 = 59$ individuals (none and occasional) in the no-group who reported lower of physical activity than each of the eight individuals in the yes-group (to the left) and 32 individuals with the same level of physical activity. Therefore, there are $8 \times [25 + 34 + \frac{1}{2}(32)] = 600$ individuals in the no-group with lower levels of physical activity than the eight individuals in the yes-group among those who reported moderate exercise. That is, the Mann-Whitney u_i-count is $u_3 = 600$. These u_i-counts for all four physical activity categories (Table 13–2) are:

- None: $u_1 = 7 \times [\frac{1}{2}(25)] = 87.5$
- Occasional: $u_2 = 7 \times [25 + \frac{1}{2}(34)] = 294$
- Moderate: $u_3 = 8 \times [25 + 34 + \frac{1}{2}(32)] = 600$, and
- Strenuous: $u_4 = 20 \times [25 + 34 + 32 + \frac{1}{2}(32)] = 2140$.

Specifically, the estimated Mann-Whitney probability estimate becomes

$$\hat{P} = \frac{\sum u_i}{n_1 n_2} = \frac{87.5 + 294 + 600 + 2140}{42(123)} = 0.604.$$

where there are $n_1(n_2) = 42(123)$ comparisons between the 165 surveyed individuals. Thus, the probability that a randomly selected person from the no-group has a lower level of physical activity than a randomly selected person from the yes-group is 0.604.

In general notation, the estimated Mann-Whitney probability from a $2 \times k$ table is

$$\hat{P} = \frac{\left[\begin{array}{l} n_{11}\left[\frac{1}{2}(n_{21})\right] + n_{12}\left[n_{21} + \frac{1}{2}(n_{22})\right] + n_{13}\left[n_{21} + n_{22} + \frac{1}{2}(n_{23})\right] \\ + n_{14}\left[n_{21} + n_{22} + n_{23} + \frac{1}{2}(n_{24})\right] + \cdots \end{array} \right]}{n_1 n_2}.$$

The Mann-Whitney estimated probability $\hat{P}$ calculated from a table of observations has the same statistical properties as already described. For the health survey data, the estimated probability of $\hat{P}$ is 0.604, and the probability $P = 0.5$ is the value expected when reported amounts of physical exercise are unrelated to the answer of the yes/no attitude question. The variance of the approximate normal distribution of $\hat{P}$ is

$$variance(\hat{P}) = \frac{variance(W)}{(n_1 n_2)^2} \approx \frac{1}{12n_1} + \frac{1}{12n_2} = \frac{1}{12(42)} + \frac{1}{12(123)} = 0.00266,$$

making the test statistic

$$z = \frac{0.604 - 0.5}{\sqrt{0.00266}} = 2.020.$$

The p-value is $P(more\ extreme\ \hat{P} \mid P = 0.5) = P(|Z| \geq 2.020 | no\ association) = 0.043$. The estimate $\hat{P} = 0.604$ is, therefore, unlikely to differ from 0.5 entirely because of random variation.

The normal distribution test statistic z is likely understated because the estimate of the variance is biased (too large). This bias results from not accounting for the reduction in variability due to the "tied" observations that are inevitable in a table. Corrections for this usually slight bias exist [31].

To emphasize that the choice of the scale can make a difference, the case–control data describing the risk of coffee consumption and the likelihood of pancreatic cancer are reanalyzed as ordinal data (Table 13–3, repeated from Chapter 2).

The previous analyses (Chapters 2) did not account for the reported number of cups of coffee consumed per day. A test of independence between case–control status and coffee consumption yields a p-value of 0.069, and the ordering of the column variables (cups of coffee) has no influence on the analytic results. An alternative to no scale for assessing coffee consumption consists of the ordered responses: *none, light, moderate*, and *heavy*. Computing the Mann-Whitney statistic for the 2×4 table in the same manner as before yields the estimate

$$\hat{P} = \frac{\sum u_i}{n_1 n_2} = \frac{144 + 8601 + 9964 + 15960}{216(307)} = 0.553.$$

Table 13–3. Pancreatic cancer and coffee consumption among male cases and controls (repeated from Chapter 3)

| | Coffee consumption (cups/day) | | | | |
	None	Light	Moderate	Heavy	**Total**
$Y = 1$ (cases)	9	94	53	60	216
$Y = 0$ (controls)	32	119	74	82	307
Total	41	213	127	142	523
$\hat{P}_j$	0.220	0.441	0.417	0.423	0.413

Thus, the probability that a randomly selected control consumes less coffee than a randomly selected case is estimated to be $\hat{P} = 0.523$. The variance of the distribution of the estimate $\hat{P}$ is

$$variance(\hat{P}) = \frac{1}{12n_1} + \frac{1}{12n_2} = \frac{1}{12(216)} + \frac{1}{12(307)} = 0.00066.$$

Again, the key value $P = 0.5$ (no case–control difference) creates the approximate normally distributed test statistic

$$z = \frac{0.553 - 0.5}{\sqrt{0.00066}} = 0.889.$$

The resulting p-value is $P(a\ more\ extreme\ \hat{P}|P = 0.5) = P(|Z| \geq 0.889|no\ association) = 0.373$. The Mann-Whitney test statistic $\hat{P}$ calculated from an ordinal variable analysis produces little evidence of an association between case–control status and reported coffee consumption.

CORRELATION BETWEEN ORDINAL VARIABLES

When pairs of numeric values are classified into a two-way table, a number of options exist to measure and assess the relationship between these two variables. In some cases, a correlation coefficient measures the degree to which a straight line reflects their association (Chapter 2). Chi-square statistics indicate correspondences between observed and theoretical values generated under specific conditions. Statistical models allow a quantitative assessment of even complex numerical associations. However, it also useful to measure the association between categorical variables when one or both variables are not numeric but ordinal. Several techniques are available to account for the ordering and, these produce a scale-free numeric measure of association. The following describes two such techniques based on a Mann-Whitney-like counting strategy.

Two similar coefficients measuring the association between ordinal variables are called a gamma-*coefficient* (γ) and *Kendall's tau-coefficient* (τ). Both coefficients produce summary values that are always between -1 and $+1$, where zero indicates exactly no association based on n not necessarily numeric pairs of observations (x_i, y_i). The calculation of these measure of association begins with counting the number of concordant and disconcordant pairs. Each of the $N = n(n-1)/2$ possible comparisons among n pairs are classified as concordant or discordant. A pair (x_i, y_i) is concordant with respect to a pair (x_j, y_j) when x_i is greater than x_j and y_i is greater that y_j, or when x_i is less than x_j and y_i is less that y_j; otherwise, the pair is discordant. Concordant–discordant determinations directly apply to ordinal variables (for example, $x_i =$ mild is less than $x_j =$ severe).

Consider a small sample of five pairs of numeric observations ($n = 5$ pairs):

$$(2, 20), (12, 1), (6, 2), (9, 7), \text{ and } (10, 14).$$

The first and second pairs are discordant because $2 < 12$ but $20 > 1$ and the fourth and fifth pairs are concordant because $9 < 10$ and $7 < 14$. The following computational table identifies the concordant (denoted c) and discordant (denoted d) pairs among 10 possible comparisons:

	(2, 20)	(12, 1)	(6, 2)	(9, 7)	(10, 14)
(2, 20)	x	d	d	d	d
(12, 1)	–	x	d	d	d
(6, 2)	–	–	x	c	c
(9, 7)	–	–	–	x	c
(10, 14)	–	–	–	–	x

The total number of concordant pairs is $C = 3$, and the total number of discordant pairs is $D = 7$ among the total $C + D = N = 5(4)/2 = 10$ possible comparisons.

The gamma-coefficient (denoted $\hat{\gamma}$) is then defined as

$$\hat{\gamma} = \frac{C}{C+D} - \frac{D}{C+D} = \frac{C-D}{C+D}$$

and $-1 \le \hat{\gamma} \le 1$. When $\hat{\gamma} = -1$, all pairs are disconcordant ($C = 0$). When $\hat{\gamma} = 1$, all pairs are concordant ($D = 0$). Otherwise the coefficient $\hat{\gamma}$ is between -1 and $+1$. In addition, for exactly unrelated variables $D = C$, the value $\hat{\gamma} = 0$. For the example values, the estimated measure of association is $\hat{\gamma} = (3-7)/(3+7) = -0.4$.

A parallel process produces estimates of association from a table constructed from ordinal categories. Consider the simplest possible table, in which observations in category A_1 are less than those in A_2, and observations in category B_1 are less than those in B_2. In symbols, the 2×2 table is

	B_1	B_2
A_1	a	b
A_2	c	d

Both values within each of the d pairs are greater than both values within all a pairs, yielding a total of $C = ad$ concordant pairs. Similarly, the values within each of the c pairs are less than one and greater than the other of the members within all b pairs, yielding a total of $D = bc$ discordant pairs. Therefore, the γ-measure of association between two binary variables classified into a 2×2 table is

$$\hat{\gamma} = \frac{C - D}{C + D} = \frac{ad - bc}{ad + bc} = \frac{\hat{or} - 1}{\hat{or} + 1}$$

where $\hat{or}$ is the estimated odds ratio. This measure of association was among the earliest proposed.

Mothers participating in a study of birth defects ($n = 758$) were classified into three categories based on reported dietary calories (Kcals) consumed per day (low, medium, and high). They were also asked about their vitamin use during pregnancy and classified into three categories (never take vitamins, took vitamins only during pregnancy, and always take vitamins). The data describing the joint distribution of these two ordinal variables are given in Table 13–4.

To measure the association between reported calories and vitamin use, the concordant and discordant pairs are again counted among all 758 individuals. Each cell in the table contributes to the total counts of the concordant or discordant pairs. Mechanically, the number of concordant pairs for an individual in a specific cell is the total of the cell frequencies that are to the right and below that specified cell. Similarly, the number of discordant pairs for an individual in a specific cell is the total of the cell frequencies to the left and below the specified cell. A comprehensive notation for the process of counting these concordant/discordant pairs of observations is difficult but the calories/vitamin example indicates the

Table 13–4. Mothers of newborn infants with birth defects ($n = 758$) classified by reported dietary calories and vitamin use

		Dietary Calories			
		Low	Medium	High	**Total**
	Never	78	69	155	302
Vitamin use	During	56	43	112	211
	Always	85	44	116	245
	Total	219	156	283	758

general pattern for any two-way table. The total number of concordant pairs is

$$C = 78(43 + 112 + 44 + 116) + 69(112 + 116) + 56(44 + 116) + 43(116)$$
$$= 54,250,$$

and the total number of discordant pairs is

$$D = 69(56 + 85) + 155(56 + 43 + 85 + 44) + 43(85) + 112(85 + 44)$$
$$= 63,172.$$

The γ-coefficient is again defined as

$$\hat{\gamma} = \frac{C - D}{C + D}.$$

Therefore, for the birth defects data, $C - D = -8922$ and $C + D = 117,422$ give the estimated coefficient $\hat{\gamma} = -8922/117,422 = -0.076$.

Kendall's ordinal τ-coefficient is not very different from the γ-coefficient. The τ-coefficient, however, takes into account the "tied" values (values in the same row or same column) that necessarily occur when data are classified into a table. The τ-coefficient is defined by the expression

$$\hat{\tau} = \frac{C - D}{\sqrt{(tr + C + D)(tc + C + D)}}$$

where tr and tc represent the number of "tied values." The value tr (same row) represents the number of pairs that are "tied" for the first value of each pair and tc (same column) represents the number of pairs "tied" for the second value of each pair. For the birth defects data (Table 13–4),

$$tr = 78(69 + 155) + 69(155) + 56(43 + 112) + 43(112) + 85(44 + 116) + 44(116)$$
$$= 60,367,$$

and

$$tc = 78(56 + 85) + 56(85) + 69(43 + 44) + 43(44) + 155(112 + 116) + 112(116)$$
$$= 71,985.$$

Based on these counts, Kendall's measure of association is then estimated by $\hat{\tau} = -8922/\sqrt{(177,789)(189,407)} = -0.049$. It is always the case that $|\hat{\tau}| < |\hat{\gamma}|$.

Table 13–5. Mothers of newborn infants with birth defects ($n = 758$) classified by prepregnancy maternal weight and vitamin use

		Prepregnancy maternal weight *(kg.)*					
		<50	50–60	60–70	70–80	>80	**Total**
	Never	58	137	125	65	49	219
Vitamin use	During	17	43	34	16	13	156
	Always	49	75	51	20	6	383
	Total	124	255	210	101	68	758

Consider another example: Table 13–5 also contains counts of mothers of newborn infants with a birth defect ($n = 758$) classified by their prepregnancy weights (<50, 50–60, 60–70, 70–80, >80 kilograms) and again classified by vitamin use during pregnancy.

For this 3 × 5 table, the ordinal measures of association are $\hat{\gamma} = -0.216$ and $\hat{\tau} = -0.142$. It is worth noting that prepregnancy weight is a numeric value classified into numeric categories, but only the ordering of the categories influences the value of the estimated coefficients (a scaleless use of a numeric variable).

One last note: When two variables are independent in the classic sense ($\hat{p}_{ij} = \hat{p}_i \hat{q}_j$, Chapter 2), both ordinal measure of association are exactly zero ($\hat{\gamma} = \hat{\tau} = 0$).

LOG-LINEAR MODELS: CATEGORICAL DATA ANALYSIS

From a broad perspective, a log-linear model applied to describe categorical data is a generalization of the classic chi-square analysis. Nevertheless, its application is not very different from most regression models, such as those already discussed, especially the Poisson model (Chapter 6). There is, however, an important distinction. Unlike most regression models, the outcome studied (dependent variable) is not viewed as a direct function of observed values (independent variables). When a log-linear model is applied to categorical data, the independent variables are not observed values, but are components of a design variable constructed to define specific relationships within a table. In other words, the design variable dictates the relationships between the model parameters and the table frequencies. As with all statistical models, the log-linear model remains a statistical tool that yields efficient summary values that frequently produce an effective description of the relationships within collected data, as well as a statistical assessment of the influences of random variation.

Independence in a Two-Way Table

An association between two categorical variables that create a two-way table is usually and optimally assessed using a chi-square test-statistic to compare theoretically generated and observed values (Chapter 2). It is, however, instructive to analyze the same two-way table employing a Poisson log-linear model. Both methods yield identical results from different perspectives.

For a two-way table, levels A_i and B_j of two categorical variables, denoted A and B, are independent when,

$$P(A_i \text{ and } B_j) = P(A_i)P(B_j)$$

or, equally, when they are additive on the log-scale then,

$$log[P(A_i \text{ and } B_j)] = log[P(A_i)P(B_i)] = log[P(A_i)] + log[P(B_j)].$$

An analogous additive relationship between the logarithms of cell frequencies of a table produces an additive log-linear regression model describing two unrelated (independent) categorical variables. Consider a 3×3 table in which the log-linear model is

$$log(cell\text{-}frequency) = log(n_{ij}) = a + r_1 R_1 + r_2 R_2 + c_1 C_1 + c_2 C_2.$$

The symbols R and C represent a design variable that identifies the rows and columns of the 3×3 table when variables A and B are unrelated. The symbols n_{ij}, as before, represents the counts of observations in the $(i, \ j)^{th}$-cell. In detail, the additive model is

	B_1	B_2	B_3
A_1	$log(n_{11}) = a$	$log(n_{12}) = a + c_1$	$log(n_{13}) = a + c_2$
A_2	$log(n_{21}) = a + r_1$	$log(n_{22}) = a + r_1 + c_1$	$log(n_{23}) = a + r_1 + c_2$
A_3	$log(n_{31}) = a + r_2$	$log(n_{32}) = a + r_2 + c_1$	$log(n_{33}) = a + r_2 + c_2$

The row and column categorical variables A and B are additive on a log-scale. Additivity of categorical variables, in the case of a log-linear model, is not different in principle from the previously discussed additive models (linear, logistic, or Poisson). Each level of one categorical variable has the same influence on the log-frequencies regardless of the levels of the other variable. The influence of A_2, for example, is r_1 for each of the three levels of variable B. Thus, as before, additivity on a log-scale is an expression for statistical independence of categorical variables.

Table 13–6.   Data from a study of the efficacy of high doses of vitamin C in the prevention of colds conducted in Canada

		$B_1 = 0$	$B_2 = 1$ to 4	$B_3 \geq 5$	Total
		\multicolumn{4}{c}{$B =$ Number of colds}			
	$A_1 =$ high dose	7	12	22	41
$A =$ vitamin C	$A_2 =$ usual dose	3	1	7	11
	$A_3 =$ placebo	10	1	8	19
	Total	20	14	37	71

Table 13–7.   Details of the design variable describing complete independence between two categorical variables in a 3 × 3 table

Notation	Data	a	R_1	R_2	C_1	C_2	Model
n_{11}	7	1	0	0	0	0	a
n_{21}	3	1	1	0	0	0	$a + r_1$
n_{31}	10	1	0	1	0	0	$a + r_2$
n_{12}	12	1	0	0	1	0	$a + c_1$
n_{22}	1	1	1	0	1	0	$a + r_1 + c_1$
n_{32}	1	1	0	1	1	0	$a + r_2 + c_1$
n_{13}	22	1	0	0	0	1	$a + c_2$
n_{23}	7	1	1	0	0	1	$a + r_1 + c_2$
n_{33}	8	1	0	1	0	1	$a + r_2 + c_2$

Data from a Canadian study of the efficacy of high doses of vitamin C on the number of colds during a winter season illustrate (a 3 × 3 table, Table 13–6). For the additive model (complete independence), the details of the design variable are described in Table 13–7. The estimation of the five model coefficients (a, r_1, r_2, c_1, and c_2) based on the logarithms of the cell frequencies (Table 13–8) is the first step.

A regression model consists of a dependent variable and a series of independent variables. The dependent variable of a Poisson log-linear model is the logarithm of the cell count n_{ij} and, to repeat, the independent variables are the components of a design variable (the rows of zeros and ones, Table 13–7). From the vitamin C data, the logarithm of the cell count $log(n_{33}) = log(8) = 2.079$ is the dependent variable, and the corresponding five independent variables are $a = 1$, $R_1 = 0$, $R_2 = 1$, $C_1 = 0$, and $C_2 = 1$ (parameter present $= 1$ and parameter absent $= 0$) making $log(n_{33}) = a + r_2 + c_2$. Furthermore, these counts are assumed to be sampled from Poisson distributions.

Nine $log(\hat{n}_{ij})$-values produce five maximum likelihood estimated model parameters (Table 13–8).

Table 13–8. Model-estimated parameters from the Canadian vitamin C data

Variables	Symbols	Estimates	Std. errors
Constant	a	2.447	0.246
Second row	r_1	−1.316	0.340
Third row	r_2	−0.769	0.278
Second column	c_1	−0.357	0.348
Third column	c_2	0.615	0.278

Table 13–9. Model-estimated and observed values (in parentheses)
from the Canadian vitamin C study data

		$B =$ Number of colds			
		$B_1 = 0$	$B_2 = 1\text{–}4$	$B_3 > 4$	**Total**
	$A_1 =$ high dose	11.55 (7)	8.08 (12)	21.37 (22)	41
$A =$ vitamin C	$A_2 =$ usual dose	3.10(3)	2.17 (1)	5.73 (7)	11
	$A_3 =$ placebo	5.35 10	3.75 (1)	9.90(8)	19
	Total	20	14	37	71

As required, these coefficients produce estimated counts that exactly conform to the model of complete independence of the vitamin C dose and the frequency of colds. For the example, the estimated log-frequency is

$$log(\hat{n}_{33}) = \hat{a} + \hat{r}_2 + \hat{c}_2 = 2.447 - 0.769 + 0.615 = 2.293,$$

and the estimated cell count becomes

$$\hat{n}_{33} = e^{2.293} = 9.901.$$

The corresponding observed count is $n_{33} = 8$. As always, the difference is a result of strictly random variation or random variation plus a systematic association. The nine model-estimated values and the nine observed values are contained in Table 13–9.

The Pearson chi-square test statistic measures the correspondence between model and observed values in the usual way. That is, nine cell comparisons yield the test statistic

$$X^2 = \sum \frac{(o_i - e_i)^2}{e_i} = \frac{(7 - 11.55)^2}{11.55} + \cdots + \frac{(8 - 9.90)^2}{9.90} = 11.036.$$

The test statistic X^2 has a chi-square distribution with the degrees of freedom equal to the number of cells in the table, minus the number of parameters in the model or $9 - 5 = 4$. The associated p-value is $P(X^2 \geq 11.035 | no\ association) = 0.026$.

This chi-square test statistic is identical to the value directly calculated from the expected values created under the hypothesis of independence ($p_{ij} = p_i q_j$, Chapter 2). For the Canadian data, for example, the estimate $\hat{n}_{33}$ is also $\hat{n}_{33} = n\hat{p}_3\hat{q}_3 = 71(37/71)(19/71) = 9.901$.

The example introduces the process of applying Poisson model techniques in conjunction with a specially constructed design variable to measure the extent of an association between categorical variables. As will be discussed, a log-linear model approach can be extended to the analysis of a wide variety of kinds of multivariate categorical data.

The nonadditive log-linear model for a 3×3 table follows the usual pattern, producing the model

$$log(cell\text{-}frequency) = a + r_1 R_1 + r_2 R_2 + c_1 C_1 + c_2 C_2$$
$$+ d_1(R_1 \times C_1) + d_2(R_2 \times C_1) + d_3(R_1 \times C_2) + d_4(R_2 \times C_2).$$

Adding four interaction terms to the model brings the total number of coefficients to nine. A 3×3 table consists of nine cells, making the model saturated. For example, the model value is

$$log(\hat{n}_{33}) = \hat{a} + \hat{r}_2 + \hat{c}_2 + \hat{d}_4 = 1.946 + 0.357 + 1.145 - 1.368 = 2.079,$$

and $e^{2.079} = 8.0$. Thus, no difference exists between the model-estimated values and the data ($X^2 = 0$). However, it is important to note that the lack of fit of an additive model can be viewed as the failure to account for interaction influences among the categorical variables. From this perspective, the magnitude of an interaction between two categorical variables indicates the extent of a statistical association. Or, the absence of an interaction indicates independence (additivity) between two categorical variables. Thus, the statistical terms *independence* and *association* are synonymous with the model properties additivity and interaction.

TABLES WITH STRUCTURAL ZEROS

Occasionally, tables are created in which specific combinations of the categorical variables cannot occur. For example, females with prostatic cancer cannot occur in a table of kinds of cancer mortality by sex, or the kinds of medication among individuals without a history diabetes cannot occur in a table of kinds of diabetic medications by personal medical history, or male–female pairs of twins cannot appear in a table of twin pairs by sex and zygosity. This absence of observations is

Table 13–10. Data on the selection for two kinds of cancer therapy drugs ($n = 78$)

	X	Y	Z	Total
A	36	5	–*	41
B	18	4	8	30
C	–*	3	4	7
Total	54	12	12	78

* = Structural zero.

different from an empty cell in a table (a random zero). These observations never occur, regardless of the sample size and are called *structural zeros*.

An example of such a situation arises in exploring the relationship between two drugs prescribed for the treatment of a specific cancer. Three choices of drugs are available for chemotherapy (called here X, Y, and Z to avoid pharmaceutical names). In addition, to reduce side effects caused by these drugs, one of a series of three other drugs is also prescribed (called here A, B, and C). In a survey of cancer specialists prescribing these drugs, it is desired to know if the choice of the cancer drug influences the choice of the second drug (independence?). The situation is complicated by the fact that drugs A and Z as well C and X are never prescribed together (contraindicated). Data from a survey of 78 physicians is given in Table 13–10.

The primary question is: Does a pattern exist associated with prescribing these two kinds of drugs? When no association exists, the two categorical variables are said to be *quasi-independent*. To address this issue, the previous additive model is used. That is, the log-linear model remains

$$log(cell\text{-}frequency) = a + r_1R_1 + r_2R_2 + c_1C_1 + c_2C_2.$$

With a slight modification of the design variable, the model parameters are again estimated using a Poisson log-linear model, accounting for the two structural zeros. The design variable describes independence (additivity) as before, but is modified by eliminating the two cells with structural zeros. Table 13–11 contains the complete details of this log-linear model.

As before, the log-frequencies are the dependent variables, and the components of the design variable are the independent variables in a Poisson log-linear model producing estimated model coefficients (Table 13–12).

The only important difference between the analysis of a complete table (Table 13–7) and a table containing structural zeros (Table 13–11) is the loss of two degrees of freedom (one for each structural zero). The analysis is based on the seven log-frequencies, instead of nine. Sums of the estimated coefficients again estimate the logarithm of the cell frequencies that perfectly conform to the

Table 13–11. A design variable for the analysis of a 3×3 table with two structural zeros describing use of two cancer therapy drugs

Notation	Data	a	R_1	R_2	C_1	C_2	Model
n_{11}	36	1	0	0	0	0	a
n_{21}	18	1	1	0	0	0	$a + r_1$
n_{31}	5	1	0	0	1	0	$a + c_1$
n_{12}	4	1	1	0	1	0	$a + r_1 + c_1$
n_{22}	3	1	0	1	1	0	$a + r_2 + c_1$
n_{32}	8	1	1	0	0	1	$a + r_1 + c_2$
n_{33}	4	1	0	1	0	1	$a + r_2 + c_2$

Table 13–12. Model-estimated parameters to evaluate the question of quasi-independence of the pattern of two cancer therapy drugs

Variables	Terms	Estimates	Std. errors
Constant	a	3.548	0.164
Row 2	r_1	–0.590	0.257
Row 3	r_2	–1.017	0.500
Column 2	c_1	–1.713	0.331
Column 3	r_2	–0.975	0.393

Table 13–13. Estimated frequencies from the quasi-independence model and observed values (in parentheses) from a survey of two cancer therapy drugs

	X	Y	Z	
A	34.74 (34)	6.26 (5)	–*	41
B	19.26 (18)	3.47 (4)	7.26 (8)	30
C	–*	2.26 (3)	4.74 (4)	7
Total	54	12	12	78

* = Structural zero.

model. Exponentiating these estimates produces model-generated cell frequencies that are exactly quasi-independent (Table 13–13).

For example, the estimated number of occurrences of the pair (Z, C) is

$$\hat{n}_{33} = e^{\hat{a} + \hat{r}_2 + \hat{c}_2} = e^{3.548 - 1.017 - 0.975} = e^{1.556} = 4.736$$

where the observed value is 4. The comparison between the seven-model and observed counts shows no apparent evidence of a nonrandom pattern. The chi-square test statistic

$$X^2 = \frac{(36 - 34.74)^2}{34.37} + \cdots + \frac{(4 - 4.74)^2}{4.74} = 0.891$$

supports the inference from the informal comparisons. The associated degrees of freedom are two (number of cell frequencies $= 7$ minus number of parameters in the model $= 5$). A formal p-value of $P(X_2 \geq 0.891 | no\ association) = 0.640$ indicates that the deviations between the model and observed values are plausibly random.

CAPTURE/RECAPTURE MODEL

A two-stage sampling scheme called *capture/recapture sampling* is occasionally applied to estimate the size of a free-living wild animal population. First, a sample of animals is captured, marked, and returned to their environment. The population now consists of two kinds of animals, marked and unmarked. Then, a second independent sample of size n is collected (recapture), and the number of marked animals is recorded (denoted x). The number of marked animals in the second sample relates to the population size. When the second sample contains a large proportion of marked animals, the population is likely small and, conversely, a small proportion of marked animals indicates the population is likely large. This simple principle is turned into an estimate of the total population size. That is, the population size (denoted N) is estimated by equating the proportion of marked animals in the population (p) to the proportion of marked animals in the sample ($\hat{p}$) or,

$$p = \hat{p} \quad \text{or} \quad \frac{m}{\hat{N}} = \frac{x}{n} \quad \text{making the estimate of population size} \quad \hat{N} = \frac{mn}{x}$$

where m represents the number of marked animals in the first sample (caught once) and x represents the number of marked animals in the second sample (caught twice) among n animals. The estimate of the population size $\hat{N}$ is unbiased only when the marked and unmarked animals have the identical probability of being caught in the second sample. Capture/recapture techniques have been used to estimate the size of such diverse populations as the number of Gray whales in the Pacific ocean and the number of wild dogs in city of Baltimore.

A less intuitive approach to the capture/recapture estimation of a population size comes from a log-linear model. A model provides a systematic method to derive the estimated population size (N) that generalizes to more complicated situations (to be discussed). Table 13–14 defines the notation and displays the additive capture/recapture log-linear model.

Table 13–14.   Notation and model for the capture/recapture estimation of a population size

	Previous notation	Table notation	Log-linear model
Caught twice	x	n_{11}	$log(n_{11}) = a + b_1 + b_2$
Caught first sample only	$m - x$	n_{12}	$log(n_{12}) = a + b_1$
Caught second sample only	$n - x$	n_{21}	$log(n_{21}) = a + b_2$
Not caught	$-*$	n_{22}	$log(n_{22}) = a$

* = Structural zero.

The estimation of the model parameters is a simple manipulation of the observed counts, because the model is saturated (three observed counts = three model coefficients). That is, the coefficients $\hat{a}$, $\hat{b}_1$, and $\hat{b}_2$ are estimated directly from the logarithms of the three cell counts (n_{11}, n_{12}, and n_{21}). Specifically, the estimate of the logarithm of the number of animals "not caught" is $\hat{a}$. Therefore, the value $e^{\hat{a}}$ is an estimate of the number of animals not caught or

$$\hat{a} = log(n_{12}) + log(n_{21}) - log(n_{11}) \quad \text{and} \quad e^{\hat{a}} = \hat{n}_{22} = \frac{n_{12}n_{21}}{n_{11}}.$$

The estimated population size then becomes the sum of the three observed counts and the estimated count $\hat{n}_{22}$ and

$$\hat{N} = n_{11} + n_{12} + n_{21} + \hat{n}_{22} = n_{11} + n_{12} + n_{21} + \frac{n_{12}n_{21}}{n_{11}}$$

$$= \frac{n_{11}(n_{11} + n_{12} + n_{21}) + n_{12}n_{21}}{n_{11}} = \frac{(n_{11} + n_{21})(n_{11} + n_{12})}{n_{11}}.$$

The estimate is identical to the previous intuitive estimate $\hat{N} = mn/x$ but illustrates an elementary application of a log-linear model that, as noted, is a widely used statistical tool as part of the analysis of categorical data in general.

An analogous multistage sampling strategy applied to human data produces estimates of population size from a series of sources or lists that identify a specific kind of individual. The principle of relating the number of times individuals are reported by a source ("caught") again produces an estimate of the population size. In this slightly more complicated case, a log-linear model again produces an estimate of the population size. For example, in a study of the birth defect spina bifida, it was desired to estimate the number of cases among African-American children in New York state. Three sources are available to identify cases, namely birth certificates, death certificates, and state rehabilitation records. A direct count of cases identified by these three sources is biased (too small) because cases not

Table 13–15. Cases of spina bifida among African-American children from three sources [birth certificates (S_1), death certificates (S_2), and rehabilitation records (S_3)]

S_3	S_2	$\bar{S}_2$
S_1	1	3
$\bar{S}_1$	8	13

$\bar{S}_3$	S_2	$\bar{S}_2$
S_1	1	8
$\bar{S}_1$	3	–

on at least one list will not be included (a structural zero). The omission of these cases biases direct estimates of the population size.

New York state data (Table 13–15) consisting of spina bifida cases who are identified by one or more of three sources (denoted S_1 = birth certificates, S_2 = death certificates, and S_3 = rehabilitation records) allow an estimate of the total number of affected children.

A number of possible relationships exist among the three sources identifying spina bifida cases, and each requires a specific model to estimate the population size. The simplest model arises when it is known (or assumed) that the sources of data are independent. An additive log-linear regression model then allows an estimate of the total number of cases of spina bifida. Specifically, the additive model is

$$log(cell\text{-}frequency) = a + b_1F_1 + b_2F_2 + b_3F_3$$

where $F_i = 1$ indicates presence and $F_i = 0$ absence from the ith list ($i = 1, 2,$ and 3). For example, the log-frequency of cases that appear on all three lists is represented by $a + b_1 + b_2 + b_3$. As before, Poisson log-linear regression techniques provide estimates of the additive model parameters based on an appropriately constructed design variable (Tables 13–16 and 13–17).

The New York state spina bifida data produce estimates of the four model parameters (a, b_1, b_2, and b_3, Table 13–18) from the seven observations (log-counts).

Of more importance, the estimated model parameters produce an estimate of the number of unobserved cases. The logarithm of the unobserved cell count n_{222} (cases not identified by any of the three sources) is estimated by $log(\hat{n}_{222}) = \hat{a} = 2.759$. The estimate $\hat{a}$ leads directly to an estimate of the number of cases not among the collected data. This estimate is $\hat{n}_{222} = e^{\hat{a}} = e^{2.759} = 15.782$. The estimated population size then becomes the number of observed cases, plus the estimated number of unobserved cases or $\hat{N} = 37 + 15.782 = 52.782$ cases. As before, the model-generated counts can be estimated for all seven cells (Table 13–19), and the goodness-of-fit of the model can be assessed.

Table 13–16. Log-linear model: the complete independence model for the estimation of the population size based on three sources of counts (sources denoted S_1, S_2, and S_3)

S_3	S_2	$\bar{S}_2$
S_1	$log(n_{111}) = a + b_1 + b_2 + b_3$	$log(n_{121}) = a + b_1 + b_3$
$\bar{S}_1$	$log(n_{211}) = a + b_2 + b_3$	$log(n_{221}) = a + b_3$

* = Structural zero.

$\bar{S}_3$	S_2	$\bar{S}_2$
S_1	$log(n_{112}) = a + b_1 + b_2$	$log(n_{122}) = a + b_1$
$\bar{S}_1$	$log(n_{212}) = a + b_2$	$-$*

* = structural zero.

Table 13–17. Details of the design variable used to estimate the parameters for a log-linear model describing three independent sources of spina bifida cases

Notation	Data	a	F_1	F_2	F_3	Model
n_{111}	1	1	1	1	1	$a + b_1 + b_2 + b_3$
n_{211}	8	1	0	1	1	$a + b_2 + b_3$
n_{121}	3	1	1	0	1	$a + b_1 + b_3$
n_{221}	13	1	0	0	1	$a + b_3$
n_{112}	1	1	1	1	0	$a + b_1 + b_2$
n_{212}	3	1	0	1	0	$a + b_2$
n_{122}	8	1	1	0	0	$a + b_1$
n_{222}	$-$*	1	0	0	0	a

* = Structural zero.

Table 13–18. Model-estimated parameters from the New York state spina bifida data

Variables	Terms	Estimates	Std. errors
Constant	a	2.759	0.453
S_1	b_1	−1.118	0.380
S_2	b_2	−1.118	0.380
S_3	b_3	−0.106	0.403

Table 13–19. Model-estimated and observed counts (in parentheses) of spina bifida cases for all eight possible combinations of the three independent sources

S_3	S_2	$\bar{S}_2$		$\bar{S}_3$	S_2	$\bar{S}_2$
S_1	1.52(1)	4.64(3)		S_1	1.69(1)	5.16(8)
$\bar{S}_1$	4.64(8)	14.20(13)		$\bar{S}_1$	5.16(3)	15.78(−)

CATEGORICAL VARIABLE ANALYSIS FROM MATCHED PAIRS DATA

The fundamental purpose of a case–control study is the comparison of the distributions of a risk factor between cases and controls (Chapters 2 and 7). For a matched-pairs categorical variables from a $k \times k$ table, the comparison between distributions of the risk factor is a comparison between the marginal frequencies. Continuing the example from Chapter 7, the comparison of case–control distributions of measures reflecting electromagnetic field (EMF) radiation exposure illustrates the use of a Poisson log-linear model applied to the analysis of categorical matched-pairs data. These EMF data are repeated in Table 13–20.

The comparison of the marginal frequencies from the case–control table is key to assessing the differences in the distributions of EMF exposure (Chapter 7). However, the marginal frequencies must accurately summarize the relationships within the table.

Two contrived examples illustrate marginal frequencies that fail to reflect the distributions associated with the row and column variables (Table 13–21) and marginal frequencies that perfectly duplicate the distributions associated with the row and column variables (Table 13–22). Clearly, the constant marginal frequencies of Table 13–21 do not summarize the row or column distributions within the table. An obvious interaction exists because the distribution of variable A is different at each level of variable B and vice versa.

Table 13–20. The case–control matched pairs array ($N = 126$ pairs, repeated from Chapter 7) displaying childhood leukemia data at three levels of EMF radiation exposure (HCC, OCC, and LCC)

		Control HCC	Control OCC	Control LCC	**Total**
Case	HCC	0	5	17	22
Case	OCC	5	5	11	21
Case	LCC	13	9	61	83
	Total	18	19	89	126

Table 13–21. An illustration of the failure of the marginal frequencies to reflect the row and column relationships (an extreme interaction)

	B_1	B_2	B_3	**Total**
A_1	10	20	30	60
A_2	20	20	20	60
A_3	30	20	10	60
Total	60	60	60	180

Table 13–22. An illustration of marginal frequencies that reflect exactly the row and column relationships (independence, or no interaction, or perfect additivity)

	B_1	B_2	B_{13}	Total
A_1	3	6	9	18
A_2	12	24	36	72
A_3	15	30	45	90
Total	30	60	90	180

Table 13–23. Counts of case–control matched pairs at three levels of EMF radiation exposure with the concordant pairs removed (structural zeros)

		Control HCC	Control OCC	ControlLCC
Case	HCC	–*	5	17
Case	OCC	5	–*	11
Case	LCC	13	9	–*

* = Structural zero.

A necessary condition for the marginal frequencies to summarize accurately the row and column distributions is the independence of the categorical variables (Table 13–22).

That is, each row of the table has the identical distribution as the row marginal frequencies, and each column of the table has the identical distribution as the column marginal frequencies. Thus, the row and column marginal frequencies accurately summarize the distributions of the categorical variables (in Table 13–22, perfectly). The row and column variables are said to be independent or have additive influences or no interaction exists.

A complicating property of matched-pairs data is that the analysis requires the exclusion of the concordant pairs of observations (Table 13–23). The question of independence of row and column variables then applies to a case–control array, with the structural zeros generated by the elimination of the concordant pairs. As before, all that is necessary to assess the question of independence (quasi-independence) of the case–control data is to modify the design variable to account for the absence of the three concordant pairs (structural zeros).

Again, the additive (quasi-independent) log-linear model (details in Table 13–24) is

$$log(cell\text{-}frequency) = log(n_{ij}) = a + r_1R_1 + r_2R_2 + c_1C_1 + c_2C_2.$$

The five model coefficients (a, r_1, r_2, b_1, and b_2) estimated from the six cell frequencies of EMF data (Table 13–23) are based on a Poisson log-linear regression

Table 13–24. Details of the additive log-linear model to assess the quasi-independence of case–control levels of EMF exposure data

Notation	Data	a	R_1	R_2	C_1	C_2	Model
n_{21}	5	1	1	0	0	0	$a + r_1$
n_{31}	13	1	0	1	0	0	$a + r_2$
n_{12}	5	1	0	0	1	0	$a + c_1$
n_{22}	9	1	0	1	1	0	$a + r_2 + c_1$
n_{13}	17	1	0	0	0	1	$a + c_2$
n_{23}	11	1	1	0	0	1	$a + r_1 + c_2$

Table 13–25. Estimated coefficients from a Poisson log-linear model describing the relationships within the case–control array of matched-pair EMF exposure data

Variables	Terms	Estimates	Std. errors
Constant	a	2.013	0.429
Row 2	r_1	−0.422	0.345
Row 3	r_2	0.559	0.424
Column 2	c_1	−0.385	0.375
Column 3	c_2	0.815	0.421

analysis (Table 13–25). These coefficients produce estimated cell-counts that are perfectly quasi-independent.

As before, directly comparing the model-generated values to the observed values indicates the fit of the additive model (quasi-independence) in the presence of structural zeros. The obvious correspondence between the estimated and observed cell counts (Table 13–26) is formally evaluated with the Pearson chi-square test-statistic, or

$$X^2 = \frac{(5 - 4.91)^2}{4.91} + \cdots + \frac{(11 - 11.09)^2}{11.09} = 0.0062.$$

The close correspondence between the data values and the model-generated values indicates that treating the case–control observations as if they are quasi-independent will almost certainly not be misleading. That is, a direct comparison of the marginal frequencies accurately reflects the case–control differences in EMF exposure.

For a 3×3 case–control array of matched-pairs data, symmetry of the cell frequencies, quasi-independence of the categorical variables, and the distribution of the marginal frequencies are related. Under the conjecture that the observed case–control data are random deviations from symmetric values (no association),

Table 13–26. Model-estimated and observed frequencies (in parentheses) of the six combinations of the three levels of EMF radiation exposure data

		Control HCC	Control OCC	Control LCC
Case	HCC	–*	5.09 (5)	16.91 (17)
Case	OCC	4.91 (5)	–*	11.09 (11)
Case	LCC	13.09 (13)	8.91 (9)	–*

* = Structural zero.

Table 13–27. Estimated and observed frequencies (in parentheses) of six combinations of the three levels of EMF exposure derived under the conjecture that the cell frequencies are symmetric (no association, Chapter 7)

		Control HCC	Control OCC	Control LCC
Case	HCC	–*	5.00 (5)	15.00 (17)
Case	OCC	5.00 (5)	–*	10.00 (11)
Case	LCC	15.00(13)	10.00 (9)	–*

* = Structural zero.

the estimated values for the EMF data are given in Table 13–27 (repeated from Chapter 7).

The likelihood ratio chi-square test statistic to assess symmetry is

$$G_S^2 = -2\sum o_{ij} \log\left(\frac{e_{ij}}{o_{ij}}\right) = -2\left[5\log\left(\frac{5}{5}\right) + \cdots + 10\log\left(\frac{10}{11}\right)\right] = 0.735$$

where e_{ij} represents values generated as if the underlying cell counts are symmetric (exactly no case–control differences) and o_{ij} represents the corresponding observed values (Table 13–27). This chi-square statistic G_S^2 (degrees of freedom = 3) is an explicit form of the log-likelihood statistic typically calculated as part of the maximum likelihood parameter estimation process (Chapters 3 and 7).

The chi-square measure of symmetry is the sum of the likelihood ratio chi-square measure of quasi-independence (denoted G_I^2) and the likelihood ratio chi-square measure of marginal homogeneity (denoted G_H^2). In symbols, this partitioned chi-square value is $G_S^2 = G_I^2 + G_H^2$.

Specifically, the quasi-independence likelihood ratio chi-square test-statistic G_I^2 (degrees of freedom = 1) is

$$G_I^2 = -2\sum o_{ij} \log\left(\frac{E_{ij}}{o_{ij}}\right) = -2\left[5\log\left(\frac{4.91}{5}\right) + \cdots + 10\log\left(\frac{11.09}{11}\right)\right] = 0.0062$$

where E_{ij} represents the values generated from the quasi-independence model (Tables 13–25 and 13–26). The likelihood ratio chi-square measure reflecting the difference between marginal distributions (homogeneity) G_H^2 becomes $G_S^2 - G_I^2$. For the EMF exposure data, the log-likelihood statistics $G_S^2 = 0.735$ and $G_I^2 = 0.006$ produce $G_H^2 = 0.735 - 0.006 = 0.729$ (degrees of freedom = 2). The degrees of freedom calculated the usual way are 3, 2, and 1, respectively. Therefore, the definitive assessment of the case–control difference in influence of EMF radiation exposure yields the p-value $= P(G_H^2 \geq 0.729 | no\ association) = 0.695$.

This partitioned chi-square statistic provides a complete description and analysis of categorical matched-pairs data classified into a 3×3 case/control array. The chi-square statistic G_H^2 addresses the fundamental case–control comparison between marginal frequencies, and G_I^2 provides assurance that observed marginal frequencies accurately summarize the distributions of the risk factor for both the cases and controls. Technically, the chi-square statistic, G_I^2, reflects the goodness-of-fit of the additive log-linear model.

QUASI-INDEPENDENCE: ASSOCIATION IN A R × C TABLE

Another example of applying a log-linear regression model to explore the association between two variables contained in a table with structural zeros (quasi-independence) arises in a study of the spread of infectious disease among pre-school children. As part of this investigation, data were collected on the physical distance between children during a "free-play" period. As part of this study, six children were observed on ten different occasions and the child closest ("nearest neighbor") was recored. The primary question becomes: Do pre-school children at play associate at random, or is there a systematic play-time association? A part of the collected data is display in Table 13–28.

Table 13–28. Number of "nearest-neighbor" contacts among six children observed on ten occasions

Child	A	B	C	D	E	F	Total
A	–*	2	2	3	3	2	12
B	2	–*	1	2	1	3	9
C	0	1	–*	1	2	4	8
D	2	3	1	–*	1	3	10
E	2	2	5	1	–*	3	13
F	1	3	2	2	0	–*	8
Total	7	11	11	9	7	15	60

* = Structural zero.

Table 13–29. Estimates of the parameters of the quasi-independence model from the pre-school contact data (6 × 6 table)

Symbol	Estimate	Std. error
a	0.500	0.501
b_1	−0.216	0.449
b_2	−0.338	0.464
b_3	−0.148	0.436
b_4	0.083	0.407
b_5	−0.252	0.467
c_1	0.407	0.492
c_2	0.387	0.492
c_3	0.219	0.513
c_4	0.021	0.544
c_5	0.711	0.467

Structural zeros occur because a child cannot be his or her own nearest neighbor. However, sixty relevant observations remain, and a quasi-independence model accurately summarizes the data when no pattern of association exists among these pre-school children during play-time. An expression for such a log-linear model is

$$log(cell\ frequency) = log(n_{ij}) = a + b_i + c_j$$

when $i \neq j$, $i = 1, 2, \cdots, 5$ and $j = 1, 2, \cdots, 5$. Log-linear model cell frequencies are generated by a combinations of the 11 parameters, a, b_i, and c_j, that are estimated from a Poisson regression model. The design variable is a direct extension of the pattern described previously for two-way tables (Tables 13–11 and 13–24), and the 30 cell frequencies (nondiagonal elements, Table 13–28) allow the calculation of the 11 model coefficients (Table 13–29).

The estimated coefficients produce model-generated cell frequencies that, as required, perfectly conform to the model (Table 13–30). For example, for children D and B, the coefficients are

$$\hat{a} = 0.500, \quad \hat{b}_3 = -0.148 \text{ and } \hat{c}_1 = 0.407, \text{ yielding}$$

$$log(\hat{n}_{42}) = \hat{a} + \hat{b}_3 + \hat{c}_1 = 0.500 - 0.148 + 0.407 = 0.759.$$

Then, the model-dictated number of "close contacts" becomes $n_{42} = e^{0.759} = 2.137$. That is, the number of "nearest-neighbor" contacts between child D and child B are calculated to be 2.137 when these ten children associate completely at random (quasi-independence). The observed number observed is 3.

Comparing the observed counts (Table 13–28) and the model-generated counts (Table 13–30) with a chi-square test statistic yields the value $X^2 = 12.943$ (degrees of freedom $= 30 - 11 = 19$) and a p-value of 0.841. Thus, the log-linear

Table 13–30. Model-estimated number of nearest-neighbor contacts among six children observed on ten occasions when no pattern of association exists (quasi-independence)

Child	A	B	C	D	E	F	Total
A	–*	2.48	2.43	2.05	1.68	3.36	12
B	1.33	–*	1.96	1.65	1.36	2.71	9
C	1.18	1.77	–*	1.46	1.20	2.39	8
D	1.42	2.14	2.09	–*	1.45	2.90	10
E	1.79	2.69	2.64	2.23	–*	3.65	13
F	1.28	1.93	1.89	1.60	1.31	–*	8
Total	7	11	11	9	7	15	60

* = Structural zero.

model analysis provides no evidence of a pattern of association among the six observed pre-school children at play.

THE ANALYSIS OF A THREE-WAY TABLE

A two-way table naturally becomes a three-way table by adding a third categorical variable. A three-way table (sometimes called a three-dimensional table) illustrates most of the issues that arise in a log-linear regression analysis applied to multidimensional tables. For the following, categorical variables are represented by A with k levels, B with l levels, and C with m levels. A table created from these variables contains $N = k \times l \times m$ cell frequencies, each denoted n_{ijk}. Table 13–31 is an example of a three-way table from a study of weight gained during pregnancy, consisting of A = two levels of weight retention 6 weeks after pregnancy ($k = 2$), B = three levels of prepregnancy weight ($l = 3$), and C = four levels of parity ($m = 4$) producing $N = 2 \times 3 \times 3 = 24$ cell frequencies (details follow).

Three-way tables are conveniently distinguished by four kinds of relationships among the categorical variables. They are:

1. When all three pairs of categorical variables are independent (denoted: $AB = AC = BC = 0$), the variables are said to be *completely independent*.
2. When two pairs of categorical variables are independent (for example, $AC = BC = 0$), the variables are said to be *jointly independent*.
3. When one pair of categorical variables is independent (for example, $AB = 0$), the variables are said to be *conditionally independent*.
4. When all three pairs of categorical variables are related but each pairwise association is not influenced by the remaining third variable, the variables are said to have *additive associations*.

Table 13–31. A sample of $n = 701$ mothers classified by weight retained 6 weeks after pregnancy (two levels), prepregnancy weight (three levels), and parity (four levels)

Prepregnancy weight 50 kilograms or less:

	Parity				
	0	1	2	≥ 3	**Total**
Retained < 20 kg	20	40	14	62	136
Retained ≥ 20 kg	5	10	3	17	35
Total	25	50	17	79	171

Prepregnancy weight between 50 and 60 kilograms:

	Parity				
	0	1	2	≥ 3	**Total**
Retained < 20 kg	29	138	17	42	226
Retained ≥ 20 kg	7	32	4	11	54
Total	36	170	21	53	280

Prepregnancy weight 60 kilograms or more:

	Parity				
	0	1	2	≥ 3	**Total**
Retained < 20 kg	23	117	22	9	171
Retained ≥ 20 kg	11	54	11	3	79
Total	34	171	33	12	250

Therefore, eight possible relationships exist within tables constructed from three categorical variables.

As with the previous log-linear regression models, the analyses involve the relationships among the log-frequencies and three categorical variables defined by a design variable. Again, the models are not a description of the observed influences of independent variables on a specific outcome variable but are made up of components of design variables that are treated as "independent variables." Thus, the model provides estimated cell frequencies (independent variable) based on values of design variables (dependent variables) to explore specific relationships among the categorical variables. The primary question becomes: What are the important (nonrandom) relationships among the categorical variables?

To illustrate, four $2 \times 2 \times 2$ tables of fictional data are created that perfectly conform to the four kinds of relationships ($k = l = m = 2$). These simplest of three-way tables have most of the properties of more extensive multidimensional tables that are not as easily described. For example, odds ratios are effective measures of association in a $2 \times 2 \times 2$ table and are less useful for higher-dimensional tables.

COMPLETE INDEPENDENCE

A log-linear regression model describing *complete independence* among three binary categorical variables is

$$log(cell\ frequency) = b_0 + b_1 F_1 + b_2 F_2 + b_3 F_3$$

where F_1 is a binary indicator variable $\{0, 1\}$ identifying the two levels of variable A, F_2 is a binary indicator variable $\{0, 1\}$ identifying the two levels of variable B, and F_3 is a binary indicator variable $\{0, 1\}$ identifying the two levels of variable C. Data displaying three binary categorical variables in a $2 \times 2 \times 2$ table that perfectly conform to a complete independence model are:

C_1	B_1	B_2	Total
A_1	1	6	7
A_2	4	24	28
Total	5	30	35

C_2	B_1	B_2	Total
A_1	5	30	35
A_2	20	120	140
Total	25	150	175

$C_1 + C_2$	B_1	B_2	Total
A_1	6	36	42
A_2	24	144	168
Total	30	180	210

From the example, when $F_1 = 1$, $F_2 = 0$, and $F_3 = 1$, the logarithm of the model cell frequency $log(n_{212})$ is represented by $b_0 + b_1 + b_3$, and the observed value denoted n_{212} is 20 (A_2, B_1, and C_2). The primary feature of a table consisting of three completely independent variables is that a table is not needed. The variables simply do not influence each other in any way. Some examples are,

$$P(A_1) = P(A_1|B_1, C_1) = P(A_1|B_2) = P(A_1|B_1, C_2) = P(A_1|C_2)$$
$$= P(A_1|B_1, C_1 + C_2) = P(A_1|\ B_1 + B_2) = 0.2.$$

The probabilities $P(B_1) = 0.143$ and $P(C_1) = 0.167$ follow a similar pattern. From another point of view, the odds ratios are 1.0 in all possible 2×2 subtables. In short, every element of the three-way table is determined by the product of three independent probabilities (for example, $n_{121} = 210(0.2)(0.857)(0.167) = 6$ or

$n_{212} = 210(0.8)(0.143)(0.833) = 20)$ because every log-frequency in the table is a sum of three coefficients. Once again, when log-values have additive relationships, the values themselves have multiplicative relationships, and vice versa. Keep in mind that these relationships are exact because artificial values are created to fit the model perfectly.

JOINT INDEPENDENCE

One of three possible log-linear models describing the *joint independence* of three categorical variables is

$$log(cell\ frequency) = b_0 + b_1F_1 + b_2F_2 + b_3F_3 + b_{12}(F_1 \times F_2) \qquad (AB \neq 0)$$

where the three indicator variables F_i are defined as before. The interaction term in the model allows for the possibility of an association, namely variable A associated with variable B. Data displaying three categorical variables that perfectly conform to the joint independence model are:

C_1	B_1	B_2	Total
A_1	1	6	7
A_2	4	48	52
Total	5	54	59

C_2	B_1	B_2	Total
A_1	4	24	28
A_2	16	192	208
Total	20	216	236

$C_1 + C_2$	B_1	B_2	Total
A_1	5	30	35
A_2	20	240	260
Total	25	270	295

A consequence of joint independence is that a single two-way table describes the only relationship relevant to the three categorical variables. In the example, variables A and C, as well as B and C, are independent ($AC = BC = 0$). A table created by adding the C_1-table and the C_2-table forms a single table that accurately reflects the AB association. That is, because the variable C is independent of variables A and B, it is not relevant to their relationship. The two subtables (C_1-table and C_2-table) are no more than multiples of the AB-table. The only difference between the tables including and excluding the variable C is the number of observations. In the example, the four elements of the two subtables are 20% of the AB-table ($59/295 = 0.2$) in the C_1-table and 80% ($236/295 = 0.8$) in the C_2-table. Thus, the variable C has no confounding influence. In terms of odds ratios,

$$or_{AB|C_1} = or_{AB|C_2} = or_{AB} = 2, \; or_{AC|B_1} = or_{AC|B_2} = or_{AC} = 1 \text{ and}$$
$$or_{BC|A_1} = or_{BC|A_2} = or_{BC} = 1.$$

A basic property of a log-linear model analysis of tabular data is apparent from this example. The two-way interaction term in the log-linear model measures the magnitude of the joint influence of two categorical variables (interaction = associated). Thus, the regression model coefficient b_{12} directly reflects the lack of independence between variables A and B. Variables A and B are independent only when $b_{12} = 0$, producing a completely additive model (model 1). Therefore, the assessment of the AB-association in a three-way table becomes a statistical assessment of the estimated regression coefficient $\hat{b}_{12}$ in the usual way.

Similar log-linear models exist where the variable A is independent of the variables B and C, and variable B is independent of the variables A and C. Specifically, the log-linear models are

$$log(cell \; frequency) = b_0 + b_1 F_1 + b_2 F_2 + b_3 F_3 + b_{23}(F_2 \times F_3)$$
$$(AB = AC = 0 \text{ and } BC \neq 0)$$

and

$$log(cell \; frequency) = b_0 + b_1 F_1 + b_2 F_2 + b_3 F_3 + b_{13}(F_1 \times F_3)$$
$$(AB = BC = 0 \text{ and } AC \neq 0).$$

Again, the extent of the pairwise association is measured by the magnitude of the interaction identified by the log-linear model coefficients, namely b_{23} or b_{13}.

CONDITIONAL INDEPENDENCE

One of the three possible log-linear models describing *conditional independence* of three categorical variables is

$$log(cell \; frequency) = b_0 + b_1 F_1 + b_2 F_2 + b_3 F_3 + b_{13}(F_1 \times F_3)$$
$$+ b_{23}(F_2 \times F_3) \quad (AC \neq BC \neq 0)$$

where the three indicator variables F_i are defined, as before. The model coefficients b_{13} and b_{23} again reflect the lack of independence. The following tables display three categorical variables that perfectly conform to the conditional independence model, where only variables A and B are unrelated $(AB = 0)$:

C_1	B_1	B_2	Total
A_1	1	6	7
A_2	4	24	28
Total	5	30	35

C_2	B_1	B_2	Total
A_1	4	96	100
A_2	40	960	1000
Total	44	1056	1100

B_1+B_2	C_1	C_2	Total
A_1	7	100	107
A_2	28	1000	1028
Total	35	1100	1135

A_1+A_2	B_1	B_2	Total
C_1	5	30	35
C_2	44	1056	1100
Total	49	1086	1135

In the case of conditional independence, two-way tables created from a three-way table by adding over the levels of either of the two variables that are independent (A or B in the example) produce summary tables that do not bias the estimation of the two-way associations. For the example tables, these kinds of tables are created by adding over the two levels of variables A or over the two levels of variable B ($AB = 0$). The underlying relationship between the two categorical variables within these collapsed tables is the same as within the three-way table but in simpler form. Specifically, for the example tables collapsed over the variable B yield

$$or_{AC|B_1} = or_{AC|B_2} = or_{AC|(B_1+B_2)} = or_{AC} = \frac{7/100}{28/1000} = 2.5$$

and collapsed over the variable A yield

$$or_{BC|A_1} = or_{BC|A_2} = or_{BC|(A_1+A_2)} = or_{BC} = \frac{5/30}{44/1056} = 4.0.$$

The strategy of collapsing tables over variables that are independent applies to tables of any dimension and is an extremely effective technique for understanding and presenting tabular data. The identification of unimportant variables is frequently a goal of statistical analysis in general. The log-linear model is a statistical tool designed to guide this strategy for categorical data.

Similar log-linear regression models exist when only variables A and C are independent ($AC = 0$) and when only variables B and C are independent ($BC = 0$). They are:

$$log(cell\ frequency) = b_0 + b_1F_1 + b_2F_2 + b_3F_3 + b_{12}(F_1 \times F_2)$$
$$+ b_{23}(F_2 \times F_3) \qquad (AB \neq BC \neq 0)$$

and

$$log(cell\ frequency) = b_0 + b_1F_1 + b_2F_2 + b_3F_3 + b_{12}(F_1 \times F_2)$$
$$+ b_{13}(F_1 \times F_3) \qquad (AB \neq AC \neq 0).$$

ADDITIVE MEASURES OF ASSOCIATION

A log-linear regression model describing *additive measures of association* for three categorical variables is

$$log(cell\ frequency) = b_0 + b_1F_1 + b_2F_2 + b_3F_3 + b_{12}(F_1 \times F_2) + b_{13}(F_1 \times F_3)$$
$$+ b_{23}(F_2 \times F_3)$$

where the three indicator variables F_i are once again defined, as before. Artificial data displaying three categorical variables that perfectly conform to an additive association model are:

C_1	B_1	B_2	Total
A_1	1	6	7
A_2	4	48	52
Total	5	54	59

C_2	B_1	B_2	Total
A_1	4	96	100
A_2	40	1920	1960
Total	44	2016	2060

In the case of additive associations, no useful two-way table is created by collapsing the three-way table by adding over the levels of either of the other variables. However, because the two-way interaction terms (measures of association) are themselves additive, they allow separate evaluations of each pairwise relationships. That is, the interaction terms do not interact. As with additivity in general, the model regression coefficients b_{12}, b_{13}, and b_{23} measure separate pairwise associations unaffected by the third variable. For example, the coefficient b_{12} indicates the magnitude of an association between variables A and B unaffected by the level of the variable C. In general, for a three-way table, the association between any pair of categorical variables can be assessed without regard to possible influences of the third variable when the measures of association are additive. To repeat, the interaction terms measure association between a pair of variables (lack of additivity), and additivity of the interaction terms guarantees that any two-way association is the same regardless of the level of the third variable. Specifically, for the example data,

$$or_{AB|C_1} = or_{AB|C_2} = 2, \quad or_{AC|B_1} = or_{AC|B_2} = 2.5 \quad \text{and} \quad or_{BC|A_1} = or_{BC|A_2} = 4.$$

The last possible log-linear model is

$$log(cell\ frequency) = b_0 + b_1F_1 + b_2F_2 + b_3F_3 + b_{12}(F_1 \times F_2)$$
$$+ b_{13}(F_1 \times F_3) + b_{23}(F_2 \times F_3)$$
$$+ b_{123}(F_1 \times F_2 \times F_3).$$

The "third-order" interaction coefficient (b_{123}) measures the degree of nonadditivity among the pairwise interaction terms. For example, the influence of the AB-term can be expressed as $[(b_{12} + b_{123}F_3) \times (F_1 \times F_2)]$ and, therefore, the degree of association between variables A and B is influenced by the level of variable C ($b_{123} \neq 0$). Including the three-way interaction terms makes the log-linear regression model saturated (parameters = number of cells in the table = 8, in the example).

Returning to the weight-retention data (Table 13–31), an inspection of the cell frequencies suggests that the level of parity does not influence the relationship between weight retention and prepregnancy weight. The ratio of the numbers of mothers in the two retention categories is nearly constant for the four levels of parity within each of the three prepregnancy weight categories. This lack of variation suggests that parity has little influence on weight retention (independence), and potentially, a much simpler table can be created by collapsing the data over the levels of the parity. The log-linear model that addresses this specific case of conditional independence is

$$log - frequency = \mu + r + w + p + r^*w + p^*w \qquad (r^*p^*w = r^*p = 0)$$

where the symbols r (retention), w (prepregnancy weight), and p (parity) represent three design variables that describe the relationships among the categorical variables within the three-dimensional table. In more detail, the design variables are:

- Weight retention (two components, $k = 2$)

Variables	Categories	Design variables
Retention (r):	<20 kg	$x = 0$
Retention (r):	≥20 kg	$x = 1$

- Maternal prepregnancy weight (three components, $l = 3$)

Variables	Categories	Design variables
Prepregnancy weight (w):	<50 kg	$y_1 = 0$ and $y_2 = 0$
Prepregnancy weight (w):	50 to 60 kg	$y_1 = 1$ and $y_2 = 0$
Prepregnancy weight (w):	>60 kg	$y_1 = 0$ and $y_2 = 1$.

- Parity (four components, $m = 4$)

Variables	Categories	Design variables
Parity (p):	parity = 0	$z_1 = 0, z_2 = 0$ and $z_3 = 0$
Parity (p):	parity = 1	$z_1 = 1, z_2 = 0$ and $z_3 = 0$
Parity (p):	parity = 2	$z_1 = 0, z_2 = 1$ and $z_3 = 0$
Parity (p):	parity ≥ 3	$z_1 = 0, z_2 = 0$ and $z_3 = 1$

Table 13–32. Estimated model coefficients from the log-linear model postulating conditional independence of parity and weight retention ($r^*p^*w = r^*p = 0$)

Terms	Estimates	Std. errors
a	2.990	0.204
r_2	−1.357	0.190
w_2	0.379	0.265
w_3	0.157	0.270
p_2	0.693	0.245
p_3	−0.386	0.314
p_4	1.151	0.229
$r_2 \times w_2$	−0.074	0.243
$r_2 \times w_3$	0.585	0.233
$w_2 \times p_2$	0.859	0.306
$w_3 \times p_3$	0.922	0.309
$w_2 \times p_3$	−0.153	0.417
$w_3 \times p_3$	0.356	0.398
$w_2 \times p_4$	−0.764	0.315
$w_3 \times p_4$	−2.192	0.407

Table 13–33. Mothers classified by weight retained 6 weeks after delivery and prepregnancy weight ($n = 701$, additive model generated values in parenthesis*)

	Less than 50 kg	50–60 kg	More than 60 kg	**Total**
Less than 20 kg	136 (130.1)	226 (213.0)	171 (190.0)	533
More than 20 kg	35 (40.9)	54 (67.0)	79 (60.0)	168
Total	171	280	250	701

* $= log(n_{ij}) = a + b_1F_1 + b_2F_2$.

The model postulates that the three categorical variables have additive associations ($r^*p^*w = 0$), and weight retention and parity are independent ($r^*p = 0$). The estimated coefficients of the log-linear model are given in Table 13–32.

The likelihood ratio chi-square test statistic of $X^2 = -2(-0.283) = 0.566$ yields a p-value of 0.999 (degrees of freedom $= 24 - 15 = 9$). From a goodness-of-fit point of view, the small log-likelihood value (large p-value) means that the model values generated under the hypothesis that parity does not influence weight retention closely correspond to the observed values. The degrees of freedom are the number of model parameters subtracted from the number of cells in the table ($24 - 15 = 9$). Because the log-linear model ($r^*p^*w = r^*p = 0$) accurately represents the relationships within the three-way table, it is not misleading and it is certainly advantageous to create the far simpler 2×3 table by combining the four parity levels and evaluating relationships between weight gained and prepregnancy weight from a two-way table (2×3).

The collapsed table (Table 13–33) is more intuitive, simplifies the evaluation, and allows a graphic representation of the association between weight retention and maternal prepregnancy weight. The analysis of a three-way table provides assurance that the two-way table relationships are not influenced by parity. That is, parity does not have a substantial influence on the retention–gain relationship.

The usual application of the chi-square test to assess the independence of weight retention (two levels) and prepregnancy weight (three levels) is straightforward (Chapter 2). The Pearson chi-square test statistic comparing the observed and expected values is $X^2 = 12.510$ (degrees of freedom = 2), and the associated p-value is $P(X^2 \geq 12.510 | no\ association) = 0.002$.

Essentially, the same result emerges from applying the log-linear model

$$log-frequency + \mu + r + w + p + r^*p + p^*w \qquad (r^*p^*w = w^*r = 0).$$

to the three-way table. The corresponding likelihood ratio test statistic is $G^2 = 11.652$ with a p-value $= 0.003$.

A visual display of a two-way table is suggested by fact that the logarithms of the cell frequencies are described by an additive model when categorical variables are independent. Geometrically, additive models produce lines separated by constant distances. The log-frequencies from Table 13–31 and the corresponding values generated by the additive model (logarithms of the values in parentheses) are plotted in Figure 13–3.

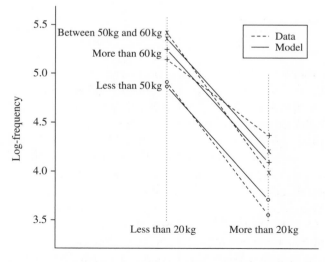

Figure 13–3. Additive model (solid lines) and observed log-frequencies (dashed lines) from the example weight retention data (Table 13–32).

The extent to which the lines generated by the logarithms of the cell frequencies are not parallel (dashed lines compared to solid lines, Figure 13–3) provides an intuitive and sometimes useful description of the lack of independence between the categorical variables. A chi-square statistic measures the lack of independence, and a plot of the logarithms of the cell frequencies potentially identifies the pattern of any dependency among the categorical variables.

The first step in describing the associations in a three-way table is to evaluate the possibility of additive pairwise associations. Analysis begins with a focus on the three-way interaction ($ABC = 0?$). When substantial three-way interactions exist, the pairwise terms of the model are not separate measures of the association between pairs of categorical variables (as noted). In other words, the association between any two variables depends on the levels of the third variable. The log-linear model regression coefficients, b_{ij}, therefore, do not directly measure the two-way associations and are not simply interpreted.

The log-likelihood value associated with a log-linear model with third-order terms removed ($b_{123} = 0$) is the key to summarization. When the log-likelihood ratio test statistic indicates that nonadditivity plays a substantial role in describing the data, separate tables are necessary to accurately assess the pairwise associations. However, when no evidence emerges that a three-way interaction plays an important role, it is usual to behave as if the pairwise interaction terms in the log-linear model provide a single, simple, and separate summary of each pairwise association (additivity).

Again dietary data serve to illustrate. From a study of birth defects and dietary risk factors [42], it was important to describe the relationships between race/ethnicity (r), vitamin use (v), and level of dietary fat consumption (f) (Table 13–34). Specifically, these data consist of 758 mothers classified by three levels of race/ethnicity (white, African-American, and Hispanic), three levels of vitamin use (as before; never used, used only during pregnancy, and used always), and two levels of reported fat consumption (below the median and above the median).

The results from applying all eight possible log-linear models are shown in Table 13–35. Of particular analytic importance are the likelihood ratio test statistics (column 5) associated with each model. The first model postulates that three-way interaction terms are unnecessary ($rfv = 0$, model 1). The log-likelihood value that reflects the difference between this model and the fully saturated model (log-likelihood $= 0$) is small and entirely consistent with random variation. The likelihood ratio chi-square test statistic $G^2 = -2(-0.656) = 1.312$ with four degrees of freedom yields a p-value of $P(G^2 \geq 1.312 | rvf = 0) = 0.859$.

In light of no evidence of a substantial three-way association, the three models formed by removing the pairwise associations one at time from the additive model reflects the separate strength and significance of each association. Thus, each model with one of the pairwise interaction terms removed ($rv = 0$ or $rf = 0$ or

Table 13–34. Mothers of infants with birth defects classified by three levels of race/ethnicity, three levels of vitamin use and two levels of dietary fat ($n = 758$)

Below median fat consumption level:

	Never	During	Always	**Total**
White	35	70	115	220
African-American	9	7	32	48
Hispanic	54	5	48	107
Total	98	82	195	375

Above median fat consumption level:

	Never	During	Always	**Total**
White	44	58	112	214
African-American	23	11	41	75
Hispanic	54	5	35	94
Total	121	74	118	383

$vf = 0$) yields a likelihood ratio evaluation of the influence of the removed term when compared to the log-linear model containing all three additive interaction terms ($rvf = 0$, model 1).

The race–vitamin analysis ($rv = 0$, model 2) shows by far the strongest association (model 2 compared to model 1, likelihood ratio test statistic = $G^2 = 112.930$ and a p-value <0.001). Similarly, the race–fat analysis ($rf = 0$, model 3) shows an important but weaker association (model 3 compared to model 1, likelihood ratio test statistic $G^2 = 8.314$ and a p-value of 0.016). And, finally the vitamin–fat analysis ($vf = 0$, model 4) shows no evidence of an important association (model 4 compared to model 1, likelihood ratio test statistic = $G^2 = 4.373$ and a p-value 0.112). All degrees of freedom equal the difference between the degrees of freedom from each of the compared models.

Other comparisons among the eight log-likelihood values in Table 13–35 yield similar results. For example, model 7 compared to model 8 also reflects the vitamin–fat association (likelihood ratio test statistic = $G^2 = -2[-61.956 - (-60.529)] = 2.872$ and a p-value = 0.238). However, the least complicated comparison is between the models that differ by only one pairwise association from the model containing all pairwise associations.

It should be noted that the linear effect terms in all eight models (r, v, and f terms) are not of analytic importance. Their magnitude is determined by the observed frequencies of the variables in the sampled data. Thus, log-linear model analysis of categorical variables (tables) is essentially a study of interactions.

Table 13–35. Summary of all eight possible log-linear models applied applied to assess the relationships among race/ethnicity, vitamin use, and dietary fat consumption

Model	Hypothesis	Log-likelihood	df^*	Test statistic	df^{**}	p-Value
Additive independence						
1.	$rvf = 0$	−0.656	4	1.312	4	0.859
Conditional independence						
2.	$rv = 0$	−57.121	8	112.930	4	< 0.001
3.	$rf = 0$	−4.813	6	8.314	2	0.016
4.	$vf = 0$	−2.842	6	4.373	2	0.112
Joint independence						
5.	$rf = vf = 0$	−6.250	8	11.188	4	0.025
6.	$rv = vf = 0$	−58.558	10	115.804	6	< 0.001
7.	$rv = rf = 0$	−60.529	10	119.745	6	< 0.001
Complete independence						
8.	$rv = rf = vf = 0$	−61.965	12	122.619	8	< 0.001

$* = df$ = degrees of freedom = 18 − (number of model parameters).
$** = df$ = difference in degrees of freedom between compared models.

The analysis of the race–vitamin–diet data illustrates the process of evaluating tabular data with log-linear models by contrasting log-likelihood values (likelihood ratio tests) to select a model that simply but usefully represents the relationships under investigation.   The likelihood values provide a guide to the selection of a single analytic model among the kinds previously described (complete independence, joint independence, conditional independence, and no interaction models). As with most other regression tools, the selected model then provides a rigorous assessment of the influence of sampling variation and, in addition, frequently produces efficient and parsimonious summary descriptions of the relationships among the observed categorical variables.

14

MISCLASSIFICATION: A DETAILED DESCRIPTION OF A SIMPLE CASE

When a binary risk factor is classified into categories created by a binary disease outcome, the resulting 2×2 table is fundamental to the study of the likelihood of disease (Chapter 1). However, the risk factor could be misclassified, the disease outcome could be misclassified, or both, making interpretation of data contained in the 2×2 table difficult and likely misleading.

EXAMPLE: MISCLASSIFICATION OF THE DISEASE STATUS

A clinical trial [43] was conducted to evaluate a specific diet (excluding methylxanthines) thought to reduced the severity of benign breast disease. The nurse who evaluated the progression of the disease, however, knew from laboratory tests whether the patient in fact complied to the diet. This knowledge possibly leads to misclassification of disease status because of a tendency to think the diet is effective, sometimes called *observer bias*. Patients on the diet could be occasionally misclassified as "improved" and patients not on the diet as "not improvement" based on either a conscious or unconscious bias of the examiner and not the actual progression of the disease.

EXAMPLE: MISCLASSIFICATION OF THE RISK FACTOR STATUS

In a case–control study of childhood leukemia, mothers were asked to recall sources of exposure to potentially toxic household materials during their pregnancy. It is possible that mothers of cases are more focused and motivated to remember such exposures than mothers of controls because of the experience of having a child with leukemia. Thus, misclassification of the exposure status (the risk factor) could possibly lead to over-reporting from mothers of cases or under-reporting from mothers of controls. Such a misclassification of the risk factor status is called *recall bias*.

In general, misclassification is undetectable, and realistic statistical corrections are rarely possible. Clearly, the best strategy is to avoid misclassification whenever possible. The following discussion of the consequences of misclassification addresses the situation in which only the disease is subject to misclassification. The misclassification of risk factor status or misclassification of both risk factor and disease outcome present essentially the same issues.

To define and explore the properties of misclassification, the disease outcome is denoted by D and the declared disease outcome by "D". For example, the true underlying probability of correctly identifying a disease is denoted $P(D)$ and the probability of the actual classification of disease status is denoted $P("D")$. When $P(D)=P("D")$, no misclassification bias is present.

Two useful terms are *sensitivity* and *specificity*. Sensitivity is defined as the probability of correctly identifying individuals with the disease among those individuals with the disease (denoted p). In symbols,

$$sensitivity = P("D"|D) = p.$$

Similarly, specificity is defined as the probability of correctly identifying individuals who are disease-free among individuals who are disease-free (denoted P). In symbols,

$$specificity = P("\overline{D}"|\overline{D}) = P.$$

These two terms have applications in a number of statistical contexts and are further developed in the following sections.

Two kinds of misclassification of disease status exist, one called *nondifferential* and the other *differential misclassification*. Nondifferential misclassification of disease status occurs when specificity and sensitivity are identical for individuals with and without the risk factor. Differential misclassification occurs when these two probabilities differ depending on the presence/absence of the risk factor. Nondifferential misclassification is more tractable statistically but rarely occurs. More frequently, like the two examples, the likelihood of misclassification is influenced by risk factor or disease status.

When misclassification is present, four outcomes occur with respect to classifying disease status. They are:

- The disease is present (D) and is stated as present ("D"),
- The disease is present (D) and is stated as absent ("$\overline{D}$"),
- The disease is absent ($\overline{D}$) and is stated as present ("D"), and
- The disease is absent ($\overline{D}$) and is stated as absent ("$\overline{D}$").

For example, when the disease is present and it is stated as present, the probability is $P(D\,and\,"D") = P("D")P(D|"D") = P(D)P("D"|D) = P(D)p$. Therefore, four probabilities with respect to misclassification of disease outcome are expressed as:

$$\bullet\,P(D\text{ and }"D") = P(D)p,$$
$$\bullet\,P(D\text{ and }"\overline{D}") = P(D)(1-p),$$
$$\bullet\,P(\overline{D}\text{ and }"D") = P(\overline{D})(1-P),\text{ and}$$
$$\bullet\,P(\overline{D}\text{ and }"\overline{D}") = P(\overline{D})P,$$

indicating the roles of sensitivity and specificity in a 2×2 table.

Tables 14–1 and 14–2 present the formal descriptions of individuals classified by disease status for those with the risk factor and those without the risk factor. To repeat, the possibility exists that the sensitivity (p) and specificity (P) differ between risk factor present and risk factor absent groups (nondifferential

Table 14–1. Risk factor present: the notation and description of the classification of disease (D)

Risk factor present

	D	$\overline{D}$	**Total**
"D"	$P(D)p$	$P(\overline{D})(1-P)$	$P(D)p+P(\overline{D})(1-P)$
"$\overline{D}$"	$P(D)(1-p)$	$P(\overline{D})P$	$p(D)(1-p)+P(\overline{D})P$
Total	$P(D)$	$P(\overline{D})$	1.0

Table 14–2. Risk factor absent: the notation and description of the classification of disease (D)

Risk factor absent

	D	$\overline{D}$	**Total**
"D"	$P(D)p'$	$P(\overline{D})(1-P')$	$P(D)p'+P(\overline{D})(1-P')$
"$\overline{D}$"	$P(D)(1-p')$	$P(\overline{D})P'$	$P(D)(1-p')+P(\overline{D})P'$
Total	$P(D)$	$P(\overline{D})$	1.0

Note: again $p' = $ sensitivity $= P("D"|\overline{D})$ and $P' = $ specificity $= P("D"|\overline{D})$.

Table 14–3.   The true and declared status with the possibility of misclassification of disease status (p and $p' =$ sensitivity and P and $P' =$ specificity)

True status

	D	$\overline{D}$
Risk factor present	A	B
Risk factor absent	C	D

Declared status

	"D"	"$\overline{D}$"
Risk factor present	$Ap + B(1 - P)$	$A(1 - p) + BP$
Risk factor absent	$Cp' + D(1 - P')$	$C(1 - P') + DP'$

misclassification or $p \neq p'$ and $P \neq P'$). Combining the these two tables creates Table 14–3, which displays the distribution of individuals classified by declared disease status ("D" or "$\overline{D}$") and risk factor status when misclassification of disease status is present. For example, the number of individuals declared to have the disease among those who have the risk factor is the sum of those individuals correctly identified as having the disease $[P(D)p]$ plus those without the disease who are misclassified as having the disease $[P(\overline{D})(1 - P)]$ (the sum of the first row in Table 14–1). The other three combinations are similar mixtures of correctly and incorrectly classified individuals (Table 14–1 and 14–2).

A FEW ILLUSTRATIONS OF MISCLASSIFICATION

Nondifferential misclassification always produces a conservative estimate of the odds ratio. It is said that "nondifferential misclassification biases the odds ratio toward the null." Two examples illustrate this attenuation of an estimated odds ratio. The unobserved underlying distribution of 1800 individuals is given in Table 14–4 labeled "TRUE STATUS" and yields an odds ratio of $or = 2.50$. Nondifferential misclassification leads to the odds ratio of 1.65 ($p = p' = 0.8$ and $P = P' = 0.9$).

When the underlying odds ratio is less than 1, nondifferential misclassification increases the observed odds ratio (Table 14–5). A "true" odds ratio of $or = 0.40$ when no misclassification is present, increases to $\hat{o}r = 0.55$ when nondifferential misclassification is present (again, $p = p' = 0.8$ and $P = P' = 0.9$).

When misclassification is differential, the observed odds ratio increases or decreases relative to the underlying odds ratio, and no general rule exists to predict the direction of this bias. Table 14–6 illustrates the situation in which the underlying odds ratio is $or = 3.5$ ($p = p' = P = P' = 1.0$) and differential misclassification ($p = 0.9, P = 0.6, p' = 0.7$ and $P' = 0.9$) produces an observed odds ratio of $\hat{o}r = 6.0$.

Table 14–4. An example of nondifferential misclassification where $p = p' = 0.8$ and $P = P' = 0.9$

True status

	D	$\overline{D}$
Risk factor present	1000	200
Risk factor absent	400	200

$or = 2.50$

Risk factor present	D	$\overline{D}$	**Total**
"D"	800	20	820
"$\overline{D}$"	200	180	380
Total	1000	200	1200
Probabilities	0.8/0.2	0.1/0.9	

Risk factor absent	D	$\overline{D}$	**Total**
"D"	320	20	340
"$\overline{D}$"	80	180	260
Total	400	200	600
Probabilities	0.8/0.2	0.1/0.9	

Declared status

	"D"	"$\overline{D}$"	**Total**
Risk factor present	820	380	1200
Risk factor absent	340	260	600
Total	1160	640	1800

$\hat{o}r = 1.65$

Table 14–5. An example of nondifferential misclassification where $p = p' = 0.8$ and $P = P' = 0.9$

True status

	D	$\overline{D}$
Risk factor present	200	1000
Risk factor absent	100	200

$or = 0.40$

Risk factor present	D	$\overline{D}$	**Total**
"D"	160	100	260
"$\overline{D}$"	40	900	940
Total	200	1000	1200
Probabilities	0.8/0.2	0.1/0.9	

Risk factor absent	D	$\overline{D}$	**Total**
"D"	80	20	100
"$\overline{D}$"	20	180	200
Total	100	200	300
Probabilities	0.8/0.2	0.1/0.9	

Table 14–5. (Continued)

Declared status

	"D"	"D̄"	Total
Risk factor present	260	940	1200
Risk factor absent	100	200	300
Total	360	1140	1500

$\hat{o}r = 0.55$

Table 14–6. An example of differential misclassification where $p = 0.9$, $p' = 0.7$, $P = 0.6$ and $P' = 0.9$

True status

	D	D̄
Risk factor present	600	400
Risk factor absent	300	700

$or = 3.5$

Risk factor present	D	D̄	Total
"D"	540	160	700
"D̄"	60	240	300
Total	600	400	1000
Probabilities	0.9/0.1	0.3/0.7	

Risk factor absent	D	D̄	Total
"D"	210	70	280
"D̄"	90	630	720
Total	300	700	1000
Probabilities	0.6/0.4	0.1/0.9	

Declared status

	"D"	"D̄"	Total
Risk factor present	700	300	1000
Risk factor absent	280	720	1000
Total	980	1020	2000

$\hat{o}r = 6.0$

It is certainly no surprise that misclassification can bias estimated summary values in a large variety of ways. Two examples demonstrate that misclassification in a 2×2 table can badly distort the underlying risk–disease relationship. In the first example (Table 14–7), an underlying interaction between a risk factor F and a variable C disappears when the data are misclassified. Specifically, when no misclassification occurs, the "true" odds ratios are $or_{DF|C} = 3.2$ and $or_{DF|\bar{C}} = 5.0$, but in the presence of misclassification both observed odds ratios become essentially equal to 1.8 ($\hat{o}r_{DF|C} = \hat{o}r_{DF|\bar{C}} = 1.8$).

Table 14–7. An example of nondifferential misclassification causing an interaction between risk factor F and variable C to disappear when $p = 0.7$, $p' = 0.9$, $P = 0.4$, and $P' = 0.8$

True status

Risk factor C present	D	$\overline{D}$	Total
Risk factor F present	900	300	1200
Risk factor F absent	290	310	600
Total	1190	610	1800

$$or_{DF|C} = 3.2$$

Declared status

Risk factor C present	"D"	$\overline{D}$	Total
Risk factor F present	$a = 810$	$b = 390$	1200
Risk factor F absent	$c = 323$	$d = 277$	600
Total	1133	667	1800

$$\hat{o}r_{DF|C} = 1.8$$

True status

Risk factor C absent	D	$\overline{D}$	Total
Risk factor F present	1000	200	1200
Risk factor F absent	200	200	400
Total	1200	400	1600

$$or_{DF|\overline{C}} = 5.0$$

Declared status

Risk factor C absent	"D"	"$\overline{D}$"	Total
Risk factor F present	$a = 820$	$b = 380$	1200
Risk factor F absent	$c = 220$	$d = 180$	400
Total	1040	560	1600

$$\hat{o}r_{DF|\overline{C}} = 1.8$$

The second example continues to illustrate the rather obvious property that misclassification can produce just about any relationship regardless of the underlying properties of the population sampled. To further illustrate (Table 14–8), for a risk–disease relationship with a "true" odds ratio of 2.5, when differential misclassification occurs, the disease occurrence and risk factor appear perfectly independent ($\hat{o}r = 1.0$).

AGREEMENT BETWEEN TWO METHODS OF CLASSIFICATION: CATEGORICAL DATA

An important assessment of accuracy arises when the same data are classified into a series of categories by two different individuals. The primary concern is the

Table 14–8. An example of nondifferential misclassification where the "true" underlying odds ratio of 2.5 appears to be 1.0 when $p = 0.9$, $p' = 0.7$, $P = 0.9$, and $P' = 0.7$

True status

	D	$\overline{D}$	Total
Risk factor present	200	400	600
Risk factor absent	100	500	600
Total	300	900	1200

$$or = 2.5$$

Declared status

	"D"	"$\overline{D}$"	Total
Risk factor present	$a = 220$	$b = 380$	600
Risk factor absent	$c = 220$	$d = 380$	600
Total	440	760	1200

$$\hat{or} = 1.0$$

ability of observers (sometimes called raters in this context) to agree on the status of the observations under investigation.

Before expanding on classification accuracy, it is useful to make a clear distinction between two variables that are associated and two variables that agree. *Agreement* means that the values of two variables are the same. In terms of data in a table, perfect agreement occurs when the two values fall in the same category (Table 14–9). *Associated* means that value of one variable predicts the value of another. Again, in terms of a table, perfect association occurs when the category of one value completely determines the category of the other (Table 14–10). More succinctly, agreement is special kind of association.

Suppose the same 40 subjects are independently classified into one of two categories by two raters. Data that illustrate this are displayed in Table 14–11.

Table 14–9. Perfect agreement and perfect association

		Rater 1		
		C_1	C_2	C_3
	C_1	10	0	0
Rater 2	C_2	0	20	0
	C_3	0	0	30

Table 14–10. No agreement and perfect association

		Rater 1		
		C_1	C_2	C_3
	C_1	0	0	20
Rater 2	C_2	10	0	0
	C_3	0	30	0

Table 14–11. Fictional data to illustrate the principles and calculation of a measure of agreement

Counts:

		Rater 1		
		C_1	C_2	**Total**
Rater 2	C_1	12	8	20
	C_2	4	16	20
	Total	16	24	40

Proportions:

		Rater 1		
		C_1	C_2	**Total**
Rater 2	C_1	0.30	0.20	0.50
	C_2	0.10	0.40	0.50
	Total	0.40	0.60	1.0

A natural measure of classification accuracy is the total proportion of subjects when both raters agree. That is, agreement is measured as the overall proportion of pairs of observations that occur in the same categories. For the example, this value is $0.30 + 0.40 = 0.70$. However, this proportion overstates the underlying classification accuracy because a portion of the 70% agreement likely occurred by chance. The extent of this random agreement can be estimated from the observed marginal frequencies. Thus, within the 70% agreement, the proportion that agree by chance is estimated as $(0.5)(0.4) + (0.5)(0.6) = 0.20 + 0.30 = 0.50$. Therefore, correcting the overall measure of agreement produces an estimate that better reflects the pure ability of two raters to accurately classify the sampled subjects. For the example, a corrected agreement is $0.70 - 0.50 = 0.20$ or 20%. It should be noted that this adjustment is only one of a number of possibilities to correct for random agreement, and no general consensus exists on the choice of methods to compensate for the influences of chance.

A popular measure of agreement within a table is called the *kappa statistic*. The kappa statistic (denoted K) is the adjusted probability of agreement divided by the probability that the agreement did not occur by chance and, for the example, this value is

$$kappa\ statistic = \hat{K} = \frac{0.70 - 0.50}{1 - 0.50} = 0.40.$$

A $k \times k$ agreement/disagreement table has the same properties as a 2×2 table. The notation for the $k \times k$ case is presented in Table 14–12, where p_{ij} represents the proportion of counts in the ij^{th}-cell. This table is always square (number of rows = number of columns) because the raters use the same categories. The ordering of the row and column categories is also the same and typically has a natural sequence. These two features produce diagonal categories (p_{ii}, $i = 1$, $2, \cdots, k$) that reflect the extent of agreement between rates.

Table 14–12.   General notation for data collected to assess agreement between two raters

		Rater 1					
		C_1	C_2	C_3	...	C_k	**Total**
	C_1	p_{11}	p_{12}	p_{13}	...	p_{1k}	q_1
	C_3	p_{21}	p_{22}	p_{23}	...	p_{2k}	q_2
Rater 2	C_3	p_{31}	p_{32}	p_{33}	...	p_{3k}	q_3
	...	...	...	...	...	...	...
	...	...	...	...	...	...	...
	...	...	...	...	...	...	...
	C_k	p_{k1}	p_{k2}	p_{k3}	...	p_{kk}	q_k
	Total	p_1	p_2	p_3	...	p_k	1.0

A kappa statistic is constructed so that when the raters agree only by chance, the value of the kappa statistic is zero ($K = 0$). The normalization of the kappa statistic by the estimated probability of nonrandom agreement produces a value such that when the agreement is perfect (all data are on the diagonal of the agreement/disagreement table), the value of the kappa statistic is 1 ($K = 1$). In addition, this specific normalization makes several measures of agreement equivalent, unifying the approach to measuring agreement [44].

The following are the components of the k-level kappa statistic:

$$crude\ accuracy = \sum p_{ii},$$
$$random\ agreement = \sum p_i q_i,$$
$$nonrandom\ agreement = 1 - \sum p_i q_i,$$
$$corrected\ accuracy = crude\ accuracy - random\ agreement = \sum p_{ii} - \sum p_i q_i, \quad \text{and}$$
$$kappa\ statistic = K = \frac{\sum p_{ii} - \sum p_i q_i}{1 - \sum p_i q_i}$$

where $i = 1, 2, \cdots, k$ = number of categories. Conceptually, the kappa statistic measures the extent of observed nonrandom agreement relative to the maximum possible extent of nonrandom agreement.

The expression for the variance of the distribution of an estimated value of the kappa statistic ($\hat{K}$) is complicated, extensive, and is not presented [45]. Statistical computing systems that produce estimates of the kappa statistic also produce estimates of its variance. Alternatively, using a bootstrap estimation approach also produces an estimated variance for an estimated kappa statistic (Chapter 8).

Two independent raters reviewed 98 images of the media of the coronary vessel. All vessels are from different individuals, and disease status was evaluated

Table 14–13. Coronary artery data: agreement between pathology scores given by two independent raters ($n = 98$ individuals)

Counts:

		Rater 1				
		C_1	C_2	C_3	C_4	**Total**
Rater 2	C_1	3	2	0	0	5
	C_2	7	14	1	0	22
	C_3	4	19	42	2	67
	C_4	0	0	1	3	4
	Total	14	35	44	5	98

Or proportions:

		Rater 1				
		C_1	C_2	C_3	C_4	**Total**
Rater 2	C_1	0.031	0.020	0.000	0.000	0.051
	C_2	0.071	0.143	0.010	0.000	0.224
	C_3	0.041	0.194	0.429	0.020	0.684
	C_4	0.000	0.000	0.010	0.031	0.041
	Total	0.143	0.357	0.449	0.051	1.000

by a visual process called *color deconvolution*. The scoring is based on a four-category scale and the resulting data are presented in Table 14–13.

The estimated kappa statistic is

$$\sum p_{ii} = 0.633, \quad \sum p_i q_i = 0.397 \quad \text{and} \quad \hat{K} = \frac{0.633 - 0.397}{1 - 0.397} = 0.391.$$

The estimated variance of the distribution of the estimate $\hat{K}$ is $variance(\hat{K}) = 0.00442$. An approximate 95% confidence interval becomes $0.391 \pm 1.960 \sqrt{0.00442} = (0.260, 0.521)$.

The kappa statistic is most often applied in a descriptive fashion to make comparisons among different situations. To provide guidance for the interpretation of these comparisons, the following has been suggested:

$\hat{K}$ greater than 0.75	excellent agreement
$\hat{K}$ between 0.75 and 0.40	fair to good agreement
$\hat{K}$ less than 0.40	poor agreement

Needless to say, these qualitative values are an attempt to be helpful and certainly do not apply in all situations.

A note of caution: The value of the kappa statistics depends on the distribution of the marginal frequencies. The same rating process can, therefore, produce rather different kappa estimates because of differences in the distributions of the variable being classified, thus complicating the comparison of kappa statistics calculated under different conditions.

DISAGREEMENT

The kappa statistic is calculated only from the total count of agreements and the marginal frequencies from the agreement/disagreement table. The pattern of disagreement, however, is also potentially a useful part of describing a classification process. To emphasize the point, Table 14–14 displays two contrived agreement/disagreement tables with the identical values of the kappa statistic ($\hat{K} =$ 0.243). However, each table has a distinctively different pattern of disagreement.

The analysis of disagreement starts with eliminating the agreement counts and focusing on the remaining table containing the $k(k - 1)$ counts where the raters disagree. Using the previous color deconvolution example, these data yield 12 counts of observer disagreement (Table 14–15). As with many statistical techniques, it is useful to compare the observed distribution of disagreement to a specific postulated pattern. Natural values to explore the pattern of disagreement are the counts estimated by assuming quasi-independence among the discordant cell frequencies (nondiagonal values). That is, it is assumed that the properties of the variable being observed are completely unrelated to the classification process thus making disagreement between raters completely random. This quasi-independence model has been previously applied to analyze matched-pairs data, associations between contraindicated drugs, and patterns of pre-school children at play (Chapter 13). A version of this log-linear model requires that all association, once the counts of agreement are eliminated, arise by chance alone and is again

$$cell\ frequency = AB_iC_j \quad \text{or} \quad log(cell\ frequency) = a + b_i + c_j$$

when $i \neq j$, $i = 1, 2, \cdots, k - 1$ and $j = 1, 2, \cdots, k - 1$. Using a design variable analogous to those described previously for two-way tables (Tables 13–9, 13–14, and 13–26), the discordant cell frequencies produce estimates of the model

Table 14–14. Two agreement/disagreement tables with the same kappa statistic ($\hat{K} =$ 0.243) but different patterns of disagreement

		Rater 1			
		C_1	C_2	C_3	**Total**
	C_1	10	25	5	40
Rater 2	C_2	5	20	25	50
	C_3	25	5	30	60
	Total	40	50	60	150

		Rater 1			
		C_1	C_2	C_3	**Total**
	C_1	10	15	15	40
Rater 2	C_2	15	20	15	50
	C_3	15	15	30	60
	Total	40	50	60	150

Table 14–15.   Previous color deconvolution data (Table 14–13) yielding 12 counts of observer disagreement and four structural zeros

		Rater 1			
		C_1	C_2	C_3	C_4
	C_1	–	2	0	0
Rater 2	C_2	7	–	1	0
	C_3	4	19	–	2
	C_4	0	0	1	–

Table 14–16.   Estimates of the parameters of the quasi-independence log-linear regression model from the coronary artery data (Table 14–15)

Symbol	Estimate	Std. error
a	−0.665	–
b_1	2.333	0.882
b_2	2.367	0.741
b_3	−0.885	1.228
c_1	1.218	0.456
c_2	−1.103	0.803
c_3	−1.732	0.770

parameters $\hat{a}$, $\hat{b}_i$, and $\hat{c}_j$ with Poisson regression tools. The seven model-estimated coefficients from the log-linear regression model applied to the coronary artery color deconvolution classification data (Table 14–15) are given in Table 14–16.

These estimated coefficients, as always, produce cell frequencies that perfectly conform to the model (Table 14–17). For example, the quasi-independent model-generated value for the category with the largest number of disagreements (third row and second column) is

$$log(frequency) = \hat{a} + \hat{b}_2 + \hat{c}_1 = -0.665 + 2.367 + 1.218 = 2.920,$$

and the model estimated value is then $e^{2.920} = 18.544$. The observed count is 19.

Goodness-of-fit is usually an issue with a statistical model. However, the primary purpose of these theoretical values is to serve as a basis for comparison to help identify patterns of disagreement. A variety of ways exist to compare the observed and model values to potentially identify any pattern. The difference $(observed - expected)$, or the contribution to the chi-square statistic $(observed - expected)^2/expected$, or simply the *signs* or *ranks* of the differences are possibilities. For the artery data, using the signs of the differences (observed values minus model-estimated counts) shows large positive differences highly associated with the diagonal of the agreement/disagreement table (Table 14–18).

Table 14–17. Coronary artery data: pathologic scores estimated as if the raters disagree completely at random (quasi-independence) and observed values (parentheses)

		Rater 1			
		C_1	C_2	C_3	C_4
	C_1	–	1.74 (2)	0.17(0)	0.09 (0)
Rater 2	C_2	5.30 (7)	–	1.76(1)	0.94 (0)
	C_3	5.49 (4)	18.54 (19)	–	0.97 (2)
	C_4	0.21 (0)	0.72 (0)	0.07 (1)	–

Table 14–18. Coronary artery data: the signs of the differences between the observed counts and the corresponding quasi-independent model values

		Rater 1			
		C_1	C_2	C_3	C_4
	C_1	–	+	–	–
Rater 2	C_2	+	–	–	–
	C_3	–	+	–	+
	C_4	–	–	+	–

That is, when disagreement occurs, the raters rarely differ by more than one category when classifying coronary artery abnormalities. This kind of association is not surprising for data collected from a clinical setting. However, in other situations, patterns of disagreement might reveal different training, skills, biases, or tendencies between the raters.

A MEASUREMENT OF ACCURACY: CONTINUOUS DATA

Clearly, the ideal strategy, as noted, is to avoid errors altogether, but since this is rarely possible, the next best strategy is to estimate their magnitude, describe their properties, and attempt to control their consequences. The assessment of the accuracy of a test to identify a condition relative to its actual existence is important in a number of situations. For example, a test to determine the presence or absence of diabetes from a biochemical assessment of the level of glucose. The following discussion first focuses on a parametric approach to describe a specialized technique to measure test accuracy followed by a description of the parallel nonparametric approach.

A statistical tool developed during World War II to analyze radar signal data, called a *receiver operating characteristic (ROC) curve*, is common today in many fields, including medical research, epidemiology, radiology, and even the social sciences. A ROC curve is a visual display of the performance of a binary classification process relative to a standard. The principal purpose is a detailed description of the unavoidable trade-off between the frequency of

Table 14–19.   The notation for the counts of the four possible outcomes of a test used to detect a disease condition

	Disease D+	No disease D–
Test positive T+	true positive $= tp$	false positive $= fp$
Test negative T–	false negative $= fn$	true negative $= tn$

Table 14–20.   Example of performance data' describing the accuracy of a test

	D+	D–
T+	$tp = 90$	$fp = 30$
T–	$fn = 10$	$tn = 70$

false-positive results (costs) and the frequency of true-positive results (benefits) from a test used to identify a specific outcome, such as one used to detect a specific pathologic condition.   In addition, like most statistical techniques, summary statistics estimated from the ROC curve are a useful description of this cost–benefit balance, especially when accompanied by a rigorous statistical evaluation of the always present influence of sampling variation.

The terminology and notation associated with the performance of a test to correctly detect a specific condition are not uniformly established.   For the following, the most common definitions are used.   A positive test is represented by $T+$ and a negative test by $T-$.   In a parallel fashion, the presence of a disease is represented by $D+$ and its absence by $D-$.   A test can be correct in two ways and incorrect in two ways (Table 14–19).

The four possible outcomes that result from declaring a disease present or absent based on a positive or negative test result are frequently summarized by the following performance measures:

- True positive fraction (sensitivity) $= tpf = \dfrac{tp}{tp+fn}$,
- False negative fraction $= fnf = \dfrac{fn}{tp+fn}$,
- False positive fraction $= fpf = \dfrac{fp}{fp+tn}$,
- True negative fraction (specificity) $= tnf = \dfrac{tn}{fp+tn}$, and
- Accuracy $= \dfrac{tp+tn}{tp+fp+fn+tn}$.

A small numeric example clarifies these measures and their notation (Table 14–20).

- True positive fraction (sensitivity) $= tpf = \dfrac{tp}{tp+fn} = \dfrac{90}{100} = 0.90$,

- False negative fraction $= fnf = \dfrac{fn}{tp+fn} = \dfrac{10}{100} = 0.10$,
- False positive fraction $= fpf = \dfrac{fp}{fp+tn} = \dfrac{30}{100} = 0.30$,
- True negative fraction (specificity) $= tnf = \dfrac{tn}{fp+tn} = \dfrac{70}{100} = 0.70$, and
- Accuracy $= \dfrac{tp+tn}{tp+fp+fn+tn} = \dfrac{160}{200} = 0.80$.

These fractions (estimated probabilities) appear in a variety of statistical contexts and are given different names. For example, in the context of hypothesis testing (Chapter 15), the probabilities $tpf = $ level of significance, $fnf = $ type I error, $fpf = $ type II error, and $tnf = $ power of the test.

Parametric Approach

The primary element of a ROC analysis is the ROC curve that graphically describes test accuracy in terms of two performance probabilities for all possible test outcomes. In other words, the resulting ROC curve is a visual display of the pattern of accuracy of a test relative to a standard, based on collected data. This curve emerges from the construction a series of 2×2 tables that contain estimates of the probabilities of a true-positive result and a false-positive result. That is, every possible value of a test is considered by selecting cut-points (denoted c) that create a positive test $(T+)$ and negative test $(T-)$, thus producing four performance probabilities (Table 14–19). Three ROC curves illustrate (Figure 14–1) test accuracy in terms of two of these performance probabilities for all values of the cut-point c. Specifically, the plot consists of a description of the pattern of the true-positive fractions ($tpf = $ sensitivity, vertical axes) and the false-positive fractions ($fpf = 1 - $ specificity, horizontal axes).

Making the parametric assumption that the variation in both the test and standard measures are accurately described by normal distributions with different mean values but the same variances, the four performance probabilities of a test at any specific cut-point can be directly calculated (Figure 14–2).The ROC curve is a plot of all possible pairs of these estimated performance probabilities (fpf, $tpf) = (1 - specificity, sensitivity)$ based on the properties of two cumulative normal distribution probability functions. A ROC analysis requires a sample of test data (n_1 observations) and a sample of standard data (n_0 observations) to estimate these probabilities.

When the test is perfectly accurate, then $tpf = 1.0$ ($fnf = 0$) and $fpf = 0$ ($tnf = 1$), and the ROC "curve" becomes the single point $(0, 1)$. On the other hand,

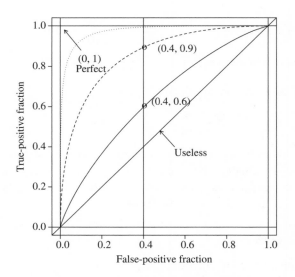

Figure 14-1. Three example ROC curves.

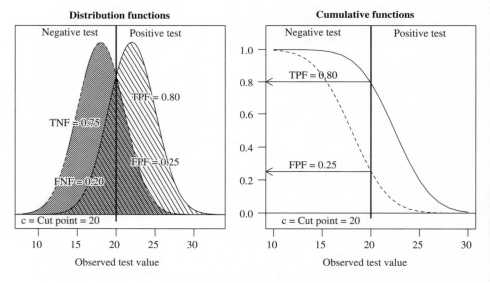

Figure 14-2. Probabilities defining the performance at the cut-point c = 20 of a test relative to a standard based on normal distributions (two versions).

when all comparisons of the true-positive and the false-positive probabilities are equal ($tpf = fpf$), then the ROC "curve" is a straight line from the point $(0,0)$ to $(1,1)$. That is, these two performance probabilities are equal for all possible situations (for all possible cut-points). Between these two extremes, the ROC curve displays the entire range of the pairs of probabilities fpf and tpf, forming a complete description of the performance of a test relative to a standard, as a curve from points $(0, 0)$ to $(1, 1)$. As the accuracy of the test increases, the ROC curve moves away from for the "useless" line toward the "perfect" upper left-hand corner (Figure 14–1). In fact, the area under the ROC curve is a measure of the overall performance of the test relative to the standard (to be discussed). For two ROC curves, the higher curve indicates better performance probabilities. For the example, at a value of fnf equal to 0.4, for the lower curve the tpf-value is 0.6 and for the higher curve, the tpf-value increases to 0.9 (the vertical line, Figure 14–1). Similarly, the higher ROC curve has the smaller fnf-values at the same tpf-values (a horizontal line).

The fundamental determinant of test performance is the difference between the test and standard measurement distributions. For a parametrically estimated ROC curve, the statistical assumptions, estimates, and interpretations are not very different from classic two-sample comparison (for example, the two-sample parametric Student's t-test). Figure 14–3 displays three ROC curves that result from two normal distributions that have different mean values and the same variances. Instead of a classic two-sample analysis, a ROC curve produces a comparison between these two distributions in terms of the performance probabilities fpf and tpf. However, most of the underlying statistical issues are the same. Also clear from the plots is the relationship between the two extreme ROC curves (perfect and useless "curves") and the distributions of the test and standard measures. When the ROC "curve" is a straight line (area under the curve $= 0.5$), the two compared normal distributions are identical. When the ROC "curve" is perfect (area under the curve $= 1.0$), the two normal distributions do not overlap. Thus, the area under the ROC curve is a direct function of the distance between the mean values of the test and standard measurement distributions in this parametric approach.

As noted, every point on a ROC curve is created by a cut-point that determines the four performance probabilities (tpf, fnf, fpf, and tnf). To further illustrate this property, Table 14–21 contains fictional data from four cut-points created from two normal distributions. The two performance probabilities from these four tables (fpf and tpf) are identified as four specific points on a continuous ROC curve (Figure 14–4). For the example in Table 14–21 and Figure 14–4, the mean of the test distribution is $\mu_t = 10$, the mean of the standard distribution is $\mu_s = 12$, and the variance of both normally distributed populations is $\sigma^2 = 4$.

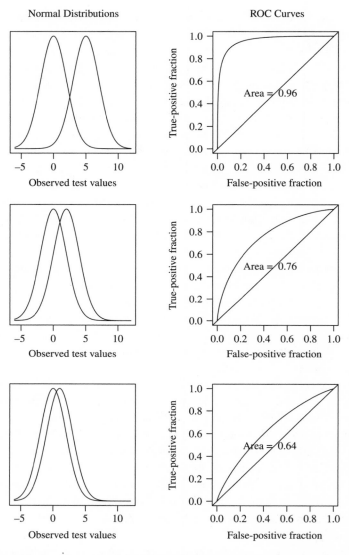

Figure 14–3. Illustration of the relationship between test and standard measure distributions and the resulting ROC curve.

From a more general point of view, the complete ROC curve is established by plotting values from two cumulative probability functions over the entire range of cut-points c. For the normal distribution approach, expressions for these

Table 14–21. Four example 2×2 tables (four cut-points c)that are the source of the estimates creating a receiver operating characteristics (ROC) curve (Figure14–4)

$c_1 = 12.8$	$D+$	$D-$	**Total**
$T+$	35	8	43
$T-$	65	92	157
Total	100	100	200

$c_2 = 10.6$	$D+$	$D-$	**Total**
$T+$	75	38	113
$T-$	25	62	87
Total	100	100	200

Table 1 (c_1): true-positive fraction $= tpf = 0.35$
Table 1 (c_1): false-positive fraction $= fpf = 0.08$

Table 2 (c_2): true-positive fraction $= tpf = 0.75$
Table 2 (c_2): false-positive fraction $= fpf = 0.38$

$c_3 = 9.4$	$D+$	$D+$	**Total**
$T+$	90	61	151
$T-$	10	39	49
Total	100	100	200

$c_4 = 8.2$	$D+$	$D-$	**Total**
$T+$	97	80	177
$T-$	3	20	23
Total	100	100	200

Table 3 (c_3): true-positive fraction $= tpf = 0.90$
Table 3 (c_3): false-positive fraction $= fpf = 0.61$

Table 4 (c_4): true-positive fraction $= tpf = 0.97$
Table 4 (c_4): false-positive fraction $= fpf = 0.80$

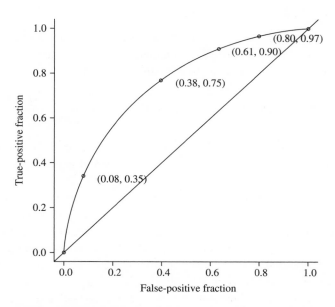

Figure 14–4. Hypothetical ROC curve illustrating the four specific performance probabilities described in Table 14–19 ($\mu_t = 10$, $\mu_s = 12$ and $\sigma^2 = 4$).

cumulative probability functions are

$$fpf = 1 - \Phi\left[\frac{c - \mu_t}{\sigma}\right] \quad \text{and} \quad tpf = 1 - \Phi\left[\frac{c - \mu_s}{\sigma}\right]$$

where μ_s represents the mean value of the normal distribution of the standard measures and μ_t represents the mean value of the normal distribution of the test measures ($\mu_s > \mu_t$). Both distributions have the same variances, represented by σ^2. The symbol $\Phi(z) = P(Z \leq z)$ denotes the value of the cumulative probability function from a standard normal distribution at the value z. For example, when $z = 1.645$, $P(Z \leq 1.645) = \Phi(1.645) = 0.95$. More simply, a ROC curve can be viewed as a plot of test *sensitivity* ($y = tpf$) against $1 - specificity$ ($x = fnf$) based on the cumulative probabilities from two normal distributions.

Two points of note: First, for the normal distribution model, the point on a ROC curve closest to perfect discrimination ($tpf = 1$ and $fpf = 0$) occurs at the cut-point at $c = (\mu_t + \mu_s)/2$. Or, this same ROC point occurs when $tpf = tnf$ (sensitivity = specificity). Second, the case in which the mean value μ_s is less than the mean value μ_t has the same properties but produces the same ROC curve with ftp and fpf values reversed.

Nonparametric Approach

As with the parametric ROC curve, the nonparametric estimate is also generated from two cumulative probability distribution functions. A nonparametric estimate of a cumulative distribution function of a variable labeled X is

$$cumulative \; probability \; distribution \; function = P(X \leq x) = \frac{number \; of \; values \leq x}{n}$$

for a sample of n observations. At each n sampled values of x, the cumulative probability is the proportion of values that are less than or equal to the value x (Chapter 8).

Mechanically, the nonparametric estimate of a ROC curve is accomplished by sorting the performance measures from low to high, regardless of whether they are from test or standard samples. Then, starting with the smallest observed value and the point $(x_0, y_0) = (0, 0)$, the first point of the ROC curve becomes $(x_0, y_0 + 1/n_0)$ if the first observation is a standard measurement, or the first point becomes $(x_0 + 1/n_1, y_0)$ if it is a test measurement where, again, n_0 represents the number of standard observation and n_1 represents the number of test observations ($n_0 + n_1 = n$). Continuing the pattern, if the observation is a standard measurement, then $x_i = x_{i-1}$ and $y_i = y_{i-1} + 1/n_0$, and if the observation is a test measurement, then $x_i = x_{i-1} + 1/n_1$ and $y_i = y_{i-1}$ for $i = 1, 2, \cdots, n$. The sequential values $fpf_i = 1 - x_i$

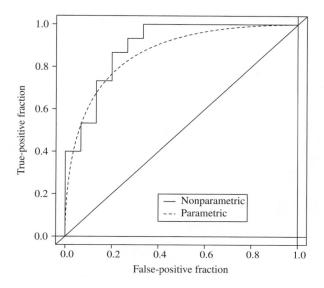

Figure 14–5. A nonparametric (solid line) and parametric (dashed line) estimated ROC curve from $n_0 = n_1 = 15$ observation (Table 14–22).

and $tpf_i = 1 - y_i$ form the nonparametric estimated ROC "curve." At the end of this section, a small example ($n = 6$) employing two specific nonparametric cumulative distribution functions is presented in detail to further illustrate the nonparametric estimation of a ROC curve. The construction of a nonparametric ROC curve parallels the previously described parametric estimate.

The data in Table 14–22 consist of the first 30 observations ($n_0 = 15$ standard and $n_1 = 15$ test values) from a larger data set (to be described and explored in detail) that illustrate the construction of both parametric (dashed line) and nonparametric (solid line) estimated ROC curves (Figure 14–5).

The parametric performance probability estimates are

$$\textit{false positive fraction} = fpf = 1 - \Phi\left[\frac{c - \bar{x}_t}{\sqrt{V}}\right] = 1 - \Phi\left[\frac{c - 3.862}{\sqrt{0.055}}\right],$$

and

$$\textit{true positive fraction} = tpf = 1 - \Phi\left[\frac{c - \bar{x}_s}{\sqrt{V}}\right] = 1 - \Phi\left[\frac{c - 4.267}{\sqrt{0.055}}\right]$$

where $\bar{x}_t = 3.862$ is the estimated mean of the test values, $\bar{x}_s = 4.267$ is the estimated mean of the standard values, and $\sqrt{V}$ is the estimated common standard deviation of the performance measurement distributions. Specifically, the estimate of the

Table 14–22. Example data ($n_0 = n_1 = 15$, ordered) to illustrate the nonparametric construction of a ROC curve (full data set to be analyzed, $n = 86$)

Observations	1	2	3	4	5	6	7	8	9	10
Measure	3.294	3.568	3.586	3.725	3.728	3.800	3.808	3.885	3.889	3.916
Test/standard*	x	x	x	x	x	x	x	x	x	x
u_i	15	15	15	15	15	15	15	15	15	15
Observations	11	12	13	14	15	16	17	18	19	20
Measure	3.924	3.943	4.003	4.011	4.067	4.071	4.200	4.204	4.212	4.246
Test/standard*	o	x	o	x	o	o	x	o	o	o
u_i	0	14	0	13	0	0	11	0	0	0
Observations	21	22	23	24	25	26	27	28	29	30
Measure	4.306	4.349	4.354	4.362	4.375	4.380	4.384	4.411	4.415	4.527
Test/standard*	x	o	o	x	o	o	o	o	o	o
u_i	8	0	0	6	0	0	0	0	0	0

* = Test measure coded = x and standard measure coded = o

Nonparametrically estimated ROC curve (Figure 14–5)

tpf_i	1.00	1.00	1.00	1.00	1.00	1.00	1.00	1.00	1.00	1.00
fpf_i	0.93	0.87	0.80	0.73	0.66	0.60	0.53	0.47	0.40	0.33
tpf_i	0.93	0.93	0.87	0.87	0.80	0.73	0.73	0.66	0.60	0.53
fpf_i	0.33	0.16	0.16	0.20	0.20	0.20	0.13	0.13	0.13	0.13
tpf_i	0.53	0.47	0.40	0.40	0.33	0.26	0.20	0.13	0.07	0.00
fpf_i	0.07	0.07	0.07	0.00	0.00	0.00	0.00	0.00	0.00	0.00

common variance σ^2 is the usual pooled estimate associated with Student's t-test where

$$V = \frac{(n_0 - 1)V_s + (n_1 - 1)V_t}{n_0 + n_1 - 2}$$

and, V_t and V_s represent the variances of the test and standard performance measurement distributions estimated from the n_1 and n_0 observations, respectively. For the example data (Table 14–22), the estimated common variance is $V = 0.055$. The values of cut-points c cover the relevant ranges of both normal probability distributions.

To emphasize the parametric and nonparametric approaches to estimating a ROC curve, Figure 14–6 shows the expected property that, as the sample size increases, these two estimates become essentially indistinguishable. That is, the

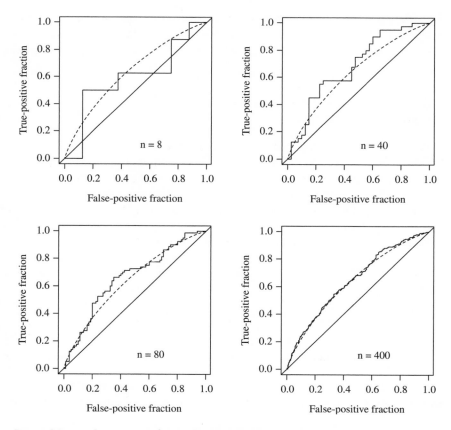

Figure 14–6. Comparison of parametric and nonparametric estimates of the ROC curve for four sample sizes ($n = 8$, 40, 80, and 400).

two estimated ROC curves converge when the test and standard measures are sampled from two normal distributions with the same variances.

The advantage of a nonparametric estimated ROC curve is that it describes the accuracy of a test relative to a standard without assumptions about the populations sampled. The disadvantage is that the results can be difficult to interpret. Examples exist where a nonparametric estimated ROC curve can be extremely misleading. In rather unrealistic situations, test values perfectly discriminate, but the ROC curve indicates the opposite. This kind of example serves as a warning that when the test and standard distributions are not normally distributed with the same variances, caution should be exercised in the interpretation, and the test and standard distributions should be carefully inspected. At a minimum, these two distributions should be estimated and plotted (Chapter 10). Another potential issue arises when two nonparametric ROC curves are compared. Unlike parametric estimation, there is no guarantee that one ROC curve lies entirely above another. The relative accuracies of two tests can depend on the region compared. For example, one ROC curve could indicate superior performance for low values of fpf but have less effective performance for high values. That is, the ROC curves cross.

A Detailed Example of the Construction of a Nonparametric ROC Curve

Statistical software certainly exists to calculate and plot a nonparametrically estimated ROC curve. However, a simple (very simple) example demonstrates the process in detail and provides additional insight into the interpretation of ROC curves in general, particularly the roles of two cumulative probability functions.

Purely hypothetical standard/test measurements (x) are:

standard ($n_0 = 3$): 24, 47, and 62; and test ($n_1 = 4$): 12, 34, 53, and 68.

These values combined into a single ordered data set ($n_0 + n_1 = n = 7$ observations) become:

	1	2	3	4	5	6	7
Source*	x	o	x	o	x	o	x
x	12	24	34	47	53	62	68

* = Test observations are coded x and standard observations are coded o

The basis of a ROC curve is two cumulative distribution functions estimated from the two sets of observations. The nonparametrically estimated cumulative

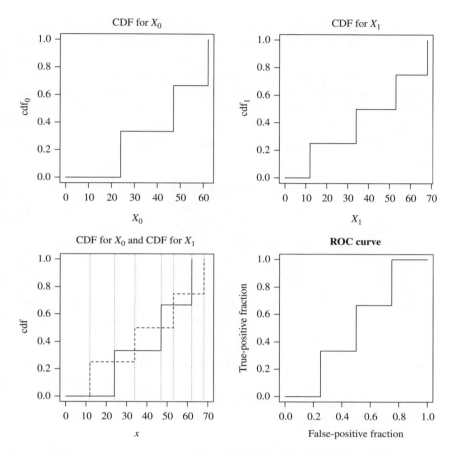

Figure 14–7. Four steps in the construction of a ROC curve (CDF = cumulative distribution function).

distribution functions for the standard and test data are:

Standard cumulative distribution function (Figure 14–7, upper left)

x	0	24	47	62
cdf_0	0.00	0.33	0.67	1.00

and the

Test cumulative distribution function (Figure 14–7, upper right)

x	0	12	34	53	68
cdf_1	0.00	0.25	0.50	0.75	1.00

As noted, ROC curves are a description of the performance probabilities calculated for a series of cut-points. In the continuous (parametric) case, every cut-point produces a different 2×2 table, which in turn produces four different performance probabilities. The estimated ROC curve, therefore, describes the performance probabilities ($x = fpf$ and $y = tpf$) as a smooth continuous curve. For the nonparametric case, the maximum number of cut-points is the total number of observations (n). That is, the n observations produce a maximum of n cut-points and, therefore, produce a maximum of n sets of different performance probabilities (2×2 tables, Table 14–19). For the example, this number is seven ($n = 7$), and the associated probabilities from the two cumulative distribution functions at each observation are:

Combined cumulative distribution functions (Figure 14–7, lower left)

	1	2	3	4	5	6	7	–
cdf_1	0.00	0.25	0.25	0.50	0.50	0.75	0.75	1.00
cdf_0	0.00	0.00	0.33	0.33	0.67	0.67	1.00	1.00

The seven cut-points (data points = cut-points = x) are identified on the plot as dotted vertical lines. The ROC curve is not plotted in terms of cumulative probabilities but in terms of false-positive values (fpf) and true-positive values (tpf). Therefore, the plotted values become $fpf = 1 - cdf_1$ (horizontal axes) and $tpf = 1 - cdf_0$ (vertical axes) and are:

ROC curve (Figure 14–7, lower right)

	1	2	3	4	5	6	7	–
$fpf(x)$	1.00	0.75	0.75	0.50	0.50	0.25	0.25	0.00
$tpf(y)$	1.00	1.00	0.67	0.67	0.33	0.33	0.00	0.00

Area Under the ROC Curve

A fundamental summary statistic calculated from a ROC analysis is the area under the ROC curve (denoted $a\hat{u}c$). This value, between 0.5 (test is useless) and 1.0 (test is perfect), has two interpretations that make it a valuable measure of overall test performance. They are:

1. The value $a\hat{u}c$ reflects the mean true-positive fraction (tpf) or mean sensitivity, and
2. The value $a\hat{u}c$ estimates the probability that a randomly selected test measurement has a smaller value than a randomly selected standard measurement.

A parametric estimate of the area under the ROC curve based on the normal distribution model is

$$a\hat{u}c = \Phi \left[\frac{\bar{x}_t - \bar{x}_s}{\sqrt{2V}} \right]$$

where, again, $\bar{x}_t$ is the estimated mean value of the test measurements, $\bar{x}_s$ is the estimated mean value of the standard measurements, and V is an estimate of the common variance. For the example data (Table 14–22), the overall performance of the test relative to the standard is summarized by the estimate

$$\widehat{auc} = \Phi\left[\frac{4.267 - 3.862}{\sqrt{2(0.055)}}\right] = \Phi[1.179] = 0.881$$

where the mean values μ_s and μ_t are estimated by the sample mean values $\bar{x}_s = 4.267$ and $\bar{x}_t = 3.862$, and the pooled estimate of the variance is $V = 0.055$.

The variance of the quantity

$$\hat{R} = \frac{\bar{x}_s - \bar{x}_t}{\sqrt{2V}}$$

is approximately

$$variance(\hat{R}) = variance\left[\frac{\bar{x}_s - \bar{x}_t}{\sqrt{2V}}\right] = \frac{1}{2}\left[\frac{1}{n_0} + \frac{1}{n_1}\right]\left(1 + \frac{\hat{R}^2}{4}\right)$$
$$= \frac{1}{2}\left[\frac{1}{15} + \frac{1}{15}\right]\left(1 + \frac{1.179^2}{4}\right) = 0.089.$$

A normal distribution-based approximate 95% confidence interval for R, calculated from the estimate $\hat{R}$, is

$$lower\ bound = \hat{A} = \hat{R} - 1.960\sqrt{variance(\hat{R})} = 1.179 - 1.960\sqrt{0.089} = 0.592$$

and

$$upper\ bound = \hat{B} = \hat{R} + 1.960\sqrt{variance(\hat{R})} = 1.179 + 1.960\sqrt{0.089} = 1.767.$$

Therefore, an approximate 95% confidence interval based on the parametric estimate $\widehat{auc}$ is

$$(\hat{A},\ \hat{B}) = (\Phi[lower\ bound],\ \Phi[upper\ bound]).$$

From the example data (Table 14–22) and the estimate $\widehat{auc} = \Phi[1.179] = 0.881$, the approximate 95% confidence interval becomes $(\Phi[0.592], \Phi[1.767]) = (0.723, 0.961)$.

The nonparametric estimated auc-value results from recognizing that the nonparametric estimated ROC curve is a display of the Mann-Whitney statistic used to compare the difference between two samples (Chapter 13). The nonparametric estimate of $a\hat{u}c$ is identical to the Mann-Whitney estimate of the probability that a randomly selected value from one sample is smaller than a randomly selected value from another sample (denoted $\hat{P}$, Chapter 13). In symbols, the Mann-Whitney probability, previously denoted $\hat{P}$, is $\hat{P} = P(T \leq S) = a\hat{u}c$, where T represents a random test measurement and S represents a random standard measurement. Therefore, the area under the nonparametric ROC curve is estimated by

$$a\hat{u}c = \frac{1}{n_0 n_1} \sum u_i \qquad i = 1, 2, \cdots, n_0$$

where u_i represents the Mann-Whitney count of the number of values in the test samples that are less than the ith-value in the standard sample. For the 30 test/standard measurements given in Table 14–22, there are 15 standard values above the smallest test value (3.294), there are 15 standard values above the second smallest test value (3.568), and so on until there are six standard values above the largest test value (4.326), yielding a total of 202 values of the standard values larger than each test value. Therefore, the probability $\hat{P} = P(T \leq S) = a\hat{u}c = 202/225 = 0.898$.

Geometrically, these counts are proportional to the height of the nonparametric ROC curve at the ith standard measure. The total area (sum) based on these counts is the area under the ROC curve and, to repeat, is exactly the value of the Mann-Whitney two-sample test statistic. For the example data (Table 14–22 and Figure 14–8), the value is $a\hat{u}c = 202/225 = 0.898$.

Or, in more detail,

$$a\hat{u}c = \frac{1}{15(15)} (10(15) + 14 + 13 + 11 + 8 + 6)$$
$$= 0.667 + 0.062 + 0.058 + 0.049 + 0.035 + 0.026 = 202/225 = 0.898.$$

The variance of the nonparametrically estimated area under the ROC curve is the variance of the Mann-Whitney test statistic given by the expression [31],

$$variance(a\hat{u}c) = [a\hat{u}c(1 - a\hat{u}c) + (n_0 - 1)(p_1 - a\hat{u}c^2)$$
$$+ (n_1 - 1)(p_2 - a\hat{u}c^2)]/n_0 n_1$$

where

$$p_1 = \frac{a\hat{u}c}{2 - a\hat{u}c} \quad \text{and} \quad p_2 = \frac{2a\hat{u}c^2}{1 + a\hat{u}c}.$$

For the example (Table 14–22), the estimated value is $a\hat{u}c = 0.898$ and its distribution has an estimated variance of $variance(a\hat{u}c) = 0.00364$.

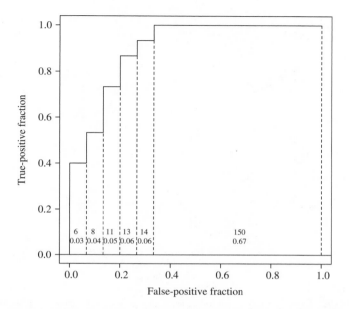

Figure 14–8. The nonparametric estimated ROC curve ($n_0 = n_1 = 15$) displaying the elements of the estimation of the area under the ROC curve (repeated from Figure 14–5).

The directly calculated approximate 95% confidence interval, based on the estimated value $a\hat{u}c = 0.898$, is

$$lower\ bound = \hat{A} = a\hat{u}c - 1.960\sqrt{variance(a\hat{u}c)}$$
$$= 0.898 - 1.960(0.060) = 0.780$$

and

$$upper\ bound = \hat{B} = a\hat{u}c + 1.960\sqrt{variance(a\hat{u}c)}$$
$$= 0.898 + 1.960(0.060) = 1.000.$$

A more extensive method using a logistic transformation improves the accuracy of the confidence interval estimation, particularly for estimated values ($a\hat{u}c$) in the neighborhood of 1.0 or 0.5.

Application: ROC Analysis Applied to Carotid Artery Disease Data

Three methods for evaluating the disease status of carotid arteries are presented to realistically illustrate the ROC curves as a technique to statistically compare test–standard accuracy. Using measured intensity of histochemical staining to

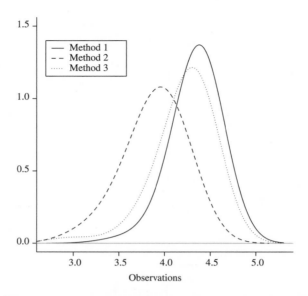

Figure 14–9. Kernel density smoothed distributions of the logarithms of the test–standard measurements (method 1, method 2, and method 3), where method 1 is the "standard" $(n_0 = n_1 = n_2 = 86)$.

characterize the disease status of carotid artery tissue produces three sets of data from 86 sampled individuals. A method called *color picking* is a computer-based scanning process that reads the color intensities pixel by pixel from slide images made into tissue micro-arrays, and this is selected as the "standard" (method 1). Two visual methods are compared to the computer method, one method called *color deconvolution* (method 2) and the other a purely visual assessment (method 3) [46].

Kernel density smoothed estimated distributions (Chapter 10) of the logarithms of the measurements from methods 1, 2, and 3 indicate that these three sets of transformed measurements likely have at least approximate normal distributions (Figure 14–9). The analysis of the logarithms of the measurements, rather than the measurements themselves, produces more symmetric and normal-like distributions that improve the accuracy of the parametric approach to estimating the performance probabilities and the area under the ROC curve and has no affect on nonparametric approach.

The parametric and nonparametric estimated ROC curves for the comparison of method 1 ("standard") and method 2 ("test") are displayed in Figure 14–10. For example, at the value $fpf = 0.5$, the value read from the plot for the level of sensitivity is $tpf = 0.87$ for both parametric (dashed line) and nonparametric (solid line) estimated ROC curves. A key performance summary of method 2 is the estimated area under the ROC curve. The mean sensitivity is estimated by $a\hat{u}c = 0.647$ (parametric) or $a\hat{u}c = 0.663$ (nonparametric). The respective approximate 95% confidence intervals are (0.566, 0.722) and (0.582, 0.744).

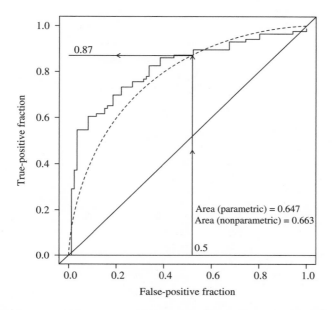

Figure 14–10. The parametric (dashed line) and the nonparametric (solid line) ROC curves (method 1 vs. method 3) from the carotid artery data.

The approximate 95% confidence intervals follow the usual pattern. For example, the nonparametric estimate $a\hat{u}c = 0.663$ produces the interval $[\hat{A}, \hat{B}] = [0.663 - 1.960(0.041), \ 0.663 + 1.960(0.041)] = (0.582, 0.744)$ where the estimated standard error is 0.041.

To contrast the accuracy of methods 2 and 3, two ROC curves are estimated (parametric and nonparametric estimates, Figures 14–11 and 14–12). Again, to improve the accuracy of the parametric approach, the logarithms of the measurements are analyzed. As before, the plot of the three curves (Figure 14–9) continues to justify applying the normal distribution model. From the comparison of the ROC curves estimated for methods 2 and 3, relative to the "standard" (method 1), the superiority of method 3 is apparent from both plots. The summary auc-estimates present strong evidence of a systematic difference. For the parametric model, the estimates are $a\hat{u}c_3 = 0.903$ [95% confidence interval $= (0.861, 0.934)$] and $a\hat{u}c_2 = 0.647$ [95% confidence interval $= (0.566, 0.722)$]. Similarly, for the nonparametric approach, they are $a\hat{u}c_3 = 0.928$ [95% confidence interval $= (0.888, 0.969)$] and $a\hat{u}c_2 = 0.663$ [95% confidence interval $= (0.582, 0.744)$]. For both parametric and nonparametric estimates, the approximate 95% confidence intervals clearly indicate that it is unlikely that the observed differences between methods 2 and 3 are due to chance alone.

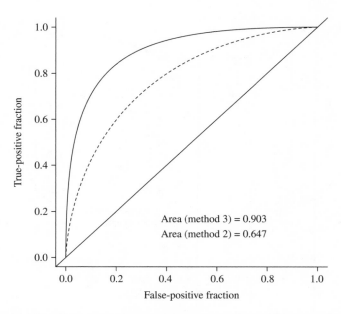

Figure 14–11. The parametric estimated ROC curves for method 2 (solid line) and method 3 (dashed line) from the $n_0 = n_1 = 86$ measurements from the carotid arteries.

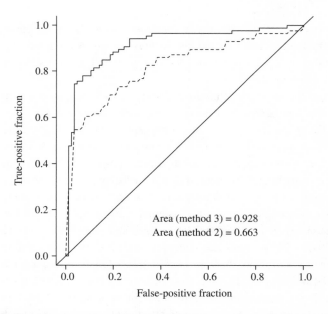

Figure 14–12. The nonparametric estimated ROC curves for method 2 (solid line) and method 3 (dashed lines) from the $n_0 = n_1 = 86$ measurements from the carotid arteries.

AGREEMENT BETWEEN TWO METHODS OF MEASUREMENT: CONTINUOUS DATA

Frequently a central issue in the comparison of two measurements made on the same subject is their consistency, particularly in the context of assessing the agreement between two clinical procedures. Perhaps, a new and less expensive method could replace the presently used method if it performs as well. Perfect agreement between two measurements, denoted x_1 and x_2, means that all values are identical ($x_1 = x_2$). A plot of these values produces a straight line with a slope of 1.0 (a 45-degree angle) with an intercept of zero. A second case arises when these values differ by a constant value. In this case, the line describing values of x_1 and x_2 has a slope of 1 but a non-zero intercept ($x_1 = x_2 + bias$). In both cases, the correlation between the two values is 1.0. The situation becomes more complicated when the observations compared are measured with error. The error variability associated with the distribution of each measurement can be equal or unequal, and it is the interplay of these factors (bias and variability) in assessing the agreement of two sets of continuous measurements that is the subject of this section. Occasionally, it is important to distinguish between the agreement between two measurements made by the same method (repeatability) and the agreement between two methods (reproducibility). The essential elements of both approaches are contained in the following.

A Statistical Model: "Two-Measurement" Model

Consider an observation denoted x_i that represents the value of the ith value sampled from a distribution, with mean value represented by μ and variance by σ_x^2. Frequently, it is also assumed that the observation has a normal distribution. In addition, the observation x_i is measured twice by the same method or by two different methods. These pairs of measurements are represented as

$$x_{i1} = x_i + e_{i1}$$

and

$$x_{i2} = x_i + e_{i2}, \qquad i = 1, 2, \cdots, n = \text{number of pairs.}$$

The distributions of the values e_{ij} have mean values of zero and variances represented by σ_1^2 and σ_2^2 and, in this context, are called *measurement error variances*. The model further requires these values to be independent of each other and independent of the observation x_i. Then, the variance of each observation x_{ij} becomes

$$variance(x_{i1}) = \sigma_x^2 + \sigma_1^2 \quad \text{or} \quad variance(x_{i2}) = \sigma_x^2 + \sigma_2^2.$$

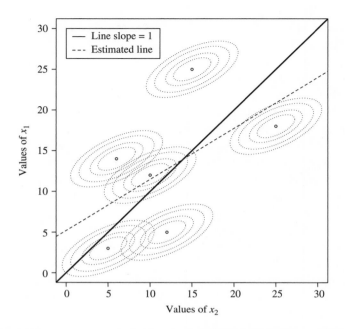

Figure 14–13. A schematic representation of joint distributions describing two measurements (six hypothetical pairs of observations x_1 and x_2 with different error variances, $\sigma_1^2 = 2$ and $\sigma_2^2 = 4$, circles).

and the covariance is

$$covariance(x_{i1}, \, x_{i2}) = covariance(x_i + e_{i1}, \, x_i + e_{i2})$$
$$= covariance(x_i, \, x_i) = variance(x_i) = \sigma_x^2.$$

Because the values x_{i1} and x_{i2} represent two uncorrelated measurements of the same quantity, their covariance is also the variance σ_x^2.

Perhaps the most sensitive issue of this statistical structure is the requirement that the error values (e) be uncorrelated with the measurements (x). It is not uncommon that the variability of a measurement is influenced by properties of the subject measured. For example, measurement error could decrease as the values measured increase. Larger values, for example, could be easier to measure accurately than smaller ones. The model is schematically displayed for six observations (Figure 14–13), with their variability visually indicated by elliptical regions (Chapter 15). In addition, Figures 14–14 and 14–15 display $n = 200$ random observations generated to exactly conform to this "two-measurement" model.

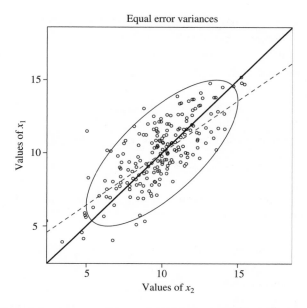

Figure 14–14. Model-generated "data" with parameters $\mu = 10$, $\sigma_x^2 = 3$, $\sigma_1^2 = 2$, and $\sigma_2^2 = 2$ (ordinary least-square line = dashed line and perpendicular least-squares line = solid line).

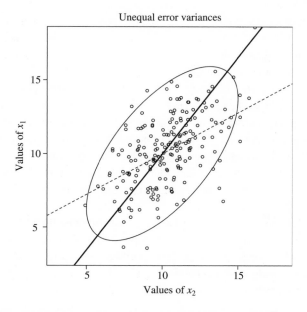

Figure 14–15. Model-generated "data" with parameters $\mu = 10$, $\sigma_x^2 = 3$, $\sigma_1^2 = 2$, and $\sigma_2^2 = 4$ (ordinary least-square line = dashed line and perpendicular least-squares line x = solid line).

Before proceeding to describe the analysis of the sampled x_1/x_2-pairs, it is necessary to provide expressions to estimate the variance components of the model. As noted, the covariance between x_1 and x_2 is the variance σ_x^2. Thus, a natural estimate of the variance of the sampled distribution is

$$estimated\ covariance = \frac{1}{n-1}\sum(x_{i1} - \bar{x}_1)(x_{i2} - \bar{x}_2) = \hat{\sigma}_x^2$$

and the two error variances are then estimated by

$$variance(e_{i1}) = \hat{\sigma}_1^2 = \hat{\sigma}_{x_1}^2 - \hat{\sigma}_x^2 \quad \text{and} \quad variance(e_{i2}) = \hat{\sigma}_2^2 = \hat{\sigma}_{x_2}^2 - \hat{\sigma}_x^2$$

where $\hat{\sigma}_{x_1}^2$ and $\hat{\sigma}_{x_2}^2$ represent the usual estimated variance (Chapter 12). Specifically, these two variance estimates are

$$variance(x_1) = \hat{\sigma}_{x_1}^2 = \frac{1}{n-1}\sum(x_{i1} - \bar{x}_1)^2 \quad \text{and}$$

$$variance(x_2) = \hat{\sigma}_{x_2}^2 = \frac{1}{n-1}\sum(x_{i2} - \bar{x}_2)^2$$

and, again, $i = 1, 2, \cdots, n = $ number of observations/pairs.

Relationships between observations made up of pairs are often effectively summarized with a correlation coefficient or an estimated straight line. When both variables are subject to random variation, an ordinary least-squares regression analysis is not appropriate. Least-squares analyses typically require the knowledge or assumption that each independent variable is a fixed value, and this is not always the case. That is, the dependent variable is required to be a value sampled from a distribution determined by the value of the independent variable. The "two-measurement" model postulates that each pair of measurements is sampled from a joint distribution. Specifically, when both observations are subject to random variation, the ordinary least-squares estimate of the slope of a summary straight line is biased. In addition, the independent and dependent variables play asymmetric roles in an ordinary least-squares regression analysis. Situations arise in which it is not clear which variable is the independent variable and which is the dependent variable. Results from a least-squares analysis generally differ depending on the choice.

The artificial data in Figure 14–14 are a sample of pairs of observations with the same error variances ($\sigma_1^2 = \sigma_2^2 = 2$ and slope $= 1.0$). That is, the observations x_1 and x_2 differ only by chance. The ordinary least-squares estimated slope (dashed line) does not have a slope of 1.0 (slope $= 0.6$). The expression for the ordinary least-squares estimated slope when both sampled observations x_1 and x_2 vary is

$$\hat{b}_1 = \frac{\hat{\sigma}_x^2}{\hat{\sigma}_x^2 + \hat{\sigma}_1^2} \qquad \text{or} \qquad \hat{b}_2 = \frac{\hat{\sigma}_x^2}{\hat{\sigma}_x^2 + \hat{\sigma}_2^2},$$

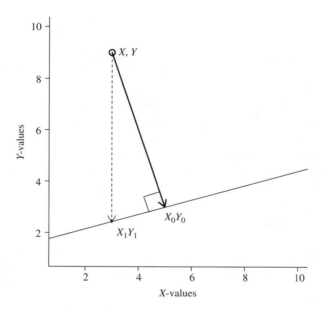

Figure 14–16. The ordinary least-squares distance (dashed line) and perpendicular least-squares distance (solid line).

depending on which member of the x_1/x_2-pair is the "dependent" variable. Therefore, the ordinary least-squares estimate of the slope will likely be less than 1.0 (illustrated in Figures 14–13, 14–14, and 14–15, dashed lines) and have different values depending on the choice of the independent and dependent variable.

An unbiased estimate of a summary line is achieved by measuring the variables x_1 and x_2, so that their influences are treated symmetrically. Figure 14–16 displays the difference between measuring the distance between a point and a line parallel to the vertical axis and measuring the distance between a point and a line by the perpendicular distance to the line. The line from (X, Y) to (X_1, Y_1) is the distance minimized by ordinary least-squares estimation to produce an estimated summary line. The line from (X, Y) to (X_0, Y_0) is the perpendicular distance and can also be minimized to produce an alternative estimated summary line. The perpendicular distance is a symmetric treatment of the pairs of observations, sometimes called an *offset*.

A line estimated by minimizing the perpendicular distances has three distinct properties when both x_1 and x_2 are randomly sampled values from a joint distribution:

1. The estimated slope of the line is unbiased. When the estimated error variances are equal ($\hat{\sigma}_1^2 = \hat{\sigma}_2^2$), the estimated slope is exactly 1.0 (Figure 14–14, solid line).
2. The intercept value is chosen so that the estimated line passes through the center of the data, namely the point ($\bar{x}_2$, $\bar{x}_1$) called the *centroid*. As with regression lines in general, such an estimated line is frequently a useful summary of the relationship between the two sampled variables.
3. The estimation process treats the two variables x_1 and x_2 in a symmetric fashion. Unlike ordinary least-squares regression analyses, the choice of the independent and the dependent variable has essentially no influence on the analytic results.

A perpendicular least-squares estimate of the slope of a summary line is sometimes called a *Deming estimate* and is also a specific application of principal components analysis (Chapter 9). An expression for the slope of a line summarizing the x_1/x_2 relationship, estimated by minimizing the perpendicular distances, is

$$\hat{B} = \frac{\hat{\sigma}_1^2 - \hat{\sigma}_2^2 + \sqrt{(\hat{\sigma}_1^2 - \hat{\sigma}_2^2)^2 + 4\hat{\sigma}_x^4}}{2\hat{\sigma}_x^2}.$$

The estimated intercept of the line becomes

$$\hat{A} = \bar{x}_1 - \hat{B}\bar{x}_2.$$

Geometrically, the estimated line can be viewed as the major axis of an ellipse surrounding the data with a centroid ($\bar{x}_2$, $\bar{x}_1$). The summary line in Figure 14–14 (solid line) has slope $B = 1.0$ because $\sigma_1^2 = \sigma_2^2$. For contrast, the summary line in Figure 14–15 (solid line) has slope $B = 1.387$ ($\sigma_1^2 = 2$ and $\sigma_2^2 = 4$). In both cases, the variance of x is $\sigma_x^2 = 3.0$. Furthermore, reversing the roles of x_1 and x_2 produces the estimated slope $1/\hat{B}$, which yields essentially the same statistical assessment. For example, test statistics constructed from $\hat{B}$ and $1/\hat{B}$ are identical when evaluated in terms of logarithms or

$$test\ statistic = \frac{log(\hat{B}) - 0}{\sqrt{variance[log(\hat{B})]}} = \frac{-log(1/\hat{B}) - 0}{\sqrt{variance[log(1/\hat{B})]}}.$$

The comparison of two measurements of hemoglobin-A_{1c} provides an illustration of the "two-measurement" model. Hemoglobin-A_{1c} is an accurate and effective measure of glucose control and is, therefore, a sensitive indicator of the severity of diabetes. Before conducting an epidemiologic investigation

Table 14–23. Hemoglobin-A1c values compared to assess the reproducibility of long-term and short-term stored samples

	Short	Long		Short	Long		Short	Long
1	5.8	5.8	11	6.6	6.6	21	5.9	6.1
2	4.9	5.7	12	5.7	6.5	22	5.7	6.0
3	6.0	6.5	13	5.4	6.4	23	5.4	5.6
4	5.4	6.0	14	6.5	6.7	24	5.6	5.7
5	7.5	7.6	15	6.0	6.0	25	5.5	5.6
6	5.7	5.9	16	12.3	12.9	26	6.2	6.2
7	5.1	5.8	17	10.9	11.2	27	7.1	7.2
8	9.6	9.7	18	6.8	6.6	28	7.0	7.1
9	5.4	5.6	19	5.8	6.8	29	7.1	7.2
10	4.8	5.6	20	5.7	6.5	30	5.9	5.9

of the relationship between diabetes and the increased risk of coronary heart disease, it was necessary to determine if long-term frozen samples yield reliable measurements [47]. In other words, the issue addressed is the reproducibility of hemoglobin-A_{1c} measurements from whole blood samples stored for more than 10 years. The data in Table 14–23 consist of a small subset of values ($n = 30$ from the original 118 observations [47]) from samples frozen and stored for a short period of time (weeks prior to long-term storage) and their corresponding long-term frozen values (years). Figure 14–17 displays these data.

For convenience, the long-term hemoglobin values are denoted x_1 and the short-term values x_2. As noted, for a symmetric treatment of the variables x_1 and x_2, the analytic results are the same regardless of this choice. The key to the analysis of the differences between members of these 30 pairs of observations is the variance estimates associated with the measurements of x_1 and x_2. These estimates for the A_{1c}-data are:

$$covariance(x_1, x_2) = \hat{\sigma}_x^2 = 2.779,$$
$$\hat{\sigma}_1^2 = \hat{\sigma}_{x_1}^2 - \hat{\sigma}_x = 2.796 - 2.779 = 0.017, \text{ and}$$
$$\hat{\sigma}_2^2 = \hat{\sigma}_{x_2}^2 - \hat{\sigma}_x = 2.879 - 2.779 = 0.100.$$

Ignoring the bias caused by the variability of the variable x_2, the ordinary least-squares estimated slope (x_1 = dependent variable and x_2 = independent variable) is

$$least\text{-}squares \ estimated \ slope = \frac{\hat{\sigma}_x^2}{\sigma_x^2 + \hat{\sigma}_2^2} = \frac{2.779}{2.779 + 0.100} = 0.965.$$

The bias in this case is slight because the variance among the observations ($\hat{\sigma}_x^2$) is substantially greater than the error variance ($\hat{\sigma}_2^2$), thus making the estimated slope essentially equal to 1.0.

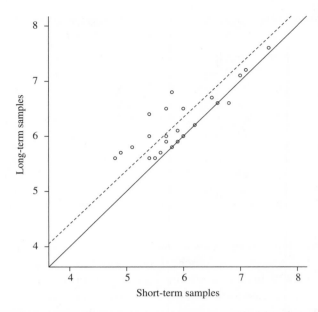

Figure 14–17. Hemoglobin-A_{1c} data compared to evaluate reproducibility of short-term and long-term storage (solid line = perfect agreement and dashed line = estimated agreement).

The correlation between two measurements made on the same subject reflects agreement in terms of the accuracy of one member of the pair to predict the other. For the "two-measurement" model, the estimated correlation coefficient (denoted $\hat{c}$) is

$$correlation\ between\ x_1\ and\ x_2 = correlation(x_1, x_2) = \hat{c} = \frac{\hat{\sigma}_x^2}{\sqrt{(\hat{\sigma}_x^2 + \hat{\sigma}_1^2)(\hat{\sigma}_x^2 + \hat{\sigma}_2^2)}}.$$

In the context of longitudinal data analysis, this estimate is the intraclass correlation coefficient when the error variances associated with both observations are the same (Chapter 12). Like the slope estimated in a least-squares regression analysis, when the variation between sampled values (σ_x^2) is much greater than both the measurement error variances (σ_1^2 and σ_2^2), the correlation coefficient is close to 1.0.

The unbiased perpendicular least-squares regression analysis from the A_{1c} data (treating x_1 and x_2 symmetrically) yields an estimated slope $= \hat{B} = 0.985$ and intercept $\hat{A} = 0.419$, producing the estimated summary line $0.419 + 0.985x_2$. The estimated slope is again essentially equal to 1.0. However, the estimated intercept is substantially different from zero. That is, the line of perfect agreement ($x_1 = x_2$) and the estimated line of agreement are close to parallel because the long-term A_{1c}

observations have consistently higher values than the short-term A_{1c} observations (Figure 14–17). An estimate of this constant difference is the intercept itself ($\hat{A} =$ 0.419). Nevertheless, the short-term values remain an almost perfect predictor of the long-term values ($x_1 \approx x_2 + 0.419 - correlation(x_1, x_2) = 0.980$).

An expression for the variance of the perpendicular least-squares estimated slope is complicated and unnecessary. Resampling the original $n = 30$ observations produces an assumption-free bootstrap estimate of the distribution of the estimated value $\hat{B}$. From this bootstrap-estimated distribution, an estimate of the variance and a confidence interval directly follow. For the estimate $\hat{B} = 0.985$ ($n = 30$), the bootstrap-estimated variance is 0.00289 (standard error = 0.054) and a bootstrap 95% confidence interval is (0.804, 1.031), based on 5000 replicate samples of the original 30 A_{1c} measurements. The similar normal-based confidence interval is $0.985 \pm 1.960(0.054) = (0.879, 1.091)$. From either a visual (Figure 14–17) or a confidence interval point of view, no apparent evidence exists that the slope of the estimated line systematically differs from 1.0.

More formally, a test statistic

$$z = \frac{-log(1/\hat{B}) - 0}{\sqrt{variance[log(1/\hat{B})]}} = \frac{-0.015 - 0}{0.054} = -0.281$$

has a standard normal distribution when $B = 1$. The resulting p-value $= P(|Z| \geq 0.281 | B = 1) = 0.389$ again indicates no evidence that the error variances are unequal ($x_1 = x_2$).

An Alternative Approach: Bland-Altman Analysis

The question of agreement between two measurements is alternatively addressed by creating two new variables and then applying ordinary least-squares regression methods. These transformed variables are the mean values $X_i = \frac{1}{2}(x_{i1} + x_{i2})$ and the differences $Y_i = x_{i1} - x_{i2}$ within each pair of observations. The transformation produces two variables that treat x_1 and x_2 in a symmetric fashion. The analytic results are the same regardless of the choice of the independent and dependent variables (X is unaffected and Y only changes in sign). Using these mean values and differences, made popular by two medical statisticians, Bland and Altman [48], is frequently referred to as a *Bland-Altman analysis*.

The bias encountered from directly applying ordinary least-squares linear regression methods is no longer an issue in the analysis of the transformed X/Y pairs. Using mean values and differences based on the observations, x_1 and x_2 converted to the pairs (X, Y) produce the expressions for a least-squares estimated line with slope of

$$estimated\ slope = \hat{B}_{Y|x} = \frac{\hat{\sigma}_2^2 - \hat{\sigma}_1^2}{2\hat{\sigma}_x^2 + \frac{1}{2}(\hat{\sigma}_1^2 + \hat{\sigma}_2^2)}$$

and intercept

$$estimated\ intercept = \hat{A} = \bar{Y} - \hat{B}_{Y|x}\bar{X}$$

where

$$\bar{X} = \frac{1}{2n}\sum(x_{i1} + x_{i2}) \text{ and } \bar{Y} = \frac{1}{n}\sum(x_{i1} - x_{i2})$$

for $i = 1, 2, \cdots, n$ and, again, n represents the number of observations (pairs). The expression for the estimated slope clearly shows that $\hat{B}_{Y|x} = 0.0$ when $\hat{\sigma}_1^2 = \hat{\sigma}_2^2$ (unbiased). The resulting summary line becomes $\hat{Y}_i = \hat{A} + \hat{B}_{Y|x}X_i$.

To illustrate, a computer-generated sample of $n = 100$ pairs of observations x_1 and x_2 ($\mu = 10$, $\sigma_x^2 = 2$, $\sigma_1^2 = \sigma_2^2 = 4$) is used to create $X = \frac{1}{2}(x_{i1} + x_{i2})$ and $Y = x_{i1} - x_{i2}$. Using these hypothetical data, the estimated slope is $\hat{B}_{Y|x} = -0.080$ ($B_{Y|x} = 0$) and intercept $\hat{A} = 0.523$ ($A = 0$). The data and the estimated line ($\hat{Y}_i = 0.523 - 0.080X_i$, dashed line) are displayed in Figure 14–18 and illustrate the unbiased nature of the regression analysis. When the variances of the variables x_1 and x_2 differ by chance alone, the estimate $\hat{B}_{Y|x}$ randomly differs from zero. To test this conjecture, an ordinary regression analysis, based on the transformed values X and Y, yields an estimate of the slope B and its variance.

Traditionally included on the plot (Figure 14–18) are the upper and lower bounds that are expected to contain 95% of the observations Y. These bounds are given by

$$lower\ bound = \bar{Y} - 1.960\sqrt{\hat{\sigma}_1^2 + \hat{\sigma}_2^2} \text{ and } upper\ bound = \bar{Y} + 1.960\sqrt{\hat{\sigma}_1^2 + \hat{\sigma}_2^2}.$$

When the distributions of the sampled values x_1 and x_2 are not badly skewed (approximately symmetric), then about 95% of the observed values of Y should lie between these bounds. When the sampled values have normal distributions, then it is expected that 95% of the observed Y-values will lie between these bounds. In neither case do these bounds form a 95% confidence interval. The bounds only identify where the Y-values are likely to be located and do not reflect the precision of an estimate.

Returning to the hemoglobin-A_{1c} data, the mean values (X) and the differences (Y) are given in Table 14–24. Using ordinary least-squares estimation-based on the 30 X/Y pairs of A_{1c} data produces the estimated slope $\hat{B}_{Y|x} = -0.015$ and intercept $\hat{A} = 0.421$ (Table 14–25). The estimated summary line becomes $\hat{Y}_i = 0.421 - 0.015X_i$. Wald's chi-square test of the estimated slope ($B_{Y|x} = 0$?)

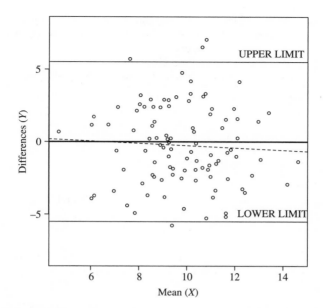

Figure 14–18. Hypothetical observations x_1 and x_2 ($\mu = 10$, $\sigma_x^2 = 2$, $\sigma_1^2 = \sigma_2^2 = 4$) used to create transformed values $X = \frac{1}{2}(x_1 + x_2)$ and $Y = x_1 - x_2$ for $n = 100$ (least squares estimate = dashed line).

Table 14–24. Values $X = \frac{1}{2}(x_1 + x_2)$ and $Y = x_1 - x_2$ where x_1 and x_2 are the observed long-term and short-term values of the hemoglobin-A_1c measurements (Table 14–23)

	X	Y		X	Y		X	Y
1	5.80	0.0	11	6.60	0.2	21	6.00	0.2
2	5.30	0.8	12	6.10	0.8	22	5.85	0.0
3	6.25	0.5	13	6.60	0.2	23	5.50	0.2
4	5.70	0.6	14	6.10	0.8	24	5.65	0.1
5	7.55	0.1	15	6.00	0.0	25	5.55	0.1
6	5.80	0.2	16	12.60	0.6	26	6.20	0.0
7	5.45	0.7	17	11.05	0.3	27	7.15	0.1
8	9.65	0.1	18	6.70	-0.2	28	7.05	0.1
9	5.50	0.2	19	6.30	1.0	29	7.15	0.1
10	5.20	0.8	20	6.10	0.8	30	5.90	0.1

yields

$$X^2 = \left[\frac{\hat{B}_{Y|x} - 0}{S_{\hat{B}_{Y|x}}}\right]^2 = \left[\frac{-0.015}{0.038}\right]^2 = 0.156,$$

with an associated p-value of $P(X^2 \geq 0.156 | B_{Y|x} = 0) = 0.703$. The same analytic results occur when the roles of x_1 and x_2 are reversed.

Table 14–25. Analysis of the transformed hemoglobin-A_1c data: regression analysis ($n = 30$) where the difference Y is the dependent variable and the mean value X is the independent variable

Variables	Symbols	Estimates	Std. errors	p-Values
Intercept	A	0.421	0.261	0.118
Slope	$B_{Y\mid x}$	−0.015	0.038	0.703

LogLikelihood $= -1.678$

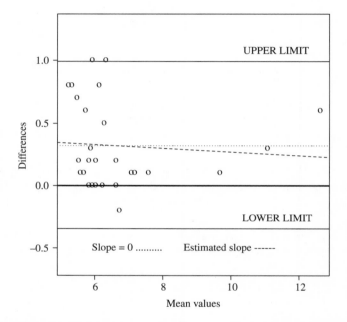

Figure 14–19. Regression analysis of $X = \frac{1}{2}(x_1 + x_2)$ and $Y = x_1 - x_2$ applied to the hemoglobin-A_{1c} data (Table 14–24).

The estimated upper and lower limits of the likely (95%) range of the observations Y contain all 30 differences (Y-values). Specifically, for the A_{1c} data, these bounds are $\overline{Y} \pm 1.960\sqrt{\hat{\sigma}_1^2 + \hat{\sigma}_2^2} = \overline{Y} \pm 1.960\sqrt{0.017 + 0.100} = 0.323 \pm 0.669$, or lower bound $= -0.345$ and upper bound $= 0.992$. As before, there appears to be a constant difference between the short-term and long-term storage values (Figure 14–19). The intercept of the estimated line summarizing the long- and short-term difference is well above zero (estimated intercept $= \hat{A} = 0.421$). However, the line is essentially horizontal, indicating again that this difference (bias) is close to constant for all values of X. Also, the plot (Figure 14–19) visually indicates that the long-term and short-term samples apparently differ by a constant value, and the statistical analysis rigorously supports this conclusion (p-value = 0.703). Again, the analysis of the A_{1c} data indicates that values from long-term storage are extremely accurate predictors of the short-term values.

ANOTHER APPLICATION OF PERPENDICULAR LEAST-SQUARES ESTIMATION

Again, the focus is on pairs of observations without a natural way to choose one member of the pair as the independent and the other as the dependent variables. For example, the likelihood of coronary heart disease is clearly the dependent variable in a study of influences of cholesterol levels. However, if the purpose is to describe the association between blood pressure and cholesterol measurements, then natural independent and dependent variables do not exist. Another example (explored further) occurs in the investigation of the birth weights of twins. Again, no clear choice of independent and dependent variables exists between the twins that make up a pair. Furthermore, the birth weight of each member of a twin pair has an associated variance, causing an ordinary least-squares analysis to produce a biased estimate of the slope of a line summarizing their association.

Consider two variables, labeled x_1 and x_2, where the variances and covariance are estimated in the usual way:

$$variance(x_1) = S_1^2 = \frac{1}{n-1}\sum(x_{i1} - \bar{x}_1)^2,$$

$$variance(x_2) = S_2^2 = \frac{1}{n-1}\sum(x_{i2} - \bar{x}_2)^2, \quad \text{and}$$

$$covariance(x_1, x_2) = S_{12}^2 = \frac{1}{n-1}\sum(x_{i1} - \bar{x}_1)(x_{i2} - \bar{x}_2)$$

where $i = 1, 2, \cdots, n$. An expression for the perpendicular least-squares estimated slope of a line summarizing the x_1/x_2-relationship is

$$\hat{B} = \frac{(S_2^2 - S_1^2) + \sqrt{(S_1^2 - S_2^2)^2 + 4S_{12}^2}}{2S_{12}}.$$

To select the line that intersects the center of the data $(\bar{x}_2, \bar{x}_1)$, the estimated intercept is $\hat{A} = \bar{x}_1 - \hat{B}\bar{x}_2$. The perpendicular least-squares estimated line $\hat{A} + \hat{B}x_2$ is then a symmetric summary of the x_1/x_2-relationship in the sense that the assessment of the estimated slope is essentially the same regardless of the selection of the independent and dependent variable. The estimated slope from the previous "two-measurement" model is a special case of this expression where $S_1^2 = \hat{\sigma}_x^2 + \hat{\sigma}_1^2$, $S_2^2 = \hat{\sigma}_x^2 + \hat{\sigma}_2^2$, and $S_{12} = \hat{\sigma}_x^2$.

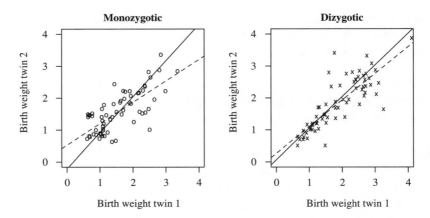

Figure 14–20. Data on $n = 131$ (66 monozygotic and 65 dizygotic pairs) twin birth weights (kilograms) classified by zygosity (solid line = perpendicular least-squares estimated line and the dashed line = ordinary estimated least-squares line).

From a study of congenital heart defects among newborn twins, data on their birth weights and zygosity (monozygotic or dizygotic pairs) were recored for 131 pairs (66 monozygotic and 65 dizygotic pairs) and serve to illustrate perpendicular least-squares estimation (Figure 14–20). Using the estimated values S_1^2, S_2^2, and S_{12} yields the perpendicular estimated slopes $\hat{B}$ and thus, the summary straight lines for monozygotic and dizygotic twins data. The standard errors associated with the estimated slopes $\hat{B}$ are estimated by bootstrap resampling of the data (replicates = 2000). Based on these estimates, no important difference appears to exist between the monozygotic and dizygotic twins in terms of the slope of the lines summarizing a linear birth weigh association. Specifically, the p-value associated with a statistical assessment of the difference is $P(|\hat{B}_{mz} - \hat{B}_{dz}| \geq 0|no\ difference) = P(|Z| \geq 0.916) = 0.359$ (Table 14–26).

The parallel analysis using ordinary least-squares estimation produces the values in Table 14–27 (for contrast). The first twin in each pair is arbitrarily selected as the independent variable for illustration purposes. The ordinary least-squares estimates are biased and are presented to emphasize that the choice of the kind of estimation (perpendicular vs. ordinary least-squares) can produce rather different results.

The statistical structure postulated to produce the perpendicular least-squares estimate $\hat{B}$ is a special case of a *structural relationship model* [49]. Explicit in this estimate is the assumption or knowledge that the variables labeled x_1 and x_2 are measured without error or, at least, the measurement error is substantially smaller than the variances associated with the sampled observations. That is, measurement error can be ignored. In symbols, the *variance*$(X + e) \approx$ *variance*(X).

Table 14–26. The perpendicular least-squares estimated slopes describing the birth weights (kilograms) from the $n = 131$ twin pairs classified by zygosity (included are bootstrap-estimated standard errors and 95% confidence interval bounds)

	$\hat{A}$	$\hat{B}$	Std. error	Lower	Upper
Monozygotic	−0.213	1.127	0.130	0.933	1.439
Dizygotic	0.066	0.989	0.076	0.843	1.127

Monozygotic twin line: $\hat{Y} = \hat{bwt}_2 = -0.213 + 1.127\ bwt_1$ and
Dizygotic twin line: $\hat{Y} = \hat{bwt}_1 = 0.066 + 0.989\ bwt_1$

Table 14–27. The ordinary least-squares estimated slopes describing the birth weights (kilograms) from the $n = 131$ twin pairs classified by zygosity (included are estimated standard errors and 95% confidence interval bounds)

	$\hat{a}$	$\hat{b}$	Std. error	Lower	Upper
Monozygotic	0.301	0.800	0.094	0.611	0.988
Dizygotic	0.379	0.818	0.069	0.680	0.957

Monozygotic twin line: $\hat{y} = \hat{bwt}_2 = 0.301 + 0.800\ bwt_1$ and
Dizygotic twin line: $\hat{y} = \hat{bwt}_2 = 0.379 + 0.818\ bwt_1$

If measurement error is an issue, then values for the error variances σ_1^2 and σ_2^2 must be found from sources other than the data. Using the ratio $\lambda = \sigma_2^2/\sigma_1^2$, the expression for the estimated slope becomes

$$\hat{B} = \frac{(\lambda S_2^2 - S_1^2) + \sqrt{(\lambda S_1^2 - S_2^2)^2 + 4\lambda S_{12}^2}}{2S_{12}}$$

and is the perpendicular least-squares estimate of the slope B. However, realistic values for the ratio of the error variances σ_1^2 and σ_2^2 are rarely available.

15

ADVANCED TOPICS

The topics in this chapter are continuations of concepts and methods previously presented. The first topic brings a new perspective to the theory and application of confidence intervals (used in most chapters). Second, smoothing techniques (introduced in Chapter 10) are again explored with an additional method that is extended to bivariate estimates and plots. A third topic adds to the discussion of the issues surrounding statistical tests. The calculation of the power of a test and sample size estimates are described for both the analysis of normal and chi-square distributed summary measures. A brief discussion of adjusting p-values to compensate for the accumulation of error due to multiple tests then ends the chapter.

CONFIDENCE INTERVALS

An estimated probability is, in many situations, called a *proportion*. In Chapter 3, the likelihood principle is discussed and, from this perspective, a proportion is the "best" estimate of a probability from data with a binomial distribution. As before, the count x, representing a number of specific events, divided by the total number of n independent events is an estimate of a underlying binomial parameter

q, denoted $\hat{q} = x/n$. A confidence interval based on the estimated probability $\hat{q}$ typically employs a normal distribution as an approximation to the binomial distribution producing two bounds, namely

$$lower\ bound = \hat{A} = \hat{q} - 1.960 S_{\hat{q}} = \hat{q} - 1.960\sqrt{\hat{q}(1 - \hat{q})/n}$$

and

$$upper\ bound = \hat{B} = \hat{q} + 1.960 S_{\hat{q}} = \hat{q} + 1.960\sqrt{\hat{q}(1 - \hat{q})/n}.$$

The interval $(\hat{A}, \hat{B})$ has an approximate 95% probability of containing the underlying parameter q. A confidence interval enhances most estimates, giving a sense of the location of the underlying parameter value and, at the same time, the width of the interval gives a sense of the precision associated with the estimated value. The confidence limits $\hat{A}$ and $\hat{B}$ are equally interpreted as bounds that identify a range of likely candidates for the underlying parameter (Chapter 3). Or, values of a parameter less than $\hat{A}$ are unlikely candidates for the parameter q because they are too small, and values of a parameter greater than $\hat{B}$ are also unlikely candidates because they are too large in light of the estimated value $\hat{q}$. Arbitrarily, but almost always, "unlikely" is defined as less than a 5% probability (likelihood <0.05). For example, when $x = 15$ and $n = 50$, then $\hat{q} = 15/50 = 0.30$. The approximate 95% confidence interval bounds constructed from this estimate are

$$\hat{A} = 0.30 - 1.960(0.065) = 0.173 \text{ and } \hat{B} = 0.30 + 1.960(0.065) = 0.427.$$

Thus, values less than 0.173 (too small) or greater than 0.427 (too large) are unlikely candidates for the underlying parameter of the binomial distribution that produced the sample estimate $\hat{q} = 0.30$, namely the parameter value represented by q. The normal distribution approximation works best when q is in the neighborhood of 0.5 and the number of sampled observations is more than 30 or so.

When the parameter q is in the neighborhood of zero or one, the binomial distribution then becomes asymmetric, and the symmetric normal distribution no longer produces accurate confidence interval bounds. The interpretation of a confidence interval as a statistical tool used to identify likely parameter values based on the sampled data then becomes the basis for construction of an accurate confidence interval when the normal distribution approximation approach fails.

An extreme example occurs when the observed sample produces zero outcomes ($x = 0$) making the estimate $\hat{q} = 0$. Specifically, during the year 1997, in west Oakland, California, no cases of colon cancer were observed ($x = 0$) among $n = 20,183$ African-American women. Clearly, the approximate normal distribution-derived bounds fail. Nevertheless, it is straightforward to determine

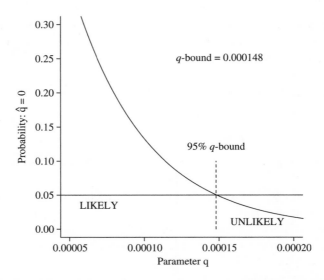

Figure 15–1. The probability that $\hat{q} = 0$ ($x = 0$) cases of colon cancer (Oakland, CA, 1977) among $n = 20{,}183$ African-American women at-risk.

the values of the parameter q that are likely and unlikely to have produced the observed value of zero. The value 30/100,000 is an unlikely candidate for the value of the parameter q (too large) because the probability of observing zero cases is small. When $q = 0.0003$, the probability that $\hat{q} = 0$ is $(1 - q)^n = 0.9997^{20,183} = 0.0023$. On the other hand, the value 3/100,000 is a likely candidate for the value of the parameter q because the probability of observing zero cases is large. When $q = 0.00003$, the probability that $\hat{q} = 0$ is $(1 - q)^n = 0.99997^{20,183} = 0.546$. A series of values of q produces a list or curve (Figure 15–1) that identifies the likelihood of the estimate $\hat{q} = 0$ ($x = 0$) for a range of values of the parameter q. A point is easily chosen that divides all possible values of q into those values likely and unlikely to have produced no cases of colon cancer.

As noted, a parameter value that makes the likelihood of an observed value greater than 0.05 is usually considered a likely value, and a parameter value that makes the likelihood of an observed value less than 0.05 an unlikely value. That is, a specific value of q (denoted q_{bound}) that divides all possible values of the parameter q into those values consistent with the data (likely) and those values inconsistent with the data (unlikely) forms a confidence interval. The bound q_{bound} is simply calculated with a computer algorithm that creates a sequence of values of $(1 - q)^n$ until this boundary value of q is found, where n represents the fixed number of sampled observations. It is the value such that $(1 - q_{bound})^n = 0.05$. Then, all values less than the bound are considered likely candidates for the unknown parameter q, and all values greater are consider unlikely candidates. For the simple case of $\hat{q} = 0$, the value q_{bound} can be found directly because

$$\text{when } (1 - q_{bound})^n = 0.05, \text{ then } q_{bound} = 1 - 0.05^{1/n}.$$

Therefore, for the colon cancer data, either method produces the bound $q_{bound} = 1 - 0.05^{(1/20,183)} = 14.842$ cases per 100,000 women (Figure 15–1). Thus, all parameter values $q > q_{bound}$ make the probability of observing $\hat{q} = 0$ less than 0.05, and all parameter values $q < q_{bound}$ make the probability of observing $\hat{q} = 0$ greater than 0.05. A confidence interval (0, 14.842) cases per 100,000 women, therefore, has a 95% probability of containing the true underlying parameter, namely q.

Consider a slightly more complicated example that employs the same principle. When $x = 2$ and $n = 50$, the estimate of q is $\hat{q} = 2/50 = 0.04$. The approximate normal-based 95% confidence interval bounds are $\hat{A} = -0.014$ and $\hat{B} = 0.094$. The negative lower bound indicates that the normal distribution is failing as an approximation. However, for $x = 2$ and $n = 50$, the 95% confidence bounds can be found by calculating the binomial probabilities for a series of values of q to locate two values that create the lower and upper bounds (denoted q_l and q_u) of a 95% confidence interval. Again, the possible values of the parameter q are divided into those values likely and those values unlikely in light of the estimate $\hat{q}$. When $\hat{q} = 0.04$ ($x = 2$ and $n = 50$), then

$$lower\ bound\ (q_l) : P(X \geq 2) = 1 - \left[\sum \binom{n}{x} q_l^x (1 - q_l)^{n-x} \right] \quad x = 0 \text{ and } 1$$

$$= 1 - \left[(1 - q_l)^n + nq_l(1 - q_l)^{n-1} \right] = 0.025$$

and, similarly,

$$upper\ bound\ (q_u) : P(X \leq 2) = \sum \binom{n}{x} q_u^x (1 - q_u)^{n-x} = 0.025 \quad x = 0, 1 \text{ and } 2$$

$$= (1 - q_u)^n + nq_u(1 - q_u)^{n-1}$$

$$+ \frac{1}{2}n(n - 1)q_u^2(1 - q_u)^{n-2}$$

$$= 0.025$$

for $n = 50$ observations and $x = 2$.

The lower bound q_l becomes 0.0049 because

$$lower\ bound\ (q_1) : \quad P(X \geq 2) = 1 - \left[\sum \binom{50}{x} 0.0049^x (1 - 0.0049)^{50-x} \right]$$

$$= 1 - [0.782 + 0.193] = 0.025,$$

and the upper bound q_u becomes 0.137 because

$$\textit{upper bound }(q_u): \ P(X \leq 2) = \sum \binom{50}{x} 0.137^x (1 - 0.137)^{50-x}$$

$$= 0.0005 + 0.005 + 0.0195 = 0.025.$$

Therefore, values of q less than the lower bound $q_l = 0.0049$ make the occurrence of $x = 2$ unlikely (too small, Figure 15–2). Similarly, values of q greater than the upper bound $q_u = 0.137$ also make the occurrence of $x = 2$ unlikely (too large, Figure 15–2). Details of the search for these values are given in Table 15–1. Thus, the bounds identify the candidates for the parameter q that are implausible because they are too small ($q_l < 0.0049$) or implausible because they are too large ($q_u > 0.137$). Or, conversely, the bounds $q_u = 0.0049$ and $q_u = 0.137$ identify the range of plausible candidates for the parameter q in light of the observed data ($x = 2$ or $\hat{q} = 0.04$).

These confidence interval bounds are not based on an approximation and can be made essentially exact using a computer search approach.

For the sake of comparison, consider the case where $x = 25$ is observed and $n = 50$, then

$$P(X \geq 25) = 1 - \left[\sum \binom{50}{x} 0.355^x (1 - 0.355)^{50-x} \right] = 0.025 \quad x = 0, 1, \cdots, 24,$$

and

$$P(X \leq 25) = \sum \binom{50}{x} 0.645^x (1 - 0.645)^{50-x} = 0.025 \qquad x = 0, 1, \cdots, 25,$$

making the 95% confidence bounds $q_l = 0.355$ and $q_u = 0.645$ based on the estimate $\hat{q} = 0.50$. Again, parameter values less than 0.355 (too small) and values greater than 0.645 (too large) are unlikely candidates for the parameter q in light of the estimate $\hat{q} = 0.5$. Using the normal approximation approach, the estimated 95% confidence interval bounds are (0.361 0.639). To repeat, both intervals describe a range of likely values of the parameter q when $x = 25$ is observed and $n = 50$.

In general, a 95% confidence interval based on the estimate $\hat{q} = x/n$ consists of finding the parameter values q_l and q_u that solve the following two expressions: Lower bound:

$$1 - \left[\sum \binom{n}{k} q_l^k (1 - q_l)^{n-k} \right] = 0.025 \qquad k = 0, 1, 2, \cdots, x - 1$$

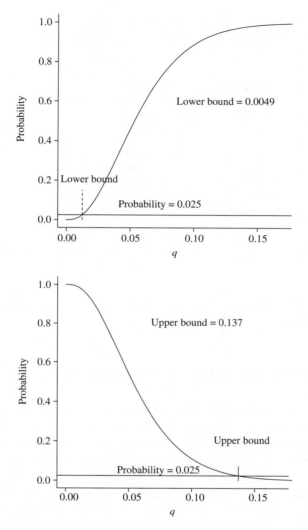

Figure 15–2. Schematic representation of the search for the upper and lower 95% confidence bounds for $x = 2$ events occurring among $n = 50$ possible outcomes ($\hat{q} = 0.04$).

Upper bound:

$$\sum \binom{n}{k} q_u^k (1 - q_u)^{n-k} = 0.025 \quad k = 0, 1, 2, \cdots, x.$$

The solutions to these two equations, q_l and q_u, can be achieved by evaluating these expressions with a trial-and-error computer strategy using the normal

Table 15–1.   An illustration of a numerical search for the lower and upper 95% confidence interval bounds when $x = 2$ and $n = 50$

Lower bound		Upper bound	
q	$(P(X \geq 2))$	q	$P(X \leq 2)$
0.0044	0.0206	0.130	0.034
0.0045	0.0215	0.131	0.032
0.0046	0.0224	0.132	0.031
0.0047	0.0233	0.133	0.030
0.0048	0.0242	0.134	0.029
q_l	0.025	0.135	0.027
0.0049	0.0252	0.136	0.026
0.0050	0.0261	0.137	0.025
0.0051	0.0271	q_u	0.025
0.0052	0.0281	0.138	0.024
0.0053	0.0291	0.139	0.023
0.0054	0.0301	0.140	0.022

approximation bounds as a starting point. Rather sophisticated algebraic solutions also exist (Chapter 7).

AN EXAMPLE OF A BIVARIATE CONFIDENCE REGION

Perhaps the most commonly estimated quantities from data are the sample mean and sample variance. As with all values estimated from data, the sample mean $\bar{x} = \sum x_i / n$ (an estimate of the parameter μ) is subject to sampling variability, estimated by $variance(\bar{x}) = S^2/n$, where $S^2 = \sum(x_i - \bar{x})^2/(n-1)$. The sample variance S^2 (an estimate of the parameter σ^2) is also an estimate and is similarly subject to the sampling variability, estimated by $variance(S^2) = 2S^4/n$. It is instructive to describe a confidence region based on these two commonly estimated values.

When a variable Z has a standard normal distribution, then Z^2 has a chi-square distribution with one degree of freedom. When Z_1 and Z_2 have independent standard normal distributions, then $Z_1^2 + Z_2^2$ has a chi-square distribution with two degrees of freedom (Chapters 2 and 12). Using these two facts, the value

$$X^2 = \frac{(\bar{x} - \mu)^2}{S^2/n} + \frac{(S^2 - \sigma^2)^2}{2S^4/n}$$

has an approximate chi-square distribution with two degrees of freedom because, for $n > 30$ or so, the estimated mean value $\bar{x}$ and variance S^2 frequently have approximate normal distributions. Thus, using the 95th percentile from a chi-square distribution with two degrees of freedom (5.991), the expression

$$X^2 = Z_1^2 + Z_2^2 = \frac{(\bar{x} - \mu)^2}{S^2/n} + \frac{(S^2 - \sigma^2)^2}{2S^4/n} = 5.991$$

forms an elliptical region that has a 0.95 probability of containing both the underlying parameters μ and σ^2, based on their estimated values $\bar{x}$ and S^2 called a *95% confidence region*. That is, the probability is approximately 0.95 that the two unknown parameters μ and σ^2 are simultaneously contained within the bounds of this region (ellipse) because $P(X^2 \leq 5.991 | degrees\ of\ freedom = 2) = 0.95$.

Consider a sample mean value of $\bar{x} = 8.0$ with an estimated variance of $S^2 = 2.0$ based on $n = 50$ observations. An approximate 95% confidence region is created from these estimated values and a chi-square distribution with two degrees of freedom (Figure 15–3). Specifically, the expression

$$P(X^2 \leq 5.991) = P\left[\frac{(8.0 - \mu)^2}{2.0/50} + \frac{(2.0 - \sigma^2)^2}{2(2.0^2)/50} \leq 5.991\right]$$

describes an approximate 95% confidence region with center at $(\bar{x}, S^2) = (8, 2)$. This confidence region, analogous to a confidence interval, has a 0.95 probability

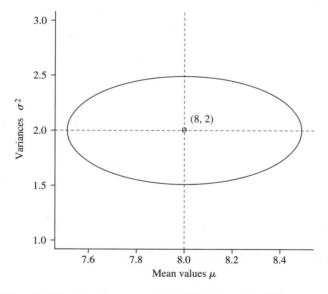

Figure 15–3.   An illustration of an approximate 95% elliptical confidence region for the mean value μ and the variances σ^2 based on the chi-square distribution and the estimated mean value $\bar{x} = 8.0$ and variance $S^2 = 2.0$ ($n = 50$).

of simultaneously containing the underlying and unknown mean value μ and variance σ^2, estimated by $\bar{x}$ and S^2. As with confidence intervals based on a single variable, the bivariate ellipse (Figure 15–3) summarizes simultaneously the possible locations of the two parameters μ and σ^2, and the size of the ellipse indicates the precision of their estimated values. Thus, the ellipse identifies likely (within the ellipse) and unlikely (not within the ellipse) pairs of parameter values μ and σ^2 based on their estimates. The axes of the elliptical confidence region are parallel to the coordinate axes, which occurs because the estimated mean and variance are independent, which is a property of the normal distribution. This bivariate confidence region is a simple case. Confidence "regions" for nonindependent estimates with more than two parameters can be estimated based on sample data but involve advanced statistical concepts and methods [41].

CONFIDENCE BAND

An important distinction exists between a series of confidence intervals and a confidence band. This distinction arises in a variety of statistical contexts. An estimated regression line illustrates the important issues.

Consider a sample of n pairs of observations $(x_i,\ y_i)$, then the least-squares estimated regression line is given by the expression

$$\hat{y}_i = \bar{y} + \hat{b}(x_i - \bar{x})$$

for $i = 1, 2, \cdots, n =$ sample size. An estimated value of y at a value x is

$$\hat{y}_x = \bar{y} + \hat{b}(x - \bar{x}).$$

The associated variance of the distribution of the predicted value $\hat{y}_x$ for the selected value x is estimated by

$$variance(\hat{y}_x) = S_{\hat{Y}_x}^2 = S_Y^2 | x \left[\frac{1}{n} + \frac{(x - \bar{x})^2}{\sum(x_i - \bar{x})^2} \right]$$

where $S_Y^2 | x = \sum(y_i - \hat{y}_i)^2 / (n - 2)$ estimates the variance of the distribution of the variable Y at the value x.

A 95% confidence interval created from the estimate $\hat{y}_x$ and its estimated variance is then

$$lower\ bound = \hat{A} = \hat{y}_x - t_{n-2}^{0.975} S_{\hat{Y}_x} \quad \text{and}$$
$$upper\ bound = \hat{B} = \hat{y}_x + t_{n-2}^{0.975} S_{\hat{Y}_x}$$

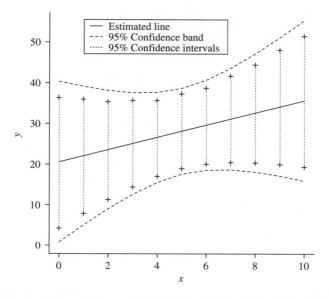

Figure 15–4. A contrast of a series of point-wise 95% confidence intervals (dotted lines) and a 95% confidence band (dashed lines) for an estimated regression line (solid lines).

where $t_{n-2}^{0.975}$ represents the 97.5% percentile for a t-distribution with $n-2$ degrees of freedom. The confidence interval $(\hat{A}, \hat{B})$ is interpreted as usual and referred to as a *point-wise confidence interval* (Figure 15–4, dotted vertical lines). Thus, the probability that the underlying value estimated by $\hat{y}_x$ is contained in the confidence interval $(\hat{A}, \hat{B})$ is 0.95. However, such confidence intervals are frequently calculated for a series of values of x, and the upper and lower bounds of these point-wise confidence intervals are connected, forming a band surrounding the estimated regression line. This band lacks a formal statistical interpretation.

A 95% confidence band based on the estimated value $\hat{y}_x$ is constructed from the bounds

$$lower\ bound = \hat{A}^* = \hat{y}_x - \sqrt{2 f_{2,\,n-2}^{0.95}} S_{\hat{Y}_x}$$

and

$$upper\ bound = \hat{B}^* = \hat{y}_x + \sqrt{2 f_{2,\,n-2}^{0.95}} S_{\hat{Y}_x}$$

where $f_{2,\,n-2}^{0.95}$ represent a 95% percentile from an f-distribution with two and $n-2$ degrees of freedom [50]. When a series of these intervals are connected (Figure 15–4, dashed line), the band formed has a 0.95 probability that the underlying regression line, estimated by the line $\hat{y}_x$, is entirely contained between the upper and lower limits. A 95% confidence band indicates a region in which straight

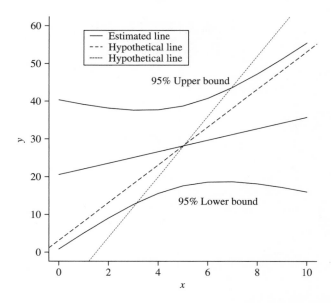

Figure 15–5. Two hypothetical lines; one line inconsistent with the data (dotted), one line consistent with the data (dashed), and the estimated line (solid).

lines are consistent with the data and in which straight lines that are not consistent (Figure 15–5).

As with a confidence interval and a confidence region, a confidence band is constructed so that the probability is 0.95 that the lower and upper limits contain the straight lines that are likely, in light of the observed data. In contrast, each point-wise confidence interval contains the parameter value estimated by $\hat{y}_x$ with probability 0.95 for a specific value of x. The probability is necessarily less than 0.95 that a sequence of such intervals simultaneously contain all such parameter values.

For this simple linear regression example, the difference in the width of a point-wise confidence "band" and the exact confidence band is approximately $S_{\hat{Y}_x}$ ($n > 30$). Therefore, the distinction between connecting a series of confidence intervals and a confidence band decreases as the sample size increases. Although in many situations connecting an easily constructed sequence of points generated by a series of point-wise confidence intervals produces an approximate confidence band, it is technically not correct.

NONPARAMETRIC REGRESSION METHODS

Regression models are certainly a fundamental statistical tool. However, situations arise where it is advantageous to describe relationships without reference to a specific model. Nonparametric regression techniques are designed specifically for this task. They produce estimates of even complicated relationships without a statistical structure (model). Thus, the properties of the resulting summary are entirely determined by the data. A description follows of one such technique, called *loess estimation*. More descriptively, the approach is also called *local linear regression estimation* or more generally, it is the specific kind of *locally weighted polynomial regression estimation*. The name loess comes from selecting letters from the more formal description "locally weighted regression smoothing." Loess estimates require extensive computation but are conceptually simple and have the particularly important feature of providing natural nonlinear and totally assumption-free descriptions of relationships within sampled data.

A special case of loess estimation is no more than a weighted moving average (Chapter 10). Specifically, an estimate of an outcome value represented by y at a specified value of x is created from the n sampled pairs of observations (x_i, y_i) and a series of weights (denoted w). An expression for this weighted average is given by

$$\hat{y}_x = \frac{\sum w(x, x_i, h) y_i}{\sum w(x, x_i, h)} \quad i = 1, 2, \cdots, n$$

where n represents the number of sampled x/y-pairs. The weights are designed so that the largest values are given to the data points y_i at the value x_i and less and less weight to points as they become further from x_i. That is, the maximum weight occurs at $x = x_i$ and subsequent weights decrease as the value $|x - x_i|$ increases.

A traditional weighting function, called a *tri-cubic function*, is

$$w(x, x_i) = \left\{ \begin{array}{ll} (1 - |x - x_i|^3)^3 & \text{for } |x_i| < 1 \\ 0 & \text{for } |x_i| \geq 1 \end{array} \right\} \quad i = 1, 2, \cdots, n.$$

In the following, another choice of weights is used. These weights are the heights of a normal distribution, with mean value equal to the observation x_i and standard deviation represented by h, evaluated at a sequence of values of x. In symbols, the weighting function for the ith observation (y_i), denoted

$$w(x, x_i, h) = \phi[x, x_i, h],$$

are the heights of the normal distribution ($\mu = x_i$ and $h = $ selected standard deviation) for a sequence of values of x. The selection of the value h determines the degree of smoothness of the estimated curve and is called the *bandwidth*

Table 15–2. Examples of two weighting functions for loess regression estimation for $x_i = 0.4$ and $h = 0.5$ and a series of values of x

x	$x_i - x$	$w(x,x_i)^*$	$w(x,x_i,h)^{**}$
−0.2	−0.6	0.482	0.388
−0.1	−0.5	0.670	0.484
0.0	−0.4	0.820	0.579
0.1	−0.3	0.921	0.666
0.2	−0.2	0.976	0.737
0.3	−0.1	0.997	0.782
0.4	0.0	1.000	0.798
0.5	0.1	0.997	0.782
0.6	0.2	0.976	0.737
0.7	0.3	0.921	0.666
0.8	0.4	0.820	0.579
0.9	0.5	0.670	0.484
1.0	0.6	0.482	0.388

* = Tri-cubic weighting function
** = Height of the normal distribution (mean value = x_i = 0.4 and standard deviation = bandwidth = $h = 0.5$)

(Chapter 10). For example, for the data value $x_i = 0.4$ (mean) and $h = 0.5$ (standard deviation), the weight $\phi[0.3, 0.4, 0.5] = 0.782$ is the height of this normal distribution at the point $x = 0.3$. Both weighting functions are illustrated in Table 15–2.

Using the classic Weinberg estimate of the proportion of dizygotic twins ($2\times$ the proportion of unlike-sex pairs), the trend in dizygotic twin births over the period 1983–2003 is summarized by a loess estimated curve (moving average) using normal distribution weights with a smoothing parameter of $h = 3$ (Figure 15–6).

Cleveland [51] suggested an extension of the weighted moving average. Instead of using a weighted average to estimate a value of a dependent variable y at a specific data value of x, a value calculated from an estimated straight line is used. For a series of values x, a series of values $\hat{y}_i$ is calculated from a series of weighted least-squares estimated regression lines using the n observed values (x_i, y_i). Again, the largest weight is given to the observation y_i at the value x_i, and subsequent weights decrease as the values of x increase in distance from the observation y_i. Technically, the quantity represented by L is minimized, thus producing weighted estimates of $\hat{a}$ (intercept) and $\hat{b}$ (slope) where

$$L = \sum (y_i - [a + b(x - x_i)])^2 \phi [x, x_i, h] \qquad i = 1, 2, \cdots, n.$$

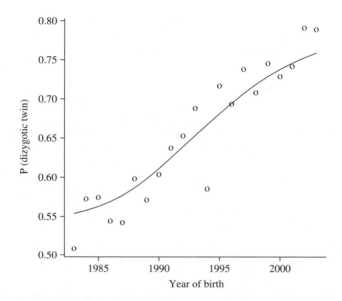

Figure 15–6. A weighted moving average curve describing the probability of dizygotic twins born in California during the period 1983–2003 ($h = 3$ and $n = 21$).

The estimated value at the specified value x_i is then the estimate from a line, namely $\hat{y}_i$. The weighting is not different from the weighting used for the moving average estimate. Expressions are available to estimate the intercept and slope of a line using a sequence of n weights. However, modern computer software is easily applied. For each observed value of x_i, a linear weighted regression analysis is performed based on the n weights $\phi[x, x_i, h]$. Then, using the resulting estimated line, a specific value $\hat{y}_i$ is calculated. This process is repeated for each value x_i, creating a series of points made smooth by the choice of the smoothing parameter h. Figures 15–7 and 15–8 depict the process. The weights w_i used to calculate the value of $\hat{y}_7$ when $x = 7$ are displayed (top) where the weights in the neighborhood of $x = 7$ have the most influence. The estimated line itself is displayed below. The second plot depicts the same process but for $x = 17$.

Weighted regression estimation applied to the previous twin data (Figure 15–6) yields an estimated curve describing again the trend in the probability of dizygotic twin births (Figure 15–9). For this relatively simple curve, the moving average (dotted line) and the loess estimate (solid line) are not substantially different.

Applying the same linear loess estimation approach to describe the probability of male twins born during the period 1983–2003 produces the smooth curve displayed in Figure 15–10 (left). Also included is a series of bootstrap loess

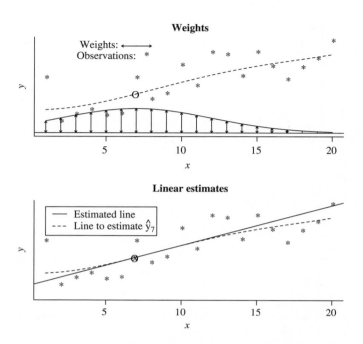

Figure 15–7. A schematic description of the weighting process using a weighted leastsquares estimated line to produce a smoothed value y at the value $x = 7$.

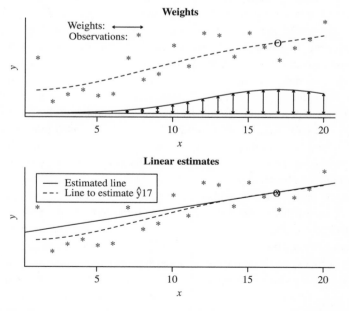

Figure 15–8. A schematic description of the weighting process using a weighted least squares estimated line to produce a smooth value y at the $x = 17$.

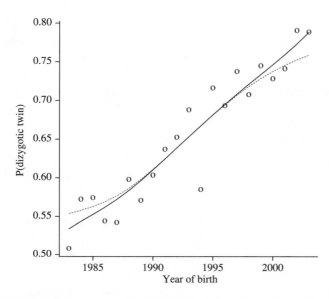

Figure 15–9. A linear loess estimated curve (solid line) and the previous weighted moving average (dotted line) describing the probability of dizygotic twins born in California during the period 1983–2003 ($h = 3$ and $n = 21$).

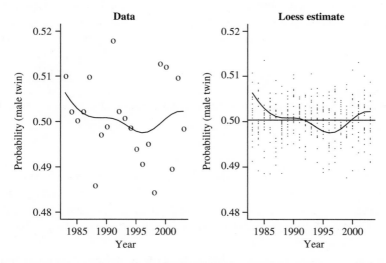

Figure 15–10. The proportion of male twins born in California during the period 1983–2003 ($h = 3$ and $n = 21$).

451

estimated lines (dots) to reflect visually the influence of sampling variation on the estimated curve (Chapter 8). The plot (right side) shows the results of bootstrap resampling of the 21 pairs of observations and estimating the curve repeatedly, yielding a series of n estimates $\hat{y}_i$ (dots) that give a sense of the influence of the associated sampling variability. This "band" of estimated values reflects the likely range of the "true" underlying relationship. For the case of males twins, the bootstrap "band" completely contains a horizontal line, indicating that the estimated curve provides no strong evidence of a systematic pattern over the 21-year period (solid line). That is, in light of the background variation, the loess estimated curve is not statistically distinguishable from a horizontal line (no apparent trend).

Occasionally plots of x/y-pairs of observations appear to have no obvious pattern upon inspection, particularly plots with a large number of points. For example, the plot of body weights and systolic blood pressures of $n = 202$ men who weight more than 200 pounds (Western Collaborative Group Study [WCGS] data, Chapters 4 and 11) appears to have no clear features (Figure 15–11). An estimated correlation coefficient of 0.131 indicates a modest upward trend that is not apparent from the plot and applies only to a straight-line summary (Figure 15–11, left). A loess estimated curve potentially identifies any systematic and nonlinear pattern between body weight and blood pressure levels (Figure 15–11, right). The loess estimated curve describing blood pressure has an essentially linear and slightly increasing association with body weight until about 230 pounds, followed by values that appear to increase at a faster rate. However, loess estimates are designed to capitalize on local variation, potentially producing apparent properties of a curve that are unimportant in light of the variability of the sampled values. On the other hand, such curves frequently suggest parametric regression models useful in further evaluating an observed pattern.

For the WCGS blood pressure data, a model suggested by the loess curve, is

$$y_i = a + bwt_i + cwt_i^2$$

and produces the estimates of a parametric representation (Table 15–3) of the influence of body weight (wt) on blood pressure levels (y_i). Supported by a test of the estimated regression model coefficient $\hat{c}$ yielding a p-value $= 0.830$, the loess estimated nonlinearity (Figure 15–11, dashed line) appears likely to be due to exploiting local random variation.

Amazingly, loess estimation produce model-free logistic-like curves from binary data. To illustrate, consider the WCGS data again, where 257 of the 3154 study participants had a coronary heart disease (CHD) event (Chapter 4). The relationship between levels of cholesterol and the presence/absence of a CHD event is shown in Figure 15–12 (dashed line). The continuous curve is a parametric

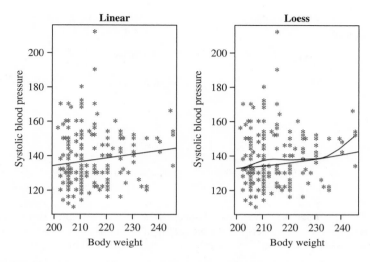

Figure 15–11. Linear and loess estimated curves describing the pattern between systolic blood pressure and body weight for $n = 202$ men who weigh more than 200 pounds (WCGS data, Chapters 4 and 11).

Table 15–3. A quadratic model describing the relationship between systolic blood pressure and body weight for $n = 202$ men who weigh more than 200 pounds (WCGS data)

Variables	Terms	Estimates	Std. errors	p-Values
Constant	a	189.448	460.173	–
wt	b	−0.683	4.195	–
wt^2	c	0.0020	0.0095	0.830

LogLikelihood $= -2670.0$

estimate from a two-parameter linear logistic model (Chapter 11, $log\text{-}odds_i = l_i = a + b(chol_i) = -5.374 + 0.0125[chol_i]$). Model-estimated probabilities of a CHD event for the entire range (0, 1) are based on cholesterol levels from 0 to 700 $mg\%$. Realistic levels of cholesterol vary over a substantially smaller range, typically between 100 and 300. A model-free loess curve describes the same cholesterol–CHD relationship over the range of the observed data and is not reasonably extended beyond the observed values (Figure 15–12, right). The two cholesterol–CHD estimated curves are similar for realistic levels of cholesterol.

One last note: rarely do high-order polynomial expressions substantially improve the overall loess estimation. Simulation studies indicate that the linear loess estimates generally out performs a weighted moving average and polynomials of order two or higher [38].

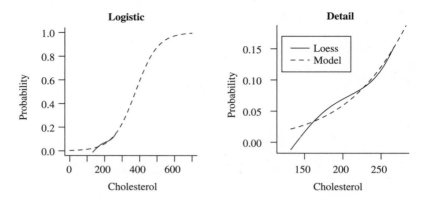

Figure 15–12. A logistic model curve (dashed line) and a loess estimated curve (solid line) describing the relationship between the probability of a coronary event and the level of cholesterol (WCGS data: CHD events = 257 and n = 3154, Chapters 4 and 11).

BIVARIATE LOESS ESTIMATION

A natural extension of the loess estimated curve is an application of the same logic and estimation process to describe a bivariate relationship. Instead of applying weighted values to estimate a line, weighted values are applied to estimate a sequence of points over a bivariate grid of values, producing an estimated surface, again made smooth by selecting specific bandwidths. The weights can have the same form as the single-variable case and are the product of one set of n weights associated with one variable and another set of n weights associated with a second variable, yielding n^2 values. These weights are incorporated, in much the same manner as the single variable estimate, into a bivariate regression estimation process. The estimated surface is then used to estimate a value, y, associated with a specified pair of values (denote x_1 and x_2). The weights, as before, emphasize the observed values in the neighborhood of the chosen grid values (x_1, x_2).

Example weights again derived from normal distributions are displayed in Table 15–4. The weights are constructed so that the maximum value (0.159) occurs at the chosen grid point of $x_1 = 0.4$ and $x_2 = 0.6$ ($h_1 = h_2 = 1.0$), and then decrease as the distance from this maximum point increases. The estimation process is repeated n^2 times and, like the linear loess estimates, a new set of weights is created and a weighted regression equation yields the estimate $\hat{y}$ for each pair of values x_1 and x_2 (n^2 estimates).

As with the single variable case, computer software is used to find the estimated parameter values that minimize the expression

$$L = \sum (y_i - [a + b_1(x_1 - x_{1i}) + b_2(x_2 - x_{2i})])^2 \phi [x_1, x_{1i}, h_1] \, \phi [x_2, x_{2i}, h_2]$$

Table 15–4. Illustration of weights for a bivariate loess-estimated surface at the data value ($x_1 = 0.4$, $x_2 = 0.6$) created from the heights of two normal distributions ($\mu_1 = 0.4$, $\mu_2 = 0.6$ with $h_1 = h_2 = 1.0$)

x_1/x_2	0.0	0.1	0.2	0.3	0.4	0.5	0.6	0.7	0.8	0.9	1.0
0.0	0.123	0.130	0.135	0.140	0.144	0.146	0.147	0.146	0.144	0.140	0.135
0.1	0.127	0.134	0.140	0.145	0.149	0.151	0.152	0.151	0.149	0.145	0.140
0.2	0.130	0.138	0.144	0.149	0.153	0.155	0.156	0.155	0.153	0.149	0.144
0.3	0.132	0.140	0.146	0.151	0.155	0.158	0.158	0.158	0.155	0.151	0.146
0.4	0.133	0.140	0.147	0.152	0.156	0.158	**0.159**	0.158	0.156	0.152	0.147
0.5	0.132	0.140	0.146	0.151	0.155	0.158	0.158	0.158	0.155	0.151	0.146
0.6	0.130	0.138	0.144	0.149	0.153	0.155	0.156	0.155	0.153	0.149	0.144
0.7	0.127	0.134	0.140	0.145	0.149	0.151	0.152	0.151	0.149	0.145	0.140
0.8	0.123	0.130	0.135	0.140	0.144	0.146	0.147	0.146	0.144	0.140	0.135
0.9	0.117	0.124	0.130	0.134	0.138	0.140	0.140	0.140	0.138	0.134	0.130
1.0	0.111	0.117	0.123	0.127	0.130	0.132	0.133	0.132	0.130	0.127	0.123

where $i = 1, 2, \cdots, n$. The estimated regression coefficients $\hat{a}$, $\hat{b}_1$, and $\hat{b}_2$ are the values that minimize the quantity L, producing a weighted estimate of a value $\hat{y}_i$ from the bivariate prediction equation estimated from the n sets of observations (y_i, x_{1i}, x_{2i}). Geometrically, the surface used to estimate the value $\hat{y}_i$ at the point (x_1, x_2) is an estimated plane and, analogous to the loess estimated line, the weights emphasize the values in the neighborhood of the point (x_1, x_2).

To illustrate bivariate loess estimation, the expression

$$y_i = 10 - 2x_{1i} + 3x_{1i}^2 + 6x_{2i} + \varepsilon_i$$

is used to produce fictional data (Figure 15–13, upper left). The expected result emerges that, when the bandwidths are made sufficiently large ($h_1 = h_2 = 5$), the estimation process essentially reproduces the model values (Figure 15–13, lower right).

Loess estimates from a pregnancy study [52] describes the bivariate relationship of maternal weight and height to the birth weight of a newborn infant. Estimated surfaces derived from $n = 1869$ mother–child pairs are displayed in four plots (Figure 15–14) with increasing bandwidths. As designed, increasing bandwidth decreases local variation. The fourth plot (bandwidths = 0.9) becomes a smooth surface, indicating an apparently complicated maternal weight–height relationship to birth weight.

Parametric analyses contrasted to nonparametric plots frequently add additional insight to the visual description. Applied to the weight–height data, an additive model containing quadratic terms suggests that maternal prepregnancy weight has an essentially linear and increasing influence on birth weight,

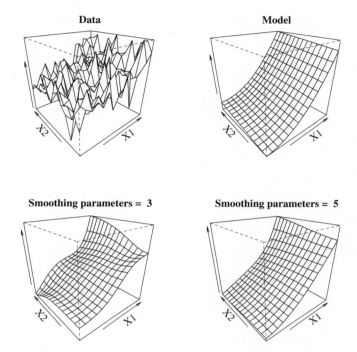

Figure 15–13.   Artificial data generated to illustrate a bivariate loess-estimated surface for two selected smoothing parameters ($h_1 = h_2 = 3$ and 5).

Table 15–5.   The coefficients of an additive nonlinear parametric model* describing the relationship between maternal weight–height and the birth weight of newborns

Variables	Terms	Estimates	Std. errors	p-Values
Constant	a	38.565	17.428	–
wt	b_1	2.588	0.780	0.001
wt^2	b_2	0.015	0.030	0.606
ht	b_3	14.211	2.049	< 0.001
ht^2	b_4	−1.042	0.219	< 0.001

* = Model: $bwt_i = a + b_1 wt_i + b_2 wt_i^2 + b_3 ht_i + b_4 ht_i^2$

whereas height has an independent (additive) nonlinear and decreasing influence (Table 15–5). However, the loess model-free estimated surface suggests that this additive relationship may not be consistent for all levels of maternal weight and height (an interaction).

Figure 15–15 displays loess estimates of the same maternal weight–height relationship to infant birth weight but for the small mothers (prepregnancy weight

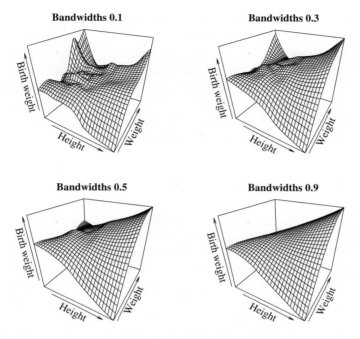

Figure 15–14. The bivariate loess plots of the maternal weight–height relationship to infant birth weight for a sample of $n = 1869$ mother–infant pairs illustrating four bandwidths.

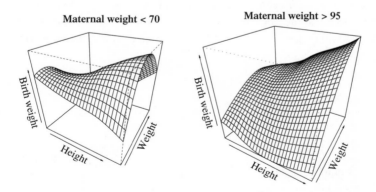

Figure 15–15. Bivariate loess estimates of the maternal weight–height relationship to birth weight for the small mothers (prepregnancy weight <70 kilograms) and for large mothers (prepregnancy weight >95 kilograms).

<70 kilograms, 25th percentile) and large mothers (prepregnancy weight >95 kilograms, 75th percentile). The data stratified into two weight categories produce plots showing less complicated but possibly different weight–height relationships to birth weight. Although the two plots appear to differ depending the maternal prepregnancy weight, it is likely that additional plotting and, perhaps, additional parametric models are necessary to make the situation entirely clear. As with the interpretation of most plots, a definitive description is not usually possible without a careful assessment of the influence of random variation.

TWO-DIMENSIONAL KERNEL ESTIMATION

Similar to a loess estimated curve, the kernel estimation process for a smooth single-variable curve (Chapter 10) is naturally extended to describe a bivariate relationship. The previously described kernel smoothing algorithm is based on combining the heights of normal distributions with mean values equal to each data point and standard deviation that establishes a bandwidth. A bivariate application uses bivariate normal distributions in much the same fashion, and the influence of the bandwidth is again determined by the choice of standard deviations. Figure 15–16 displays a circular bivariate normal distribution (one of a variety of kernel distributions) and its associated probability contours.

The following figures (Figures 15–17 and 15–18) illustrate the kernel smoothing process for a small ($n = 5$) set of values: $(x_i, y_i) = (-2, -4)$, $(-5, -7)$, $(0, 2)$, $(5, 3)$, and $(-4, 0)$. Each kernel bivariate normal distribution has a mean of (x_i, y_i), one for each of the five data points (Figure 15–17). For small bandwidths, the bivariate normal distributions essentially locate each of the five points (bandwidth = 1.0, Figure 15–18). As the bandwidths increase (standard

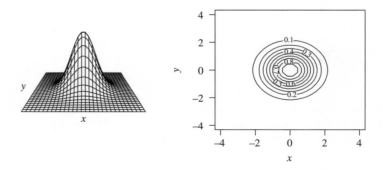

Figure 15–16. A single bivariate circular normal distribution and it, corresponding probability contours ($\mu_x = \mu_y = 0$, $\sigma_x = \sigma_y = 1$, and $\sigma_{xy} = 0$).

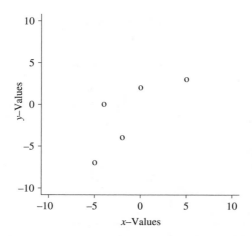

Figure 15–17. Five points used to construct the illustration in Figure 15–18.

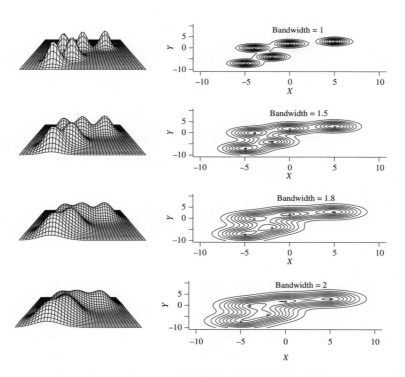

Figure 15–18. The five points in Figure 15–17 smoothed by four increasing bandwidths that reduce detail and produce more parsimonious displays of the bivariate relationship.

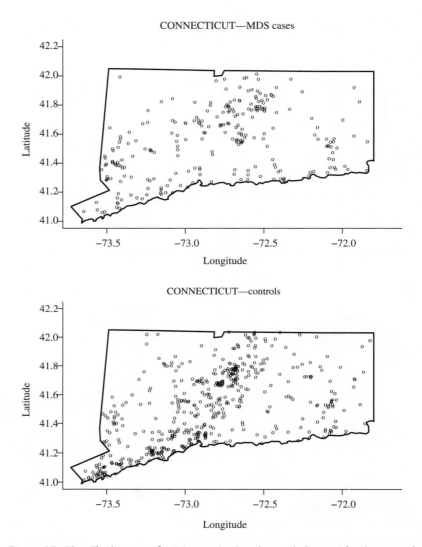

Figure 15–19. The location of MDS cases (top) and controls (bottom) for the state of Connecticut, years 2001–2003 (*n* = 255 observations for both case and control groups).

deviations of the bivariate normal distributions increase), these continuous kernel distributions representing each data value increasingly overlap. Thus, when combined, an increasingly smooth bivariate surface emerges (bandwidths = 1.0, 1.5, 1.8, and 2.0, Figure 15–18).

Case–control data collected to study the spatial distribution of myelodysplastic syndrome (MDS, formerly know as preleukemia) provide an example of bivariate kernel estimation. The state of Connecticut cancer registry reported the locations of 255 MDS cases occurring during the years 2001–2003. To estimate the spatial distribution of the adult population of Connecticut, a sample of 255 random control subjects were selected from U. S. census data. These bivariate distributions are displayed in Figure 15–19.

To estimate the case and control bivariate distributions, each location is summarized by a bivariate normal distribution with a bandwidths of 0.09. Combining these 255 kernel distributions with mean values at each of the observed 255 locations produces case and control plots (Figure 15–20) displaying smooth estimated bivariate distributions (surfaces) of the MDS frequencies of the cases and controls. Also included are their corresponding contour plots. Similar to single-variable density estimation, the extent of clustering is proportional to the

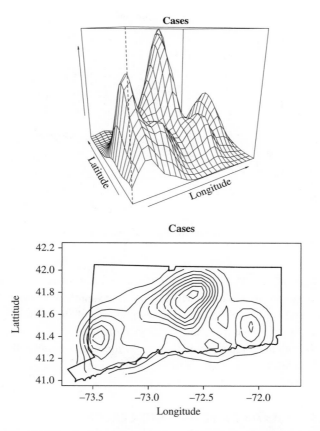

Figure 15–20.   The kernel smoothed distribution of MDS cases (bivariate representation) and their corresponding contour plot.

Controls

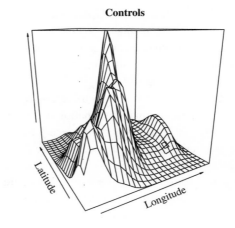

Controls

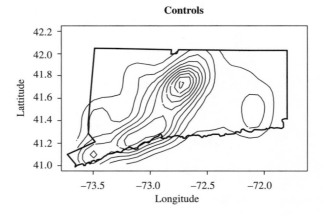

Figure 15–20.   (Continued)

height of the surface. The most striking case–control difference is an apparent
the concentration of incidence of MDS cases in the southwest corner of the state.
Further detailed spatial analysis and an assessment of the influence of random
variation on the smoothed distributions is certainly necessary. However, bivariate
kernel smoothing techniques immediately spotlight case–control differences and
provide a definite starting point for further discussion and analysis.

STATISTICAL TESTS AND A FEW OF THEIR PROPERTIES

Statistical tests are conducted to choose between one of two specific hypotheses.
The following discussion of these tests addresses a few of the issues surrounding the
formal comparison of these two hypotheses, with the primary goal of providing

a better conceptual basis for interpreting the results from statistical tests when applied to data.

Power of a Specific Statistical Test: The Normal Distribution Case

The probabilities that a statistical test yields the correct answer results from a comparison of two hypotheses. As might be expected, the focus of the comparison is a specific statistical summary (denoted X) such as:

- $X = \bar{x}$ (sample mean),
- $X = \hat{p}$ (sample proportion),
- $X = \hat{p}_1 - \hat{p}_2$ (difference between two sample proportions), or
- $X = \hat{or}$ (estimated odds ratio).

First, a hypothesis is postulated that only random variation influences the difference between an observed summary value X and a theoretically specified value. A second hypothesis is then created that postulates, in fact, a systematic influence caused by the observed difference. This second hypothesis allows the consequences of the choices made to establish the first hypothesis to be evaluated. In the language of statistical testing, the first hypothesis is called the *null hypothesis* (denoted H_0) and the second hypothesis is called the *alternative hypothesis* (denoted H_1). The incorrect choice of the null hypothesis is described in terms of an error probability called a *type I error* (denoted α). The incorrect choice of the alternative hypothesis is also described in terms of an error probability called a *type II error* (denoted β). The *power of the test* is defined as the probability a systematic influence is identified when one exists (denoted $1 - \beta$). That is, correctly choosing the second hypothesis.

Calculations to determine the power of a test begin with the premise that the summary statistic X has at least an approximate normal distribution with mean value $= \mu_0$ and variance $= \sigma_0^2/n$. The notation μ_0 and σ_0^2/n represent the mean and the variance of the distribution of the summary statistic X, calculated from n observations. The essence of the null hypothesis is that any difference observed between a summary value X and the postulated mean value μ_0 is due entirely to the random variation described by σ_0^2/n. The likelihood that this difference arose by chance alone is calculated from normal distribution probabilities with the mean value μ_0 and variance σ_0^2/n. Based on this null hypothesis, a criterion is created providing a clear choice between the inference that *the data provide no evidence of a systematic influence* and *the data produce evidence of a systematic influence*. The probability that a random difference will be declared as systematic ($\alpha =$ type I error) produces this criterion. Thus, the criterion (denoted c_0 and commonly called the *critical value*) for a sample of size n is given by

$$c_0 = z_{1-\alpha}\sigma_0/\sqrt{n} + \mu_0$$

where $z_{1-\alpha}$ represents the $(1 - \alpha)$-percentile of a standard normal distribution. Therefore, an observed value of the summary X less than c_0 produces "no evidence of a systematic influence" and an observed value of X greater than c_0 produces "evidence of a systematic influence." The probability of a type I error (α) can be set at any value but is almost always chosen to be $\alpha = 0.05$, making $z_{1-\alpha} = z_{0.95} = 1.645$, and the critical value becomes

$$c_0 = 1.645\sigma_0/\sqrt{n} + \mu_0$$

where μ_0 is the mean value and $\sigma_0/\sqrt{n}$ is the standard deviation of the postulated normal distribution of the summary value X. Thus, the critical value c_0 is the 95th percentile of the normal distribution associated with null hypothesis, making $P(type\ I\ error) = P(X \geq c_0|\mu_0\ and\ \sigma_0) = \alpha = 0.05$. Notice for this formal procedure, the statistical test yields only one of two decisions—likely random and likely not random. Further evidence that might be gain from the data is not considered.

The alternative hypothesis postulates that the distribution of the test statistic X has again at least an approximate normal distribution with mean value μ_1 ($\mu_1 > \mu_0$) and variance σ_1^2/n. This hypothesis provides an opportunity to assess the consequences of inferring that no systematic influences exist based on the critical value c_0. Specifically, the power of the test is $1 - \beta = P(Z \geq z_\beta)$ and is the probability that an observed value of the summary X exceeds the critical value c_0 when a systematic influence exists. Technically, the value z_β represents the β-level percentile of the normal distribution associated with the alternative hypothesis or $P(X \leq c_0|\mu_1\ and\ \sigma_1) = P(Z \leq z_\beta) = \beta$, where $z_\beta = \sqrt{n}(c_0 - \mu_1)/\sigma_1$. The probability is then β, that a systematic difference is incorrectly declared random (*type II error*) and, conversely, the complementary probability is $1 - \beta$, that a systematic difference is correctly identified by the statistical test. Figure 15–21 displays the comparison of these two hypothesis-generated normal distributions and indicates the roles of the two kinds of error probabilities for the case where α is set at 0.05, causing $\beta = 0.30$.

In short, for the test statistic X, a power calculation consists of determining the 95th percentile (c_0) from postulating that X has a normal distribution with mean value μ_0 and variance σ_0^2/n. Then, calculate the probability that this percentile is exceeded, based on postulating that X has a normal distribution with mean value μ_1 and variance σ_1^2/n. When the situation requires $\mu_1 < \mu_0$, the calculations are not different in principle but -1.645 replaces 1.645 in the determination of the 5% type I error rate.

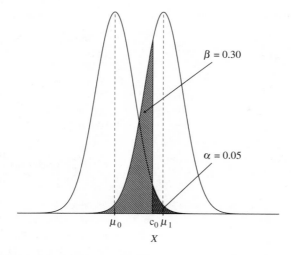

$\beta = 0.30$

$\alpha = 0.05$

$\mu_0 \quad c_0 \, \mu_1$

X

Figure 15–21. A schematic display of the two normal distributions illustrating the calculation of the statistical power $(1 - \beta)$ for an α-level $= 0.05$ statistical test.

Four summary statistical measures

single mean	single proportion	two proportions	odds ratio
$X = \bar{x}$	$X = \hat{p}$	$X = \hat{p}_1 - \hat{p}_0$	$X = \hat{or}$

serve as examples of the application of this normal distribution-based power calculation (Table 15–6).

The power calculation for an odds ratio (denoted *or*) is a special case of comparing two sample proportions. A baseline probability (denoted p_0) and a selected odds ratio determine a second probability (denoted p_1). A comparison between the baseline probability and this second probability produces the power to correctly identify a systematic influence reflected by an odds ratio.

More specifically, a baseline probability p_0 and the selected odds ratio *or* are related because

$$or = \frac{p_1/(1 - p_1)}{p_0/(1 - p_0)},$$

and solving for p_1 gives

$$p_1 = \frac{p_0 or}{1 + p_0(or - 1)}.$$

It is the comparison of p_0 to p_1 that yields the power of a test to detect an odds ratio that systematically differs from 1.0. The power associated with a series of selected odds ratios that results from comparing p_0 to p_1 is illustrated in Table 15–6.

Table 15–6. Four specific examples of power calculations

Mean values: $X = \bar{x}$
$\mu_0 = 10 \qquad n = 25$
$\sigma_0^2 = 50 \quad \sigma_1^2 = 50$
$c_0 = 12.326$

μ_0	μ_1	power
10	10.0	0.050
10	10.5	0.098
10	11.0	0.174
10	11.5	0.280
10	12.0	0.409
10	12.5	0.549
10	13.0	0.683
10	13.5	0.797
10	14.0	0.882

Two proportions: $X = \hat{p}_0 - \hat{p}_1$
$p_0 - p_1 = 0 \qquad n_0 = n_1 = 50$
$\sigma_0^2 = 2p(1-p)^*$
$\sigma_1^2 = p_0(1-p_0) + p_1(1-p_1)$

$p0$	$p1$	$p1 - p0$	power
0.1	0.10	0.00	0.050
0.1	0.14	0.04	0.151
0.1	0.18	0.08	0.310
0.1	0.22	0.12	0.497
0.1	0.26	0.16	0.673
0.1	0.30	0.20	0.811
0.1	0.34	0.24	0.905
0.1	0.38	0.28	0.958
0.1	0.42	0.32	0.984

*Note: $p = (p_0 + p_1)/2$

Single proportion: $X = \hat{p}$
$p_0 = 0.5 \qquad n = 25$
$\sigma_0^2 = p_0(1 - p_0)$
$c_0 = 0.664$

p_0	$p1$	power
0.5	0.50	0.050
0.5	0.52	0.074
0.5	0.54	0.106
0.5	0.56	0.146
0.5	0.58	0.196
0.5	0.60	0.255
0.5	0.62	0.323
3.5	0.64	0.399
0.5	0.66	0.481
0.5	0.68	0.566

Odds ratio: $X = \hat{or}$
$p_0 = 0.1 \qquad n_0 = n_1 = 50$
$\sigma_0^2 = 2p(1 - p)$
$\sigma_1^2 = p_0(1 - p_0) + p_1(1 - p_1)$

$p0$	or	$p1$	power
0.1	1.0	0.100	0.050
0.1	1.4	0.135	0.134
0.1	1.8	0.167	0.252
0.1	2.2	0.196	0.386
0.1	2.6	0.224	0.516
0.1	3.0	0.250	0.631
0.1	3.4	0.274	0.727
0.1	3.8	0.297	0.802
0.1	4.2	0.318	0.859
0.1	4.6	0.338	0.901

The comparison of two normal distributions generated by the null and alternative hypotheses also allows a sample size calculation. Instead of calculating the power of a statistical test, a specific level of power is selected. Based on the selected value, it is then possible to calculate the number of observations necessary to attain the power for a α-level type I error. Specifically, when the power $1 - \beta$ is selected, the expression

$$n = \frac{(z_{1-\alpha}\sigma_0 + z_{1-\beta}\sigma_1)^2}{(\mu_0 - \mu_1)^2}$$

yields the sample size necessary to achieve that power at the selected level α. The values $z_{1-\alpha}$ and $z_{1-\beta}$ represent the $1 - \alpha$ and $1 - \beta$ percentiles of a standard normal distribution.

For example, in the case of an odds ratio $X = \hat{or}$, when the baseline probability is $p_0 = 0.10$ and $or = 3$, then $p_1 = 0.25$ and

$$n = \frac{[1.645(0.537) + 1.282(0.527)]^2}{(0.10 - 0.25)^2}$$

$$= \frac{2.430}{0.0225} \approx 109 \quad (\sigma_0 = 0.537 \; and \; \sigma_1 = 0.527)$$

where the selected error probabilities are $P(type \; I \; error) = \alpha = 0.05$ ($z_{0.95} = 1.645$) and $P(type \; II \; error) = \beta = 0.10$ ($z_{0.90} = 1.282$). Thus, 109 observations from each of two compared samples yield a probability of at least 0.90 of detecting a systematic influence with an odds ratio measure of association of $or = 3$ or greater when one exists.

It should be noted that, in realistic situations, the test statistic X has only an approximate normal distribution. In addition, sample size and power calculations are based on a series of conjectures about the distributions sampled (μ_0, σ_0, μ_1, and σ_1), and accurate values for all four parameters are rarely available, particularly for μ_1 and σ_1^2. Furthermore, the selection of the two error rates (α and β) is rather arbitrary. So, at best, power and sample size calculations are approximate. The resulting values of $power = 1 - \beta$ or sample size $= n$, therefore, are primarily useful as guidelines for selecting among possible data collection strategies. A more fundamental limitation of power calculations is that most collected data involve multivariate measurements, at least several different summary values, and a number (sometimes a large number) of statistical tests. Although power calculations exist for a few kinds of multivariable situations, they are based on a series of usually nonverifiable assumptions and produce complex and not easily interpreted results.

POWER OF A STATISTICAL TEST: THE CHI-SQUARE DISTRIBUTION CASE

Power calculations derived from comparing two normal distributions apply to summary statistics such as mean values, proportions, and odds ratios. A second approach is useful for calculating the power or a sample size for the analysis of tabular data. These calculations depend on the probabilities derived from comparing two chi-square distributions. Nevertheless, the previous pattern of creating a critical value, c_0, under one set of conditions (null hypothesis) then assessing the consequences of this choice under a second set of conditions

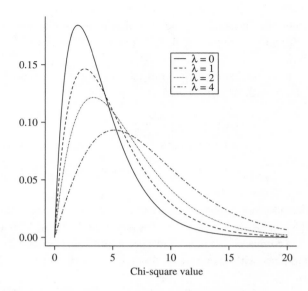

Figure 15–22.   A display of the four chi-square distributions with degrees of freedom $\gamma = 4$ and noncentrality parameters $\lambda = 0$, 1, 2, and 4.

(alternative hypothesis) is again used to calculate the power of the test or calculate a sample size.

The most familiar chi-square distribution is defined by one parameter, namely its degrees of freedom. More generally, a chi-square probability distribution is defined by two parameters, the familiar degrees of freedom (denoted γ) and a parameter called the *noncentrality parameter* (denoted λ). For most application of a chi-square distribution, the noncentrality parameter is unnecessary and set to zero ($\lambda = 0$) because it does not play a role in the typical statistical test. The noncentrality parameter λ is, however, the key to power and sample size calculations based on a chi-square test statistic. Figure 15–22 displays four chi-square distributions with degrees of freedom $\gamma = 4$ and noncentrality parameters of $\lambda = 0$, 1, 2, and 4.

Almost always, the calculation of exact probabilities from a noncentral chi-square distribution ($\lambda \neq 0$) requires a computer algorithm. However, two easily applied normal distribution-based approximations exist. Either approximation is usually sufficient for power (sample size) calculations because approximate values are generally all that are needed. Noting that the mean value of a noncentral chi-square distribution is $m = \gamma + \lambda$ and its variance is $2(m + \lambda)$ gives, for any chi-square distribution test statistic X^2, a transformed value

$$Z = \frac{X^2 - m}{\sqrt{2(m+\lambda)}}$$

or, a more accurate value,

$$Z = \frac{\left[X^2/m\right]^{1/3} - (1-f)}{\sqrt{f}}$$

where $f = 2(m+\lambda)/(9m^2)$. The transformed values Z have approximate standard normal distributions (mean value $= 0$ and variance $= 1.0$) in both cases and produce approximate probabilities associated with a noncentral chi-square statistic X^2 for specified values of γ and λ. An exact noncentral chi-square cumulative probability distribution (solid line) and the two approximations are displayed in Figure 15–23 for degrees of freedom $= \gamma = 2$ and noncentrality parameter $= \lambda = 4$ (dashed lines). For example, when $X^2 = 10$ and $\gamma = 2$ and $\lambda = 4$, then

$$z = \frac{10 - (2+4)}{\sqrt{2(2+4+4)}} = 0.894,$$

and $P(X^2 \leq 10 | \gamma = 2 \ and \ \lambda = 4) = P(Z \leq 0.894) = 0.814$ or, the value of f is 0.0617 making

$$z = \frac{[10/(2+4)]^{1/3} - 0.938}{\sqrt{0.0617}} = 0.996$$

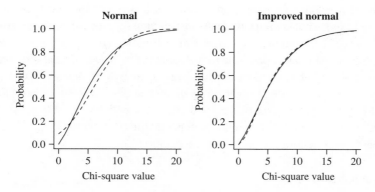

Figure 15–23. Two normal-based approximations (dashed line) for the noncentral chi-square distribution (solid line) where $\gamma = 2$ and $\lambda = 4$ (mean value $= m = 6$ and variance $= 20$).

and $P(X^2 \leq 10 | \gamma = 2 \ and \ \lambda = 4) = P(Z \leq 0.996) = 0.840$. The exact probability is 0.831.

For the calculation of power $(1 - \beta)$, the noncentrality parameter is determined by the comparison of two probability distributions, one generated under the null hypothesis (denoted p_{i0}) and another generated under an alternative hypothesis (denoted p_{i1}). The noncentrality parameter reflects the difference between these two probability distributions and is given by the expression

$$\lambda = n \sum \frac{(p_{i1} - p_{i0})^2}{p_{i0}} \qquad i = 1, \ 2, \ \cdots, \ k$$

where k probabilities are compared and n represents the sample size. This parameter is the value of a chi-square test statistic that results from comparing k theoretical values generated by a null hypothesis to k theoretical values generated by an alternative hypothesis. Instead of the usual chi-square comparison of k theoretical values to k observed probabilities $\hat{p}_i$ (p_{i0} versus $\hat{p}_i$), a second set of theoretical probabilities (p_{i1}) replaces the observed values (p_{i0} versus p_{i1}), producing a theoretical noncentrality parameter λ. This parameter is the value of the chi-square statistic when the comparison is between the postulated null and alternative probability distributions.

Once the noncentrality parameter is determined, a power calculation follows the previous pattern but for categorical data two chi-square distributions are compared. A critical value c_0 is created from the central chi-square distribution ($\lambda = 0$) for a selected type I error probability (α). That is, it is postulated that all observed differences between the theoretical probability distribution and the data occur by chance alone ($p_{i0} = p_{i1}$). The critical value c_0 is the $(1 - \alpha)$-level percentile ($1 - \alpha = 0.95$) of a central chi-square distribution ($\lambda = 0$) with γ degrees of freedom. Then, the consequence of this test of the null hypothesis is evaluated using a noncentral chi-square distribution ($\lambda \neq 0$), where λ summarizes the "distance" between the two theoretical distribution ($p_{i0} \neq p_{i1}$). Figure 15–24 displays a plot similar in principle to the comparison of two normal distributions (Figure 15–21) but applied to the comparison of two chi-square distributions ($\gamma = 6$; $\lambda = 0$ and 6) with the probability of a type I error $= \alpha = 0.05$ producing a probability of a type II error $= \beta = 0.60$. That is, the 95th percentile is $c_0 = 14.8$ (critical value) when $\lambda = 0$ and the 60th percentile ($\beta = 0.60$) when $\lambda = 6$, and the degrees of freedom are six in both cases ($\gamma = 6$).

Three Applications

Data generated by two binary variables are encountered in a variety of situations, particularly in genetic applications. Consider a binary variable denoted $Y = \{0, 1\}$ and a second binary variable denoted Y' sampled from the same probability

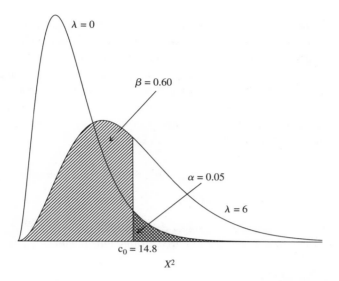

Figure 15–24. A schematic display of two chi-square distributions ($\gamma = 6$; $\lambda = 0$ and 6) for the calculation of the statistical power ($1 - \beta$) for the α-level = 0.05 statistical test.

Table 15–7. The joint probability distribution of two binary indicator variables Y and Y' sampled from the same probability distribution where $p = P(Y = 1) = P(Y' = 1)$

	$Y = 1$	$Y = 0$	Probability
$Y' = 1$	$p^2 + \varepsilon$	$p(1-p) - \varepsilon$	p
$Y' = 0$	$p(1-p) - \varepsilon$	$(1-p)^2 + \varepsilon$	$1 - p$
Probability	p	$1 - p$	1.0

distribution. The joint probability distribution of these two variables is described in Table 15–7, where p represents the probability that Y or Y' equals 1.0 [$P(Y = 1) = P(Y' = 1) = p$]. Thus, the correlation between Y and Y' is

$$\phi = correlation(Y, Y') = \frac{covariance(Y, Y')}{\sqrt{variance(Y)\ variance(Y')}} = \frac{\varepsilon}{p(1-p)},$$

sometimes called the *phi-correlation*. In genetics, the correlation coefficient ϕ is a measure of inbreeding, a measure of Hardy-Weinberg disequilibrium, or the probability that a pair of twins is monozygotic and applies as well to a wide range of nongenetic data. The correlation coefficient ϕ measures the association between two variables, as usual, by a value between −1 and +1.

Consider a power calculation where $Y = 1$ represents the inheritance of allele A and $Y = 0$ represents the inheritance of allele a. If a simple mendelian genetic trait is in Hardy-Weinberg equilibrium (alleles assort independently), then the distribution of the three genotypes AA, Aa, and aa is p^2, $2p(1-p)$, and $(1-p)^2$, where p is the probability of inheriting the allele A. For example, the probability of an AA-individual is $P(Y = 1 \ and \ Y' = 1) = P(Y = 1)P(Y' = 1) = p^2$. Therefore, the hypothesis that the alleles are inherited randomly ($\phi = \varepsilon = 0$) produces the null probability distribution

$$p_{AA} = p_{10} = p^2, \quad p_{Aa} = p_{20} = 2p(1-p) \quad \text{and}$$
$$p_{aa} = p_{30} = (1-p)^2.$$

The Pearson chi-square test statistic X^2 applied to compare the observed distribution of the three genotypes ($\hat{p}_i$) to their theoretical values (p_{i0}) is

$$X^2 = n \sum \frac{(\hat{p}_i - p_{i0})^2}{p_{i0}}$$
$$= \frac{[n_{AA}/n - p^2]^2}{p^2} + \frac{[n_{Aa}/n - 2p(1-p)]^2}{2p(1-p)} + \frac{[n_{AA}/n - (1-p)^2]^2}{(1-p)^2}$$
$$= n \left[\frac{[\hat{p}_1 - p_{10}]^2}{p_{10}} + \frac{[\hat{p}_2 - p_{20}]^2}{p_{20}} + \frac{[\hat{p}_3 - p_{30}]^2}{p_{30}} \right]$$

where the observed frequencies of these genotypes are denoted n_{AA}, n_{Aa}, and n_{aa}, and $n = n_{AA} + n_{Aa} + n_{aa}$ is the total subjects observed. The test statistic X^2 has an approximate-square distribution with one degree of freedom ($\gamma = 1$) and the noncentrality parameter is $\lambda = 0$ when $\varepsilon = 0$ (equilibrium).

Non-zero values of ε or ϕ measure the extent of disequilibrium (nonrandomness) among the three genotypes (Table 15–7). The alternative hypothesis that the inheritance of alleles is not random ($\varepsilon \neq 0$), therefore, produces the alternative probability distribution

$$p_{AA} = p_{11} = p^2 + \varepsilon, \quad p_{Aa} = p_{21} = 2p(1-p) - 2\varepsilon \quad \text{and}$$
$$p_{aa} = p_{31} = (1-p)^2 + \varepsilon.$$

The chi-square noncentrality parameter of the test statistic X^2 becomes

$$\lambda = n \sum \frac{(p_{i1} - p_{i0})^2}{p_{i0}} = n \left[\frac{\varepsilon}{p(1-p)} \right]^2 = n\phi^2$$

where n represents the total number of pairs sampled, and the theoretical distribution p_{i1} replaces the observed values (denoted $\hat{p}_i$) in the chi-square statistic.

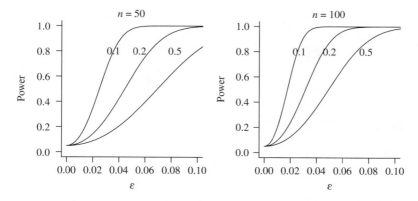

Figure 15–25. Example power curves for a chi-square test to assess Hardy-Weinberg equilibrium (random assortment) for allele frequencies $p = 0.1$, 0.2, and 0.5 for two sample sizes $n = 50$ and $n = 100$.

Therefore, the $\alpha = 0.05$ level critical value is $c_0 = 3.841$ or $P(X^2 \geq 3.841 | \gamma = 1 \ and \ \lambda = 0) = 0.05$. The power of this test statistic to detect allele frequencies that are not in equilibrium ($\varepsilon \neq 0$, disequilibrium) is then given by a noncentral chi-square distribution with one degree of freedom ($\gamma = 1$) and a noncentrality parameter of $\lambda = n\phi^2$. Specifically, it is the probability that a value from the noncentral chi-square test statistic X^2 exceeds the critical value $c_0 = 3.841$.

The power to detect genetic disequilibrium is illustrated (Figure 15–25) for a range of possible values of ε (0 to 0.1) and three selected allele frequencies p (0.0, 0.2, and 0.5) for two sample sizes $n = 50$ and $n = 100$. In general, an expression for the power of this chi-square assessment of genetic equilibrium is

$$power = 1 - \beta = P(X^2 \geq 3.841 | \gamma = 1 \text{ and } \lambda = n\phi^2).$$

For data contained in a $2 \times k$ table, an issue is frequently the assessment of a specific trend across a series of categories. For example, the likelihood of pancreatic cancer associated with increasing consumption of coffee is assessed for a linear trend in Chapter 2. In this situation, a power calculation might be a valuable guide to data collection decisions. The normal distribution approach to the comparison of postulated slopes provides a power or sample size calculation. A chi-square assessment based on the comparison of two postulated probability distributions provides an alternative calculation of the power associated with identifying a specific trend within a table. Consider, the choice between a series of constant probabilities and a series of increasing probabilities for data classified into k categories. For example, the categories $x_i = 0$, 1, 2, and 3 ($k = 4$) produce

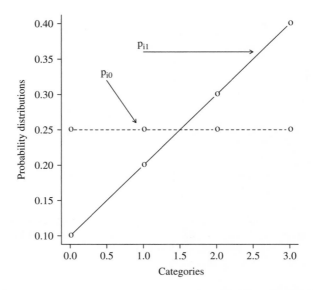

Figure 15–26. Two probability distributions (p_{i0} and p_{i1}) postulated to generate a power calculation for a comparison of four constant values to four increasing values.

two postulated probability distribution (again, denoted p_{i0} and p_{i1}) where

$$p_{i0} = \frac{1}{k} \quad \text{and} \quad p_{i1} = 0.1 + 0.1x_i$$

or, expressed in a table, the distributions are:

x_i	0	1	2	3
p_{i0}	0.25	0.25	0.25	0.25
p_{i1}	0.10	0.20	0.30	0.40

The probabilities p_{i0} and p_{i1} are displayed in Figure 15–26.
The test-for-trend Pearson chi-square test-statistic is

$$X^2 = n\sum \frac{(\hat{p}_i - p_{i0})^2}{p_{i0}}$$

and has an approximate central chi-square distribution ($\lambda = 0$) with $\gamma = k - 1$ degrees of freedom, where $\hat{p}_i$ represents the estimated probability associated with the ith cell ($i = 1, 2, \cdots, k$ and $n =$ total number of observations) and no trend exists ($p_{i0} = 1/k$). For the 2×4 table and a sample size of $n = 50$, the noncentrality parameter for this comparison (p_{i1} versus p_{i0}) is

$$\lambda = n\sum \frac{(p_{i1} - p_{i0})^2}{p_{i0}} = 50\left[\frac{(0.10 - 0.25)^2}{0.25} + \cdots + \frac{(0.40 - 0.25)^2}{0.25}\right] = 10.0.$$

The critical value is $c_0 = 7.814$, based on the distribution p_{i0} and a central chi-square distribution with $k - 1 = 3$ degrees of freedom ($\gamma = 3$ and $\lambda = 0$) and $\alpha = 0.05$. The alternative hypothesis (p_{i1}), that a linear trend exists with slope of 0.1, yields the probability of $1 - \beta = 0.761$. That is, the probability that the chi-square test statistic X^2 exceeds the critical value 7.814 is

$$power = 1 - \beta = P(X^2 \geq 7.814 | \gamma = 3 \text{ and } \lambda = 10.0) = 0.761$$

from a noncentral chi-square distribution ($\gamma = 3$ and $\lambda = 10.0$). Thus, the power of the chi-square test is $1 - \beta = 0.761$ and is the probability that a trend will be identified with a sample of 50 observations when it exists.

The comparison of two theoretical probability distributions also produces a sample size calculation for a chi-square analysis for data distributed into a series of k categories. One such case involves the comparison of a distribution with increasing probabilities (p_{i1}) to a distribution with a "threshold" pattern (p_{i0}). The following two probability distributions illustrate (Figure 15–27):

x_i	0	1	2	3
p_{i0}	0.15	0.25	0.30	0.30
p_{i1}	0.10	0.20	0.30	0.40

The question then becomes: What size sample is necessary to detect reliably a difference between these two distributions?

A chi-square distribution with degrees of freedom equal to three and a noncentrality parameter of zero describes the distribution of the Pearson test statistic X^2 applied to four categories of observations and provides the critical value $c_0 = 7.814$ for $\alpha = 0.05$, because $P(X^2 \geq 7.814 | \gamma = 3 \text{ and } \lambda = 0) = 0.05$. The noncentrality parameter for a sample size of $n = 100$ is

$$\lambda = n\sum \frac{(p_{i1} - p_{i0})^2}{p_{i0}} = 100\left[\frac{(0.15 - 0.10)^2}{0.10} + \cdots + \frac{(0.30 - 0.40)^2}{0.40}\right] = 6.0.$$

The probability that a chi-square test based on 100 observations identifies a difference between the two postulated distributions is then

$$power = 1 - \beta = P(X^2 \geq 7.814 | \gamma = 3 \text{ and } \lambda = 6.0) = 0.518.$$

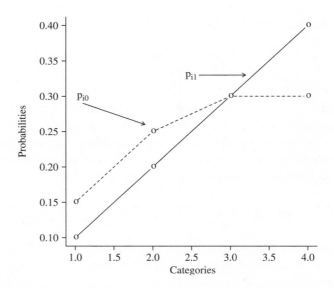

Figure 15–27. Two probability distributions postulated to generate a sample size calculation for identifying a difference between distributions of p_{i0} (linear) and p_{i1} (threshold).

Unlike the sample size calculation based on comparing two normal distributions, the chi-square sample size calculation does not have an explicit expression that directly yields a sample size n for given error probabilities α and β. However, sample size values can be sequentially increased and the power calculated until a value is found that gives the desired power. For the example, the critical value from a chi-square distribution (degrees of freedom = $\gamma = 3$) remains $c_0 = 7.814$ ($\alpha = 0.05$); then, starting at $n = 100$, the sample size necessary for a power of $1 - \beta = 0.80$ becomes

n	100	125	150	180	181	182
λ	6.00	7.50	9.00	10.80	10.86	10.92
$1 - \beta$	0.518	0.623	0.711	0.796	0.798	0.801

Therefore, a sample size of $n = 182$ produces a power of 0.80. Formally, the power of the chi-square test is

$$1 - \beta = P(X^2 \geq 7.814 | \gamma = 3 \text{ and } \lambda = 10.92) = 0.801$$

when the sample size n is set at 182.

Table 15–8. A 2×2 table description of the false discovery rate

	Declared not significant "$H-$"	Declared significant "$H+$"	**Total**
True null hypothesis ($H-$)	a	b	n_1
not true null hypothesis ($H+$)	c	d	n_2
Total	m_1	m_2	n

MULTIPLE STATISTICAL TESTS: ACCUMULATION OF TYPE I ERRORS

The classic Neyman-Pearson statistical test is designed to evaluate a single test statistic using a critical value specifically selected to produce a predetermined probability of a type I error. When two such statistical tests are conducted, each with a type I error rate of α, the probability of one or more errors is greater than α. When the two tests are independent and the type I error rate is set at 0.05 for each test, the probability of an error is *P(at least one type I error)* $= 1 - (1 - 0.05)^2 = 0.098$. Furthermore, for 20 independent tests, the probability of one or more type I errors is *P(at least one type I error)* $= 0.642$, and for 40 tests it is 0.871. This overall type I error rate is called the *family-wise error rate*. Clearly, as the number of tests increases, the family-wise error rate increases.

From another perspective, this property of increasing error probability is reflected by a measure called the *false discovery rate (fdr)*. A false discovery rate is the probability that a true null hypothesis (denoted $H-$) is among the tests declared as nonrandom (denoted "H+"). That is, a truly random result is among the tests declared as nonrandom. In symbols,

$$false\ discovery\ rate = fdr = P(H-\,|\,"H+").$$

For a more details, consider Table 15–8, where the false discovery rate is $fdr = b/(b+d) = b/m_2$.

A false-positive probability, as before (Chapter 14), is the probability that a test result will be declared as positive when in fact it is not (b/n_1 from Table 15–8). The specific relationship between the fdr and a false-positive probability (Bayes' theorem) is

$$fdr = P(H-\,|\,"H+") = \frac{P("H+"|H-)P(H-)}{P("H+")} = \frac{false\text{-}positive \times P(H-)}{P("H+")}.$$

Thus, the fdr is partially determined by the frequency of true-positive tests $[P(H+) = 1 - P(H-)]$ among a series of statistical tests. From example, for a test with sensitivity of 0.99 (type I error $= 0.01$) and specificity of 0.99 (type II error $= 0.01$), then

$$P(H+) = 0.1, \text{ yields a } fdr = 0.083,$$
$$P(H+) = 0.01, \text{ yields a } fdr = 0.500, \text{ and}$$
$$P(H+) = 0.001, \text{ yields a } fdr = 0.909.$$

In situations where the number of true-positive tests are rare, the fdr becomes close to 1.0. From the point of view of increasing family-wise error rates or false discovery rates, it is certainly important to consider the consequences of conducting a number of tests.

Several important nonstatistical issues arise in the interpretation of results from conducting a series of statistical tests. Complete discussions are found throughout the statistical, epidemiological, and medical literature ([50], [53] and [54]). Here, a few issues are briefly noted to indicate, but do not resolve, the delicate considerations concerning the control of the accumulation of type I errors associated with a series of statistical tests in a sensible and useful way.

First, it is rarely clear what constitutes the family for the calculation of a family-wise error rate. The determination is not statistical. A common practice is to define a family as all tests relevant to a specific publication or analysis. However, tests that were performed and not included, tests that occurred in previous research, and even future tests could also be candidates for inclusion. It is occasionally suggested that the number of tests in the lifetime of a statistician is a consideration. The inescapable truth was stated by statistician Ruppert Miller when he wrote, "There are no hard-and-fast rules for where the family lines should be drawn, and the statistician must rely on his own judgment for the problem at hand" [50].

In many situations, data are collected and analyzed to understand the relative role of one variable or a specific set of variables. Each variable is important and the statistical tests are not usefully considered as a single entity. For example, the variables in the Western Collaborative Group Study (WCGS) data (height, weight, blood pressure, age, smoking exposure, cholesterol, and particularly behavior type, Chapter 11) were each measured to identify and compare their specific roles in the likelihood of a coronary heart disease event. It would not be satisfactory to conduct a series of tests and state that the probability of one or more type I errors was less that 0.05. The questions of importance, such as the influence of behavior type on the likelihood of a coronary event, would not be directly addressed, which was the purpose of the collecting the data in the first place. On the other hand, modern genetic analysis can consist of the statistical comparisons among a large series of single nucleotide polymorphisms, where a global null hypothesis that all observed results occurred by chance alone is potentially valuable. Or, in the analysis of micro-array data, limiting the family-wise error is undoubtedly important. Controlling the family-wise error rate should be part of an analysis when a large, sometimes a very large, number of tests are conducted among more or less equivalent comparisons with no specific analytic focus. In these situations, a bounded likelihood of one or more type I errors is reassuring in the interpretation of the positive results. Like the selection of an appropriate family of tests, determining the balance between a focus on individual tests that make up an analysis or a focus on overall results observed from many tests is again essentially a matter of judgment.

Another difficult issue concerning a specific test result among a large number of tests is the dependency of its interpretation on the number of tests conducted. Consider a test that identifies a significant difference associated with a single variable. When this test is included among a series of tests as part of a procedure to control the family-wise error rate, the significance of this particular result is unavoidably reduced. It is, therefore, difficult to make a clear inference. It can be reasonably argued that the number of other tests, some that are not even related to the original test result, should not influence a specific inference. When a test statistic is significant based on a single test, but is not significant when adjusted for the presence other tests in the analysis, it is then not clear which result should be reported. At the extreme, one cannot envision a physician saying, "your cholesterol level is dangerously high but do not worry because it is not significant when accounting for the other 20 tests we conducted."

Three popular methods are presented to explore the "multiple testing problem" among a variety of suggested possibilities for controlling the accumulation of type I errors incurred from conducting a large number of statistical tests [54]. These methods are the Bonferroni and Holm approaches and a procedure that controls the false discovery rate.

A result from elementary probability theory (*addition theorem*) is

$$P(A \ or \ B) = P(A) + P(B) - P(A \ and \ B)$$

where A and B represent two events. When these events are $A = \{$type I error from test 1$\}$ and $B = \{$type I error from test 2$\}$, for two statistical tests the probability of one or more type I errors is

$$
\begin{aligned}
P(one \ or \ more \ type \ I \ errors) =\ &P(\{type \ I \ error \ on \ test \ 1\} \\
&or \ \{type \ I \ error \ on \ test \ 2\}) \\
=\ &P(error \ on \ test \ 1) + P(error \ on \ test \ 2) \\
&- P(errors \ on \ both \ tests).
\end{aligned}
$$

Furthermore, it follows that

$$P(one \ or \ more \ type \ I \ errors) \ < \ P(error \ on \ test \ 1) + P(error \ on \ test \ 2).$$

When this family-wise error probability is generalized to k events, it is called *Boole's inequality* or, in a statistical context, *Bonferroni's inequality*. Thus, for k events,

$$P(A_1 \text{ or } A_2 \text{ or} \cdots \text{or } A_k) < P(A_1) + P(A_2) + \cdots + P(A_k).$$

When A_i represents the occurrence of a type I error for the ith statistical test among a series of k tests. When $P(A_i) = P(type\ I\ error) = \alpha$ for the k statistical tests, the family-wise error rate is less than $k\alpha$ or

$$P(A_1 \text{ or } A_2 \text{ or} \cdots \text{or } A_k) < \alpha + \alpha + \cdots + \alpha = k\alpha.$$

In addition, if, instead of selecting an error rate of α, each "test-wise" error rate is set at α/k, then

$$P(A_1 \text{ or } A_2 \text{ or} \cdots \text{or } A_k) < \frac{\alpha}{k} + \frac{\alpha}{k} + \cdots + \frac{\alpha}{k} = k(\frac{\alpha}{k}) = \alpha,$$

or

family-wise error rate $= P(one\ or\ more\ type\ I\ errors) < \alpha$

for all k tests and is usually referred to as the Bonferroni inequality. In other words, when a series of type I error probabilities are set at α/k, the family-wise error rate for all k-tests is less than α. Table 15–9 presents a series of 20 ordered fictional p-values (column 2) generated by 20 tests. Directly applying the Bonferroni inequality to achieve a family-wise error rate of less than 0.05, the significance level of each observed p-value is compared to $\alpha/k = 0.05/20 = 0.0025$, leading to four significant tests. The family-wise error rate is less than 0.05.

Another popular approach consists of calculating an *adjusted p-value*. Adjusted values are directly compared to the selected family-wise error rate α. For the Bonferroni approach, the adjusted p-value is the originally calculated p-value multiplied by the number of tests or $k \times p_i$, where p_i represents one of the k levels of significance (p-values $= p_i$ and $i = 1, 2, \cdots, k$, Table 15–9). The adjusted p-values are then compared to α, and the null hypothesis is rejected when the adjusted value kp_i is less than α. Both unadjusted and adjusted p-values yield identical results. Note the convention (Table 15–9) of reporting the smaller of the adjusted p-value or 1.0 for each test.

An extension of the Bonferroni method that also maintains a specific family-wise error rate is called the *Holm method*. The Holm method bounds the overall type I error at α and is less conservative and more powerful than the Bonferroni approach. By less conservative, it is meant that the Holm method never rejects fewer tests than the Bonferroni approach. The Holm procedure follows the pattern of the Bonferroni procedure, except that the observed p-values are compared to the significance level α divided by $k - i + 1$, where i again indicates the ith p-value

Table 15–9. Twenty hypothetical p-values to illustrate three methods of adjustment (Bonferroni, Holm, and false discovery) for the accumulation of type I errors

		Adjusted p-values		
	p-Value	Bonferroni	Holm	fdr
1	0.000	0.002	0.002	0.002
2	0.000	0.010	0.010	0.005
3	0.001	0.020	0.018	0.007
4	0.002	0.040	0.034	0.010
5	0.003	0.060	0.048	0.012
6	0.004	0.080	0.060	0.013
7	0.010	0.200	0.140	0.029
8	0.020	0.400	0.260	0.050
9	0.030	0.600	0.360	0.067
10	0.040	0.800	0.440	0.080
11	0.050	1.000	0.500	0.091
12	0.100	1.000	0.900	0.167
13	0.200	1.000	1.000	0.308
14	0.300	1.000	1.000	0.429
15	0.400	1.000	1.000	0.533
16	0.500	1.000	1.000	0.625
17	0.700	1.000	1.000	0.824
18	0.800	1.000	1.000	0.889
19	0.900	1.000	1.000	0.947
20	0.950	1.000	1.000	0.947

in the ordered set of k tests under consideration. In addition, these comparisons only continue until the first nonrejected hypothesis. The Holm approach controls the family-wise error rate because $\alpha/(k-i+1) \leq \alpha/t$, where t represents the number of the hypotheses that are true, again making the family-wise error rate less than α.

Consider a small example. The five p-values are observed: $0.001, 0.01, 0.02,$ $0.03,$ and 0.04. These values are compared to $0.05/(5-i+1)$ or $0.01, 0.0125,$ $0.0167, 0.025, 0.05$. The Holm's criterion produces two significant values (0.001 and 0.01). Note that 0.04 is less that the point 0.05 but the comparisons stops at the first nonsignificant comparison, namely $0.02 > 0.0167$.

Also similar to the Bonferroni method, the adjusted p-value is $(k-i+1) \times p_i$ for the ith p-value. For the p-values ($k = 20$ tests) in Table 15–9, the Holm-adjusted p-values produce the same results as the Bonferroni approach. That is, comparing the Holm-adjusted p-values to 0.05 also yields four significant tests. It is not unusual that these two procedures produce similar numbers of significant tests.

Table 15–10. The correlation coefficients, their corresponding p-values (ordered), and adjusted p-values for all possible combination of the nine CHD variables (Chapter 11)

	Variable	Variable	Correlation	p-Value	Bonferroni	Holm	fdr
1.	systolic	diastolic	0.772	0.000	0.000	0.000	0.000
2.	height	weight	0.533	0.000	0.000	0.000	0.000
3.	weight	diastolic	0.296	0.000	0.000	0.000	0.000
4.	weight	systolic	0.254	0.000	0.000	0.000	0.000
5.	age	systolic	0.167	0.000	0.007	0.006	0.001
6.	cholesterol	chd	0.163	0.000	0.011	0.009	0.002
7.	age	diastolic	0.139	0.002	0.065	0.054	0.009
8.	systolic	chd	0.135	0.003	0.094	0.075	0.012
9.	diastolic	cholesterol	0.128	0.004	0.155	0.120	0.017
10.	systolic	cholesterol	0.122	0.006	0.230	0.173	0.023
11.	age	chd	0.119	0.008	0.274	0.198	0.025
12.	a/b	chd	0.112	0.012	0.428	0.298	0.036
13.	smoke	chd	0.104	0.020	0.727	0.485	0.056
14.	diastolic	chd	0.102	0.023	0.828	0.529	0.059
15.	cholesterol	smoke	0.096	0.032	1.000	0.708	0.074
16.	height	height	−0.095	0.033	1.000	0.708	0.074
17.	smoke	a/b	0.093	0.038	1.000	0.768	0.081
18.	age	cholesterol	0.089	0.047	1.000	0.893	0.087
19.	height	cholesterol	−0.089	0.048	1.000	0.893	0.087
20.	age	a/b	0.088	0.048	1.000	0.893	0.087
21.	weight	smoke	−0.082	0.068	1.000	1.000	0.117
22.	systolic	a/b	0.079	0.076	1.000	1.000	0.125
23.	weight	chd	0.064	0.155	1.000	1.000	0.242
24.	diastolic	a/b	0.059	0.186	1.000	1.000	0.275
25.	diastolic	smoke	−0.059	0.191	1.000	1.000	0.275
26.	cholesterol	a/b	0.057	0.202	1.000	1.000	0.280
27.	weight	a/b	0.043	0.340	1.000	1.000	0.453
28.	age	weight	−0.034	0.442	1.000	1.000	0.569
29.	height	a/b	0.033	0.466	1.000	1.000	0.572
30.	systolic	smoke	0.032	0.477	1.000	1.000	0.572
31.	height	chd	0.019	0.673	1.000	1.000	0.781
32.	height	systolic	0.017	0.712	1.000	1.000	0.800
33.	height	smoke	0.015	0.736	1.000	1.000	0.802
34.	height	diastolic	0.009	0.836	1.000	1.000	0.876
35.	weight	cholesterol	0.008	0.851	1.000	1.000	0.876
36.	age	smoke	−0.005	0.911	1.000	1.000	0.911

Controlling the false discovery rate is unlike the Bonferroni and Holm methods. In fact, the fdr-method does not directly involve a type I error rate but controls the expected proportion of errors among the rejected null hypotheses, the *false discovery rate*. The application, however, is Bonferroni-like and consists of rejecting the ith null hypothesis among k tests when

$$p - value \ for \ the \ i^{th}\text{-}test = p_i \leq \frac{i}{k}q$$

where q represents a chosen level of control. A sophisticated statistical proof shows

$$the \ false \ discover \ rate = P(H - |"H+") \leq q$$

for all k tests provided that the tests are independent [53]. The adjusted p-values are $(k/i) \times p_i$ for the fdr-procedure. Assuming the p-values in Table 15–9 are independent, then the fdr-method leads to declaring eight tests as notable when the level of control is set at $q = 0.05$.

To illustrate these three methods of controlling the accumulation of type I errors, Table 15–10 consists of the 36 correlation coefficients among all possible pairs of the nine variables used in the analysis of the risk of coronary heart disease (WCGS data; men less than age 50, Chapters 4 and 11). These p-values result from $k = 36$ t-tests of the hypothesis that these correlation coefficients differ from zero by chance alone. When each p-value is compared to $\alpha = 0.05$, ignoring the accumulation of type I errors, then 20 tests would be declared significant. At the α-level of $0.05/36 = 0.0014$, the application of the Bonferroni method produces six significant tests. The Holm method also produces six significant tests, and the fdr-method produces 12 notable tests. The fdr approach is approximate, at best, because these tests involve the same nine variables among the 36 estimated correlation coefficients and are, therefore, undoubtedly not independent.

REFERENCES

References frequently refer to textbooks that give a general description, which is likely more valuable for readers focused on application. Readers who wish to pursue a topic in more detail can find the original papers in these cited texts.

1. Selvin, S. (2008) *Survival Analysis for Epidemiologic and Medical Research: A Practical Guide.* Cambridge: Cambridge University Press.
2. Kang, H. K., Mahan, C. M., Lee, K. Y., Magee, C. A., and Selvin, S. (2000). Prevalence of gynecologic cancers among women Vietnam Veterans. *Journal of Occupational and Environmental Medicine.* **42**:1121–27.
3. Simpson, E. H. (1951). The interpretation of interaction in contingency tables. *Statistical Society: Series B.* **12**:238–41.
4. Bishop M. M. Y., Fienberg, S. E., and Holland, P. W. with the collaboration of Light, R. J. and Mosteller, F. (1975). *Discrete Multivariate Analysis: Theory and Practice.* Cambridge, MA: MIT Press.
5. Agresti, A. (1990). *Categorical Data Analysis.* New York: John Wiley and Sons.
6. Freeman, D. H., Jr. (1987). *Applied Categorical Data Analysis.* New York: Marcel Dekker, Inc.
7. MacMahon, B, et al. (1981). Coffee consumption and pancreatic cancer. *New England Journal of Medicine* **11**:630–33.
8. Breslow, N. E. and Day, N. E. (1987). *Statistical Methods in Cancer Research*, Vol. 2. Oxford: Oxford University Press.
9. Bithell, J. F., and Steward, M. A. (1975). Prenatal irradiation and childhood malignancy: a review of British data from the Oxford study. *British Journal of Cancer* **31**:271–87.

10. Woolf, B. (1955). On estimating the relation between blood group and disease. *Annals of Human Genetics* **19**:251–53.

11. Mantel, N., and Haenszel, W. (1959). Statistical aspects of the analysis of data from the retrospective studies of disease. *Journal of the National Cancer Institute* **22**:719–48.

12. Selvin, S. (2001). *Epidemiologic Analysis: A Case Oriented Approach* Oxford: Oxford University Press.

13. Poole, C. (1987). Beyond the confidence interval. *American Journal of Public Health.* **77**:195–99.

14. Thomas, W. D. (1987). Statistical criteria in the interpretation of epidemiologic data. *American Journal of Public Health.* **77**:191–94.

15. Letters to the Editor. (1986). *American Journal of Public Health.* **76**:237 and **76**:581.

16. Rosenman, R. H., Brand, R. J., Jenkins, C.D., et al. (1975). Coronary heart disease in the Western Collaborative Group study. *Journal of the American Medical Association.* **223**:872–77.

17. Rosenman, R. H. Brand, R. J. Sholtz, R. I., and Friedmen, M. (1976). Multivariate prediction of coronary heart disease during 8.5 year follow-up in the Eastern Collaborative Group Study. *American Journal of Cardiology* **37**:903–10.

18. Rosenman, R. H., Friedmen, M., Straus, R., et al. (1970). Coronary heart disease in the Western Collaborative Group study: a follow-up of 4.5 years. *Journal of Chronic Diseases.* **23**:173–90.

19. Ragland, D. R., and Brand, R. J. (1988). Coronary heart disease mortality in the Western Collaborative Group Study. *American Journal of Epidemiology.* **1217**:462–75.

20. Yiming, Z., Zhang, S., Selvin, S., and Spear, R. (1990). A dose response relationship for noise-induced hypertension. Proceedings of the 7th International Symposium on Epidemiology and Occupational Health, Japan. *British Journal of Industrial Medicine.* **48**:179–84.

21. Hosmer, D. W. Jr., and Lemeshow, S. (1989). *Applied Logistic Regression.* New York: John Wiley and Sons.

22. Schlesselman, J. J. *Case-Control Studies.* (1982). New York: Oxford University Press.

23. Robert, E., Harris, J. A., Robert, O., and Selvin, S. (1996). Case-control study on maternal residential proximity to high voltage power lines and congenital anomalies in France. *Pediatric and Perinatal Epidemiology.* **10**:32–38.

24. Jewell, N. P. (2004). *Statistics for Epidemiology.* New York: Chapman & Hall/CRC.

25. Ury H. K. (1975). Efficiency of case-control studies with multiple controls per case: continuous or dichotomous data. *Biometrics.* **31**:643–49.

26. Wertheimer, N., and Leeper, E. (1979). Electrical wiring configuration and childhood cancer. *Epidemiology.* **109**:272–84.

27. Ma, X., Buffler, P. A., Selvin, S., Wiencke, J. L., Wiemels, J. L., and Reynolds, P. (2002). Day-care attendance and the risk of childhood acute lymphoblastic leukemia. *British Journal of Cancer.* **86**:1419–24.

28. Lilienfeld, D. E., and Stolley, P. D. (1994). *Foundations of Epidemiology* New York: Oxford University Press.

29. Feller, W. (1950). *An Introduction to Probability Theory and Its Application.* New York: John Wiley and Sons.

30. Cochran, W. G. (1954). Some methods for strengthening the common X^2 test. *Biometrics.* **10**:417–51.
31. Lehmann, E. L., and D. Abrera H. J. M. (1975). *Nonparametrics: Statistical Methods Based on Ranks.* New York: McGraw-Hill International Book Company.
32. Hoaglin, D. C., Mosteller, F., and Tukey, J. W. (1983). *Understanding Robust and Exploratory Data Analysis.* New York: John Wiley and Sons.
33. Hoaglin, D. C., Mosteller, F., and Tukey, J. W. (1985). *Exploring Data Tables, Trends, and Shapes.* New York: John Wiley and Sons.
34. Boots, B. N., and Getis, A. (1988). *Point Pattern Analysis.* London: Sage Publications.
35. Hand, D. J., and Taylor, C. C. (1987). *Multivariate Analysis of Variance and Repeated Measures.* New York: Chapman and Hall.
36. Grunbaum, B. W. (1981). *Handbook for Forensic Individualization of Human Blood and Bloodstains.* Berkeley: University of California.
37. Johnson, R. A., and Wichern, D. W. (1998). *Applied Multivariate Statistical Analysis.* New Jersey: Prentice Hall.
38. Bowman, A. W., and Azzalini, A. (1997). *Applied Smoothing Techniques for Data Analysis: The Kernel Approach with S-Plus Illustrations.* Oxford: Clarendon Press.
39. Shaw, G. M., Carmichael, S. L., Nelson, V., Selvin, S., and Schaffer, D. M. (2003). Food fortification with folic acid and twinning among California infants. *American Journal of Medical Genetics* **119A**:137–40.
40. Harrell, F. E. Jr. (2001). *Regression Modeling Strategies: With Applications to Linear Models, Logistic Regression, and Survival Analysis.* New York: Springer.
41. Scheffe, H. (1959). *The Analysis of Variance.* London: John Wiley and Sons.
42. Carmichael, S. L., Shaw, G. M., Schaffer, D. M., and Selvin, S. (2004). Dieting behavior and risk of neural tube defects. *American Journal of Epidemiology.* **158**:1127–31.
43. Ernster, V. L., Mason, L., Goodson, W. H., Edwards, E. A., Sacks, S., Selvin, S., Dupuy, M. E., and Hunt, T. K. (1982). Effects of caffeine-free diet on benign breast disease: A randomized trial. *Surgery* **3**:263–67.
44. Fleiss, J. L. (1981). *Statistical Methods for Rates and Proportions.* New York: John Wiley and Sons.
45. Bishop, Y. M. M., Fienberg S. E., Holland, P. W., with collaboration of Light, R. J. and Mosteller, F. (1975). *Discrete Multivariate Analysis: Theory and Practice.* Cambridge, MA: MIT Press.
46. Halushka, M., Cornish, T. C., Selvin, S., and Selvin, E. (2009). Validation and quantitative analysis of protein expression in vascular tissue microarrys. *Cardiovascular Pathology* **1**; (12):11.
47. Selvin, E., Coresh, J. Jordahl, J. Bolands, L., and Steffes, M. W. (2005). Stability of haemoglobin A1c (HbA1c) measurements from frozen whole blood samples stored for over a decade. DOI **10**:1464–5491.
48. Bland, M. J., and Altman, D. G. (1999). Measuring agreement in method comparison studies. *Statistical Methods in Medical Research* **8**:135–60.
49. Kendall, M. G., and Stuart, A. (1967). *The Advanced Theory of Statistics*, Vol. 2 Inference and Relationship, 2nd Edition. New York: Hafner Publishing Company.
50. Morrison, D. F. (1967). *Multivariate Statistical Methods.* New York: McGraw-Hill Book Company.

51. Cleveland, W. S., and Devlin, S. J. (1988). Locally weighted regression: an approach to regression analysis by local fitting. *American Statistical Association* **83**:596–610.
52. Abrams, B., and Selvin, S. (1995). Maternal weight gain pattern and birth weight. *Obstetrics and Gynecology* **86**(2):163–69.
53. Benjamini, Y., and Hochberg, Y. (1995). Controlling the false discovery rate: A practical and powerful approach to multiple testing. *Journal of the Royal Statistical Society. Series B (Methodological).* **57**(1):289–300.
54. Dudoit, S., Shaffer, J. P., and Boldrick J. C. (2003). Multiple hypothesis testing in microarray experiments. *Statistical Science* **18**(1):71–103.

INDEX